D1538654

the whole mind

the whole mind

THE DEFINITIVE GUIDE TO
COMPLEMENTARY TREATMENTS FOR
MIND, MOOD, AND EMOTION

LYNETTE BASSMAN, PH.D.

New World Library
Novato, California

New World Library
14 Pamaron Way
Novato, CA 94949

Cover design: Peri Poloni / Knockout Design
Cover photograph: Tony Stone Images
Text layout and design: Margaret Copeland, Terragraphics
Editorial: Becky Benenate

Library of Congress Cataloging-in-Publication Data
The whole mind : the definitive guide to complementary treatments for mind,
mood, and emotion / edited by Lynette Bassman.
p.   cm.
Includes bibliographical references.
ISBN 1-57731-050-0 (pbk. : alk. paper)
1. Mental illness — Alternative treatment. 2. Mind and body therapies.
I. Bassman, Lynette, 1959-
Rc480.515.W48   1998   97-31585
616.89'1—dc21   CIP

First printing, June 1998
Printed in Canada on acid-free paper
ISBN 1-57731-050-0
Distributed to the trade by Publishers Group West
10 9 8 7 6 5 4 3 2 1

Dedication

This book is dedicated to all people who have suffered with untreated or inadequately treated mental illnesses, and to those health professionals who can find within themselves the ability to risk being open to new (and old) healing wisdom.

Acknowledgments

First, I would like to thank the authors who contributed to this book. They are all very busy yet gave their time so that their knowledge could come to light.

I am grateful to my husband, Larry Bassman, for understanding that I had to do this, and for being a source of so many kinds of support through the long years of preparing this book. My son, Jonah Bassman, was often my inspiration.

Eugene Herman taught me about thinking and seeing things in unconventional ways, and about being bold and daring, all qualities that were necessary in bringing this project to fruition. Betty Herman taught me about being steady, reliable, and organized, and about creating something useful with very few resources. Merle Molofsky was instrumental in helping me believe I could do this. Janee Albert served as a consultant and sounding board. Sam Faith taught me how to write.

Thanks to all the secretaries, assistants, and office managers of many of the contributors, who sent faxes, answered telephones, and sometimes put my messages on the top of the pile. None of us could do what we do without you.

There are many people who helped me along the way by leading me to the people who wrote the chapters of this book. I can't mention you all by name, but I want you to know how much I appreciate your help.

And finally, I owe sincere gratitude to my clients, who have taught me about the benefits and the limitations of psychotherapy and psychopharmacology.

Table of Contents

Lynette Bassman, Ph.D.

Editor's Preface

About fifteen years ago, my father died of cancer, the man I thought I was going to marry told me he was gay, I moved to New York City, and started graduate school to begin a career change (from the food business to counseling). It was a time of enormous change in my life and I became chronically ill with a collection of symptoms that baffled the medical doctors I went to see. My symptoms included fatigue, dizziness, pain in my joints, severe and frequent migraines, and occasional stabbing pains in my abdomen. The most troubling of my symptoms, however, was a worsening of the depression that I had struggled with from the age of eight. Throughout my childhood and adolescence, I lacked confidence, felt I was different than other children, had trouble sleeping, was socially withdrawn, and found very little pleasure in anything other than reading and eating. I didn't like to play but did enjoy reading for hours. As a child I often wished that I had never been born. My father suffered from what may have been a form of bipolar disorder — a depression that alternates with periods of elated moods and extreme and provocative behavior. My mother was quiet and somewhat unemotional. At the time, both my parents were emotionally unavailable and overlooked what was going on with me.

A few years before I moved to New York, I suffered my first severe episode of depression. My first year of college was lonely and painful for me, and after a series of crushing rejections I became suicidal. I actually developed a plan to kill myself, and called it off only seconds before driving my car into a concrete abutment. When I stumbled home that night, I cried more loudly than usual and my parents took notice and became involved. I returned to college a few weeks later under the condition that I seek counseling. As it turned out, my therapist was quiet, strained, unpleasant, and unhelpful to me. (She may have been ill at the time — she died of cancer a few years later.) I can't recall much about the few sessions I had with her, but I do know that the experience didn't help me with my emotional pain.

As luck would have it, I made friends with several students who had transferred to the school that year. Making a few new friends seemed to turn the tide. Although my self-esteem and social skills were still very poor, I was beginning to have a good time in college, and even managed to learn a few things.

I spent my junior year studying in Israel, and although I loved it there, my depression would come and go. Because I had left most of my friends behind, I was often lonely and did not feel a part of the group of students who were in Israel with me. I made some bad decisions about relationships in an effort to cope with my loneliness.

After a few weeks of living in Jerusalem, I developed the first of my physical symptoms: I was dizzy, and had pretty severe joint pains. The headaches that had troubled me on and off since I was a young child became more frequent. Despite the moderate climate, I often felt cold. At midyear, I moved to a small town in the Negev Desert. I felt much better there, physically and mentally, especially once the rainy season ended. I took up running and lost a lot of the weight I had been gaining. I changed my diet, and began living on the delicious fruits, vegetables, and fresh-baked whole-grain breads that were available there. I felt very comfortable with the desert climate, and absorbed in my work. I enjoyed getting to know the culture and the language. The depression and the physical pains subsided and didn't surface again until I moved back to New York to attend graduate school two years later. In retrospect, it seems likely that something about the city environment was the culprit for at least some of my physical symptoms.

Back in New York, my daily life was a struggle. I went through the motions of living, and again, the only pleasure I experienced was from eating and reading novels. It took all my effort to get to class and complete my assignments in a cursory way. I felt drained and hopeless. I underwent many medical tests and examinations at the university's health service (considered to be an excellent facility) and after having a few very frightening diagnoses suggested that didn't quite seemed to fit, the physicians threw up their hands and suggested that I see a psychotherapist — implying that my problems were "all in my head" and not "real."

I was already seeing a psychotherapist for my depression, my emotions, my thinking, and what I now understand to be issues relating to my spirituality. My therapist, although cool and nonverbal, was helpful to me. He was somewhat baffled, however, by my symptoms and kept suggesting that I see a physician.

Because my health care providers didn't understand what was happening with me they had little help to offer. I began to feel I was beyond help. It isn't easy when people you are accustomed to respecting as authority figures give up on you. I was desperate and willing to try anything. In fact, I felt that I had to try something new and different if I wanted to go on living. By this time, I felt so sick that I did not know if I would be able to complete my master's degree let alone go on for a doctoral degree. My life was so intolerable at this point that suicide, again, seemed the only way out. I toyed with a plan to gather enough pills, but lacked the knowledge about how to actually achieve a lethal dose rather than just making myself more sick.

Luckily, one day a friend suggested that I see his chiropractor who was trained in applied kinesiology. I figured I had nothing to lose and I went to see him. This doctor was not baffled by my symptoms. He did not think I was crazy. Nor did he feel a need to come up with one simple name for all of what was wrong with me, but saw it instead as a complex interaction of chemical toxicity, food allergy, yeast overgrowth, stressed adrenal glands, and various other imbalances. With the combination of his treatment, the nutritional supplements he recommended, and the dietary changes I made at his suggestion, I began to feel better. I had more energy, my headaches weren't as severe and became less frequent, and the depression lessened and was more bearable. The joint pain and abdominal pain were gone and the suicidal ideas stopped. I felt that I was taking more responsibility for my life, and this helped me emotionally as well.

A year or two later, I began a program of vision therapy to work on correcting my vision — I had always felt uncomfortable with the glasses I had worn since fourth grade. This was a powerful experience for me. It raised a lot of emotional issues that had not been raised through traditional psychotherapy

— issues relating to body image and how I use my body and my eyes to filter experiences. I was able to work through the emotional issues with vision exercises, and I believe that by coming to terms with these issues, I was able to correct my nearsightedness. I felt lighter, more energetic, and began to enjoy life. I fell in love, got married, completed a very difficult internship, wrote my dissertation, and got my first job as a psychotherapist.

My life was really turning around. From time to time, however, I would still lapse into occasional depression, and had some persistent negative thought patterns and low self-esteem. I found a psychotherapist who was warm, wise, and intuitive, and helped me with a lot of the remaining depression, low self-esteem, and dysfunctional thinking. But there was still a lasting core of depression in me that wouldn't go away. I was now at a time in my life when I was trying to decide whether to have a baby, and I felt that the depression was too powerful an interference in a decision of such importance.

I decided to seek the help of a classical homeopath. Within a few months of beginning my treatment the depression had lifted considerably. I felt optimistic and empowered enough to make important life decisions, and I now have a wonderful three-year-old son.

I use exercise, good nutrition, and relaxation and cognitive therapy techniques as tools to combat the short periods of depression that I still occasionally suffer from. Regular applied kinesiology treatments keep my health in balance, plus I use flower essences, herbs, and Chinese medicine for specific emotional and physical health issues as needed. Meditation, T'ai Chi, and Qigong (pronounced: *chi kung*) have been tremendously helpful to me also. I plan to tackle some remaining blocks to my happiness and further growth with a body-oriented therapy like Rubenfeld Synergy, Network Spinal Analysis, or Rolfing. I am sure that I will find my way back into traditional talk therapy during difficult times in the future.

As a practicing psychologist, I have observed that many other people have had similar experiences with chronic physical and psychological health problems. I have also noticed that the kinds of problems people bring to psychotherapy aren't always best treated by psychotherapy and/or medications alone. I have discovered when clients make use of complementary healing arts, therapy often progresses more fruitfully and more rapidly.

I put this book together because as both a *consumer* of mainstream and alternative health services and as a *provider* of psychotherapy services, I am convinced that something more than traditional psychotherapy can be offered to people suffering from mental or emotional issues. I want others who want to enhance their emotional well-being to know there are alternatives or complimentary treatments available. Although I am deeply impressed with what psychotherapy and medications can do, I am also convinced that they are not the *only* path to emotional wellness. Complementary therapies should not have to be a last resort when all else fails. Instead they should be considered along with mainstream treatments — with all available information being considered before deciding which treatments to use.

Information about alternative treatments for emotional problems is not always easy to find and has never been collected and presented in a form that allows easy comparisons. I was lucky to stumble upon such gifted and helpful healers when I needed them, but most people have no idea that there are any alternatives or adjuncts to psychotherapy and medication, and wouldn't know how to make decisions about them if they wanted to.

I am concerned that there aren't research studies confirming the effectiveness of all of the healing arts in this book, but I am also very concerned anytime information is withheld from people. My purpose for putting together this book is to provide you with information on thirty-six healing modalities, inform you of the research that has been done so far, and then let you decide how to make use of that information for your own emotional wellness or that of your loved ones.

I have asked experts in each of these healing modalities to write clear and understandable chapters about what they do and how it can help people who want to enhance their emotional wellness. I have asked them to include case studies, brief explanations of the underlying philosophies, research citations where they exist, information about choosing a reputable practitioner, and resources for learning more. When you are in emotional pain, or just wanting to achieve more of your potential, you need easy access to crucial information. This book is designed to give you that information in a format that is clear and easy to read.

PART 1

Getting Ready to Choose

Lynette Bassman, Ph.D.

Introduction

INFORMED CONSENT?

Before surgery can be performed in the United States, doctors are required to tell the patient about the procedure, its potential benefits, drawbacks, and side affects, the consequences of refusing the procedure, and other treatments available. A permission form must be signed by the patient before surgery is performed. This is called "informed consent." Informed consent is also required within the mental health field before psychotherapy can proceed and before psychotropic medication can be given.

It is my belief that psychotherapy and psychopharmacology patients are routinely cheated out of their right to *truly* informed consent. Rarely, if ever, are mental health consumers given information about other treatments available. Most mental health clinicians do not believe that alternatives to mainstream psychotherapy (psychoanalytic, gestalt, behavioral, cognitive, and so on), and medications exist. This is not true. There are many alternative healing approaches that offer help for those who suffer from the full range of emotional symptoms.

This book gives you access to information you need to be truly informed.

WHO SAYS WHETHER TREATMENT IS EFFECTIVE?

Some health care professionals demand that a new treatment be proven effective by certain standard kinds of research before that treatment is made available to patients. But many of the treatments in this book cannot be tested by these methods, or have not yet been studied in this way due to the lack of financial support for research. This does not mean that they are not effective. In some cases, thousands of years of experience attest to their usefulness. Many of the approaches that were once viewed with distrust and ridicule, later are shown to be effective, and become advocated by the same scientific community that had condemned them earlier. Chapter 2, on the politics of health care, explains the problems with research on alternative healing practices.

Despite the lack of double-blind studies, I believe that consumers have a right to learn about these treatments. In this book, some of the top clinicians and researchers of each major healing art clearly summarize the treatment so that you can make judgments about its merits. Perhaps this book will get policy makers and practitioners to start talking more openly about these approaches, and help to find creative ways to verify their effectiveness.

THE ROLE OF PSYCHOTHERAPY AND PSYCHOPHARMACOLOGY

The goal of psychotherapy is to reduce symptoms of emotional distress by either changing the behaviors that lead to the problem (for example, learning new social skills so that relationship difficulties are reduced), changing the troublesome thoughts that precede unpleasant emotions (such as learning to tell yourself about your accomplishments instead of your failures, to increase self-esteem), or by achieving insight into the underlying causes of a symptom (for example, what childhood experiences interfered with the acquisition of social skills). Psychotropic medications aim to reduce or eliminate symptoms by altering brain chemistry (for example, affecting brain chemicals that cause the brain to produce delusional thinking).

Inherent in these approaches are basic assumptions about the causes of emotional problems. Most psychotherapists assume that emotional problems stem from having learned maladaptive behaviors, from negative patterns of thought, or from having emotional blockages that prevent, distort, or delay normal development. Psychopharmacologists believe that emotional symptoms are caused primarily by incorrect signals being sent within the brain due to improper functioning of neuro-transmitters. Despite the different assumptions of these approaches, both appear to be effective. Often, both can be combined, with excellent results.

In some cases, however, neither psychotherapy nor medication is effective. Psychotherapy sometimes takes too long, and the cost in human suffering is too high during that time. Talking about problems might not be the preferred approach for people with particular personalities, learning styles, or cultural backgrounds. Often psychotropic medications cause side-effects that some people feel outweigh the benefits. Medications might not be right for people with some health problems or religious beliefs. In many of these cases, holistic approaches can provide solutions. Alternative therapies, when used at the same time as psychotherapy or medication, can sometimes accelerate the results, intensify the process, or otherwise assist in overcoming the problems.

Many complementary treatments are based on different assumptions about the causes of psychological problems. For example, mental illnesses might be caused by nutritional deficiencies, environmental sensitivities, allergies, blood sugar problems, fungal overgrowth, functional endocrine imbalance, biorhythm disturbances, or blocked energy pathways. Treating these causes with natural remedies, physical manipulations, detoxification, and other procedures sometimes provides a more direct, and therefore more effective approach.

Special Note To Current And Future Researchers

There is a great need for innovative research methods to evaluate the effectiveness of the healing arts featured in this book. Our current methods for measuring the outcomes of medical and mental health treatments simply are not adequate for evaluating the complexity of holistic treatment techniques. We need ways of looking at the effects of the entire complex treatment, since it is usually impossible to isolate single components of the therapeutic effect.

If you are a health professional or a statistician, or are thinking of becoming one, then consider directing your creativity toward this challenging and potentially rewarding field. Graduate program directors and educators can be instrumental in helping students realize that this need exists, and preparing them to take on the challenge. I would love to hear from people who want to be involved in this kind of research.

Psychotherapy and holistic approaches can usually be combined with excellent results. Following are some of the ways that psychotherapy and additional approaches can work together:

- Psychotherapy can help a person catch up on delayed development. Once a holistic therapy has resolved the physical symptoms underlying an emotional problem psychotherapy can be used to help a person catch up on social development. If a person has experienced fear, depression, or delusions for a number of years, he or she may have missed opportunities to develop normally. For instance, a person who has been depressed and withdrawn during adolescence might have missed learning social skills. This person needs to learn how to interact socially once the depression has been treated by holistic means such as homeopathy or ayurveda — the traditional health care system in India.

- Psychotherapy can help a person to unlearn maladaptive behaviors once a psychological problem has been resolved. It can also offer opportunities for learning and experimenting with more adaptive behaviors. For example, the learning-disabled child who finds it hard to maintain attention in a classroom setting becomes the class clown to gain acceptance. This serves him or her well under the circumstances, but as an adult, if the cause of the apparent disability is removed (maybe through vision training or environmental medicine), the behavior creates its own social problems and may not be helpful anymore.

- Psychotherapy can be useful in reframing life goals once good health has been restored. When burdened with health problems for a number of years many people develop poor self images and pessimistic ideas about their future. Psychotherapy can be a very good place to try out new ideas about the self.

- Psychotherapy can help with processing traumas that might be uncovered through techniques such as massage or Network Spinal Analysis. For instance, during a massage therapy or bodywork session, a person may suddenly remember an accident or some kind of abuse that occurred to that body part in the past. These memories can be sudden and distressing. Psychotherapy is a very good way of beginning to sort out the feelings to which these memories give rise.

- Psychotherapy can help people adopt healthy self-care behaviors. A major tenet of the holistic approach is prevention. Lifestyle changes are made before symptoms develop, so that good health can be maintained. Making these lifestyle changes can be difficult. Food is often used as a coping mechanism, and a change in diet can feel emotionally threatening. Beginning an exercise program may force an individual to confront a poor body image or to re-sort his or her priorities in ways that can be painful. Psychotherapy can help resolve these issues and help make lifestyle changes before illness manifests.

- Psychotropic medications can help overcome symptoms so severe that they disable the patient or threaten his or her safety. A person suffering from severe depression may not be able to get out of the house, or carry out the most basic activities of daily living. The treatment regimens required by some of the holistic approaches may demand visits to the office of the practitioner, the regular consumption of nutritional supplements, meditation, exercise, dietary changes, or hands-on contact by the practitioner. These are activities that, ironically, may be impossible for the people who need them the most. Medication may serve as a means for restoring adequate functioning, so that people can take a more active role in regaining and maintaining good health. There are times when it is advisable to have a consultation with a psychiatrist to determine whether medication is needed, and to take it if it is recommended. Many of the holistic healing arts in this book can be used while taking medication. Be sure to check with both practitioners.

HOW TO USE THIS BOOK

The first section of this book provides background information that can be helpful in understanding the later chapters about holistic healing arts. The chapters in Part One teach you about the politics of health care from a theoretical perspective and from the perspective of a parent of a mentally ill child. The chapter by Stanislav Grof raises some intriguing questions about the basic assumptions on which our current mental health care system is based. Part Two contains summaries of thirty-six different healing arts, so you can decide which, if any, is right for you. The topics chosen give you a comprehensive sampling of the alternatives and additions to psychotherapy and medication that are currently available. I have included only healing arts that are not psychotherapies or techniques commonly used in psychotherapy today. There are many innovative systems of psychotherapy available, and one of them may be right for you, but it would take another book to describe them in detail.

Well-established, comprehensive treatment systems are included, as are new, experimental approaches that perhaps serve best as additions or complements to other modes of treatment. Space limitations prevented the inclusion of some approaches (particularly in the area of bodywork, where so many exist), and a lack of demonstrated effectiveness prevented other approaches from appearing here. Some of them are so new that not enough data exist yet to evaluate them adequately, though they may eventually prove to be extremely valuable. It is possible that other approaches are valuable but unknown to me, or are practiced by so few clinicians that you would be unlikely to find one in your area. In a few cases, I was unable to find a practitioner to write a chapter on a given healing art. It is strongly recommended that you keep an eye on the periodical literature for up-to-date information about emerging approaches. The decisions about what to include in the book were difficult, and the choices were not clear. For example, psychic healing, chelation therapy, and the Feldenkrais Method are techniques that I might have included if I had unlimited time, space, and resources.

This book is intended not as an endorsement of any particular approach, but as a source of information that can be used to make decisions about your health care. Taking responsibility for your own health is an important step toward mental health. This book is also intended to bring emerging treatment methods to light, so that public policy makers can begin a dialogue with holistic practitioners, and encourage further research and development of promising approaches.

It is important to make any health care decision with prudence and with appropriate scrutiny of the approach and of the treatment provider. It is strongly suggested that you get a thorough assessment, diagnosis, and recommendation from a licensed psychologist, psychiatrist, social worker, or mental health counselor. Listen carefully to their assessment of the severity of your condition, and consider pursuing conventional treatments before alternative ones. Some mental health problems are so painful, and may involve destructive behavior, and some of the holistic approaches take so long to effect change, that you may decide that mainstream approaches make the most sense for you at this stage of your life. If you are feeling suicidal or out of control, immediately seek psychotherapy and/or psychotropic medication. The alternative treatments will still be there for you when you are feeling stronger.

Keep in mind that in traditional "talk psychotherapy," you may encounter uncomfortable feelings as you learn unpleasant truths about yourself and your life. As this information surfaces, it is natural to feel like running from the therapy and/or the therapist. Analyzing, understanding, and working through these feelings can be a very valuable experience. But this process takes patience. Try to determine if your dissatisfaction with psychotherapy is due to these natural feelings of resistance, or to the fact that psychotherapy is not right for you at this time.

If you have decided that psychotherapy or medication are not the right treatment plan for you, or that you want to add a complementary therapy to your current treatment, a decision is needed about which approach to pursue. The table at the end of my introduction is a good place to start. It lists all of the healing arts covered in this book, and the conditions for which each one can be helpful. Before making a decision it is important to carefully read and evaluate the treatment approaches, and to take advantage of the resources, books, and articles referred to at the end of each chapter. Do not rely on your initial gut reaction to one approach. Instincts are important, and often guide you to the therapies that are right for you, but read several chapters, and compare them. Be sure to consider the time frame for results, the type of contact with the healer, what you will be asked to do for yourself between visits, and the costs of treatment. Try to avoid the temptation of seeing any of the treatments as a quick fix for symptoms that probably took years to develop. Real wellness takes time and your participation in the process.

This book is packed with information. Some people may feel overwhelmed by this, and may want to avoid making any decisions right now. This could be especially true if you are suffering from fatigue, depression, anxiety, or any kind of confused thinking. If that is the case, ask a trusted friend, a family member, or your psychotherapist to help you sort out what is right for you. It may be helpful to take it slowly, reading only one chapter per week, taking time to digest the information before proceeding. Remember that any new body of information is unfamiliar until you spend some time with it. The information in this book might represent a fundamentally different view of the world than the one you are accustomed to. Give yourself a chance to get familiar with the new ideas in this book, and don't judge yourself harshly if it takes a while to absorb them.

Once a decision is made about what healing approach to pursue, you must next decide which practitioner to work with. Many of the authors have provided specific information on how to locate various practitioners skilled in the approach discussed. However, it is always important to achieve the correct match between you and the healer. In most of the holistic healing arts, the patient is more involved in treatment than with allopathic medicine, and the doctor/patient relationship is more collaborative. It is important, therefore, that you feel comfortable with the healer and that the healer be willing to take the time to explain the procedures so that you can make good decisions about your own care. Following are some suggestions for finding the right practitioner. I also strongly recommend the book *Five Steps to Selecting the Best Alternative Medicine* by Mary and Michael Morton for a thoughtful and detailed approach to this subject. *The Encyclopedia of Alternative Health Care* by Kristin Gottschalk Olsen also offers a wealth of helpful information about forming a partnership with your health care providers.

- Ask someone you know for a referral. Ask them what the practitioner is like, and how he or she works.

- Call the practitioner and ask questions you have about what he or she does and how it is done. Carefully observe how open the practitioner is while speaking to you, how clearly the practitioner communicates, and how you feel. If your gut reaction is a negative one, do not go see this person. Have similar conversations with a few other practitioners, and keep careful notes about your reactions. This will help you pick the one that seems the best for your needs and personality. It should be noted that some practitioners feel strongly about the prospective patient's right to ask questions and give special training to their office staff who handle these phone calls. Speaking with a member of the office staff is not necessarily a sign of the doctor's lack of caring.

- Ask the practitioner about his or her experience in treating the condition for which you are seeking help. Ask if any of his or her patients would agree to speak with you. This may not be possible, due to the confidentiality between doctor and patient.

- Ask the practitioner if he or she has written any books, articles, or pamphlets about his or her work, and whether he or she gives any talks or workshops. Follow up on these, as they are excellent ways to get a better feel for how the practitioner works.

- Clarify financial issues at the outset. Ask about any additional lab costs, nutritional supplements, or other expenses. Ask about the practitioner's history of reimbursement by insurance companies.

- After all the reading and talking is done, wait at least one week before making an appointment, unless your symptoms are too severe to wait. This will give you a chance to make a more rational decision, instead of reacting to your desire to get well immediately.

- Before your first visit, develop realistic expectations about the results. Most alternative approaches do not produce rapid results. It probably took many years to develop your symptoms, and it will take a while to get over them.

- During the first visit, ask as many questions as you want. Again, notice how the practitioner responds. If you do not like the way he or she responds to you, then discuss this with the practitioner. If he or she is not responsive to your concerns, leave.

- If you do not feel good about the practitioner after the first visit, and/or don't feel that you can follow through with the person's recommendations, do not go back. You may choose to send the practitioner a letter summarizing your reasons, providing feedback that may be helpful to him or her for the future.

- It is important that you carry out your part of the treatment (such as taking nutritional supplements as recommended, performing exercises, relaxation techniques, and dietary changes). If you do not pursue the treatment as recommended, you will not have an opportunity to evaluate its effectiveness.

Some of the approaches detailed in this book lend themselves to use in combination with other approaches, while some do not. For example, while getting treatment for environmental toxicities, massage therapy may be very helpful in clearing out the system. While using applied kinesiology to rebalance the system, Alexander technique lessons can enhance the process. Vision

A NOTE TO PSYCHOTHERAPISTS AND PSYCHIATRISTS

As clinicians living and practicing at this exciting time in history, we have the opportunity to prepare ourselves to be more effective at what we do by incorporating alternative healing approaches into our work. This can be very satisfying, and also very frightening. When all of your training has taught you one way of doing things, it may be difficult to think of changing. It is my belief that we will serve our clients better, and will enliven our own professional careers by choosing to seek training in one or more of the approaches detailed in the book. I plan on becoming a homeopath, because that approach is very appealing to me and would combine well with the kind of psychological work I already do. Other clinicians might choose a body-work method, or flower essence therapy, or become proficient in the use of herbs, and so on. Each chapter offers resources to find out about training opportunities. We can also serve our clients well by being familiar with the adjunctive therapies they are using, so we can help them integrate that work with their psychotherapy. Many clients I have treated have told me that their previous therapist was not respectful of the other healing work they were doing. Some therapists saw a client's involvement in holistic healing as a sign of pathology. I believe it is time to move beyond those kinds of judgments. There are indications that a substantial percentage of the population is using these therapies. They can't all be crazy.

training and some of the bodywork approaches might complement each other well. However, combining Ayurveda and Chinese medicine might render both techniques less effective. Some nutritional supplements might actually interfere with homeopathic treatment. It is best to ask the practitioners themselves for their recommendations about which approaches to use in conjunction, and which ones to avoid combining.

Finally, keep in mind that as you discover and resolve the physical causes of your emotional problems, there may be adjustments that need to be made in your lifestyle, self-concept, and coping mechanisms. Psychotherapy can help you make these changes more quickly and effectively. It is important that your psychotherapist be well versed in the holistic approach, and that he or she be open to understanding the healing approach you have chosen.

By picking up this book, you have taken an important step toward achieving emotional well-being. In addition, you have taken a step toward changing our health care system from the expensive, high-tech, authoritarian, mechanistic one we now have to a new system that will be holistic, will make appropriate use of technology and of ancient wisdom, and will place control of your health back into your own hands. I wish you well in your search for emotional well-being.

HOW TO LEARN MORE

Gottschalk Olsen, K. *The Encyclopedia of Alternative Health Care.* New York: Pocket Books, 1989.

Morton, M. and M. Morton. *Five Steps to Selecting the Best Alternative Medicine.* Novato, CA: New World Library, 1996.

Table 1. Conditions and goals for which each healing art can be helpful

	Depression	Anxiety	Schizophrenia, Psychoses	Addictions	Eating Disorders	Learning, Memory	Trauma, Abuse	Personality Disorders	Confusion, Brain Fog	Irritability	Self-Actualization	Spiritual Growth	Overall Health	Other
Alexander Technique	x	x		x	x	x	x		x	x	x	x	x	chronic pain
Applied Kinesiology	x	x	x	x	x	x			x	x	x		x	
Aromatherapy	x	x		(can help with difficult times in recovery process)	x	x	x	x	x	x	x	x	x	
Ayurveda	x	x	x	x	x	x	x	x	x	x	x	x	x	pain, stress disorders
Biofeedback	x	x		x	x	x			x		x		x	
Bonny Method of GIM	x	x		x	x	x	x	x		x	x	x	x	
Child Brain Development				(to anti-convulsant drugs)		x			x	x	x	x	x	brain injury
Chinese Medicine, Acupuncture	x	x	x	x	?	x	x	x	x	x	x	x	x	
Creative Arts Therapies	x	x	x	x	x	x	x	x	x	x	x	x	x	developmental delays, mental retardation, physical disabilities, behavior disorders, self-expression, (dance and music therapy: autism)
Ecopsychology	x	x	x	x	x		x		x	x	x	x	x	alienation/isolation
Edgar Cayce Approach	x	x	x			x			x	x	x	x	x	
Environmental Medicine	x	x	x	x	x	x	x	x	x	x	x		x	aggression, vulgarity, social withdrawal, fatigue
Exercise Therapy	x	x		x					x		x		x	
Flower Essence Therapy	x	x	(under supervision)	x	x	x	x	(under supervision)	x	x	x	x	x	environmental sensitivity, child development, job performance, men's and women's issues, death and dying
Food and Mood	x	x		x	x	x	x		x	x	x		x	
Herbs I: Holistic Approach	x	x		x	?	x			x	x	x	x	x	
Herbs II: Prescriptive, Self-Care Approach	x	x	x	x	x	x	x	x	x	x			x	
Homeopathy	x	x	x			x	x	x	x	x			x	speech disorders, sleep disorders, psychosomatic disease

(Note: "?" indicates that some practitioners of this type can help some patients with this condition. Ask a potential practitioner whether he or she has training and experience in treating it, and whether he or she thinks the treatment can be beneficial to your condition.)

	Depression	Anxiety	Schizophrenia, Psychoses	Addictions	Eating Disorders	Learning, Memory	Trauma, Abuse	Personality Disorders	Confusion, Brain Fog	Irritability	Self-Actualization	Spiritual Growth	Overall Health	Other
Light Therapies	x		(only if seasonal pattern exists)	x	x									
Macrobiotic Diet	x	x	x	x	x	x	x	x	x	x	x	x	x	immunity, free thinking
Martial Arts	x	x		x	x	x	x	x	x	x	x	x	x	
Massage Therapy	x	x		x	x	x	x		x	x	x	x	x	relationship issues, closed head injury
Meditation and Prayer	x	x		x		x	x	x	x	x	x	x	x	
Naturopathy	x	x		x	x	x	x	x	x	x	x	x	x	ADD, ADHD, OCD
Network Spinal Analysis													x	body awareness, ability to listen to one's "inner voice," adaptation to stress, increased life enjoyment, increased compassion
Orthomolecular Psychiatry	x	x	x	x		x			x		x		x	
Past Life Therapy	x	x		x	x	x	x			x	x	x		self-esteem, phobias, dissociative states, grief and loss, relationships, sexual problems, mothering issues
Polarity Therapy	x	x	?	x	x	x	x	?	x	x	x	x	x	enhance function and performance
Rolfing®	x	x		x	x	x	x	x	x	x	x	x	x	
Rubenfeld Synergy®	x	x		x	x	x	x		x	x	x	x	x	creative performance, head injury
Shamanism	x	x		x		x	x	x	x	x	x	x	x	
Sound Therapy	x	x				x	x			x	x	x	x	relaxation
Therapeutic Touch	x	x	x	x	x	x			x	x	x	x	x	
Trager Approach®	x	x	x	x	x	x	x	x	x	x	x	x	x	any condition of muscular restriction, weakness, or imbalance; optimal growth and development
Vision Therapy						x		x	x	x	x	x	x	headaches, visual blur, double vision, loss of place when reading, reading retention
Yoga	x	x		x		x			x	x	x	x	x	

Lynette Bassman, Ph.D.

1 Understanding Alternative Healing Modalities:

Basic Concepts

Following is an introduction to some of the basic concepts underlying many of the healing arts presented in this book. Reading this chapter can aid you in making the transition to a new way of thinking about your health, and assist you in creating the kind of health you want.

PSYCHOSOMATIC VS. SOMATOPSYCHIC

There was a time when the body and mind were seen as one unit, without any meaningful separation between them. It was obvious that each part of that unit affected every other part. In the past one hundred years or so, we have gotten away from that way of thinking. But lately, we are beginning to return to that view, called "holistic." Perhaps the biggest change taking place in health care today is the recognition that body and mind are connected. Evidence of this shift is offered in the recent PBS television series and accompanying book, *Healing and the Mind*, narrated by Bill Moyers. This series examines how thoughts and emotions are now seen to affect areas of physical health which were formerly thought of as functioning independently. *Healing and the Mind* looks at different survival rates for cancer patients who were involved in group therapy and other forms of emotional expression and support. It also looks at meditation, group therapy, and dietary change as integral to reversing heart disease. It is significant to note that this holistic approach to regaining cardiac health, pioneered by Dean Ornish, M.D., has recently gained acceptance to the point that it is now reimbursable by many insurance plans. It is now common to recognize the role of "stress" (meaning emotional stress) in many illnesses, including asthma, diabetes, and colitis. People with chronic pain can attend clinics where they can learn to reduce their experience of pain through the use of imagery, hypnosis, and biofeedback.

This recognition of the effect of the *mind* on the *body* is called "psychosomatic" medicine, and is a major step toward restoring the holistic view of health. Unfortunately there is less recognition about the other side of the coin: "somatopsychic" medicine, the effect of the *body* on the *mind*. This book details many different healing modalities that purport to heal, reduce, or relieve mental ills by treating imbalances in the physical body. It is important to bear in mind that the use of the terms "mind" and "body" and "somatopsychic" and "psychosomatic" are misleading, because they do not accurately portray the fully integrated reciprocal nature of the relationships involved. For example, in the case of chronic headache pain, an individual may experience pain as a result of an allergic reaction or a sensitivity to frequently eaten foods. However, food sensitivities are closely related to problems of digestion. Problems of digestion are often caused or exacerbated by emotional distress. An individual with chronic headaches and digestive disturbances may not feel motivated to be around people, and so, might develop faulty social skills and poor self-esteem. This in turn may cause the individual to develop physical symptoms to aid in the avoidance of awkward and emotionally risky social interactions. And so on. In no case does the causality go in one direction only (mind influencing body or vice versa). The causality and the influence process is mutual, as you will see from reading the chapters that follow, and from carefully examining your own life.

ALLOPATHIC VS. HOLISTIC

People born and raised in the United States and Europe in this century are familiar with a model of health and illness that sees the body as similar to a machine. When we are ill, we believe that the machine is broken, and needs to be fixed. We go to the doctor (the mechanic) and he or she uses skills and diagnostic tools such as blood tests and x-rays to determine which part is defective. The doctor prescribes medication, surgery, bed rest, or a special diet, and we expect a speedy recovery, and often get it. Frequently, each part of the body is treated separately, perhaps even by different doctors (we bring our defective heart to a cardiologist, our reproductive system failures to a gynecologist or urologist, etc.), and a problem in one body part is often not seen as having any connection to the other parts. Certainly the mind (believed to be located in the head) bears little relationship to any parts below the neck. In this century, and until quite recently, this has been the only officially recognized health care system practiced. According to Melvyn Werbach (1986), this system grew out of the invention of the microscope, which later allowed the origin of disease to be traced to the cell. This led to the formulation of the "doctrine of specific etiology," which held that illness can be categorized into different diseases, and that each disease has a unique and primary cause. This form of medicine is called "allopathic."

In recent years, there are some signs that this mechanistic view of health care is giving way to a "new" view: holistic health. The holistic view sees the body as being a fully integrated system, with all of the parts working together to maintain health. However, if we look back to the time before this century, and as far back as Hippocrates' time, we realize that the holistic view of health is not at all new. In fact, it has been the dominant view throughout history, and across most cultures, with the exception of the Western developed countries in the last one hundred years or so. Even in the United States, folk cultures (our grandmothers' remedies) have maintained vestiges of the holistic, natural ways of healing.

THE BODY'S INNATE ABILITY TO HEAL

People who believe in the holistic view of health believe that the body has the ability to heal itself and to maintain health even when conditions are not ideal. For instance, the body has systems for protecting itself from harm, and detoxifying our systems when they are poisoned; vomiting and diarrhea are natural responses for expelling offending toxins. Swelling of an injured limb and spasms of its muscles immobilize it and protect it from further damage, thus allowing it to begin to mend. The body is able to fight invading organisms by raising our body temperature to make an inhospitable environment for the organism. When faced with conflict that is too emotionally stressful to deal with, our defense mechanisms come into play to help us avoid becoming overwhelmed by the information. These systems are complex and subtly interconnected. We cannot look at any one functioning part of the body in isolation from the other parts, because they don't work in isolation. If we do view it that way, we are likely to misunderstand and interfere with the healing process rather than facilitate it.

If allowed to function naturally, these systems will usually keep us healthy. The symptoms (swelling, fever, denial) are seen as the normal functioning of our bodies and minds as they work to maintain health. According to this view, it would be a mistake to take aspirin to reduce fever, because that would allow the offending organism to proliferate. You would not want to suppress vomiting if you have eaten food tainted with salmonella. It would also not make sense to take an antianxiety medication because that would not allow you to process distressing information at a rate that is right for you. However, nature's ways sometimes lead to effects that do not seem acceptable, and that make us want to intervene. For example, a broken bone will mend, but perhaps the limb will not be straight, so we may choose to splint the limb. A high fever may kill a dangerous organism, but may also lead to brain damage, so we may choose to bring down the fever. Part of the skill of the holistic healer is knowing when and to what degree to intervene, and when to allow the body's own processes to take over.

In Chinese, there is one character that expresses the two ideas "crisis" and "opportunity." This is indicative of a worldview that is inherently holistic and that recognizes that physical symptoms are part of a process of growth rather than a problem to be removed. For instance, many people, after experiencing a major loss of some kind, will come down with a cold or the flu. This can be seen as one more misfortune heaped on top of the initial loss, or it can be seen as the body's way of slowing you down and encouraging you to properly mourn the loss rather than continuing with your regular schedule and burying the feelings. If we fail to recognize the connections between the cold and the grieving, and take a cold pill to reduce symptoms and get back to usual activities, then we have lost the opportunity to process the loss, and further (and perhaps more severe) physical symptoms may force us to deal with our emotions at a later time.

CUMULATIVE STRESS THEORY

"Stress" has become a very popular word lately, and it is usually used to describe a feeling of being overwhelmed by demands that are placed on us, for example, being overwhelmed by the amount of work there is to do, or being upset about a relationship that is not as rewarding as we would like.

There is a growing recognition that stress is a factor in the cause or exacerbation of a number of physical ills. However, this popular use of the term robs it of the rich and complex meaning that was intended by Hans Selye who first brought the term into use in the health care field in 1956. By "stress" Selye meant "the wear and tear in the body caused by life at any one time." The implication is that many things, not just emotional factors, have the effect of challenging the body's balance or homeostasis. Thus, it is not just a demanding boss that causes stress, but also extreme hot or cold, the impact of your feet on the ground when you walk, the effect of caffeine in your morning coffee, the excitement you feel when seeing your lover after a long separation, the microorganisms in the air when somebody sneezes, and the bewilderment you feel when dramatic life events fundamentally challenge your worldview. All of these stressors, and many more, challenge the body to produce an appropriate response so that balance can be maintained.

A main tenet of Selye's theory is that stress is essential to life, and is inevitable. Without it, we would function inadequately, and eventually, die. All living organisms respond to stimuli. For example, our bones respond to weight-bearing exercise by laying down additional calcium. Osteoporosis may result when a person does not adequately stress his or her bones through exercise, leading to a lack of bone density. If a child lacks opportunities to experience the minor trials and tribulations of human interaction on the playground, in the classroom, or at home, he or she may be unprepared to cope with the emotional pain of more significant traumas later in life.

Selye went on to explain that hormone-mediated defensive processes in the body help us respond to the challenges of everyday life. Sometimes these responses are inadequate or excessive. And sometimes there are so many stressors that we deplete the body's ability to cope with them. Disease is the result.

Many of the holistic healing modalities presented in this book aim to reduce the number of stressors to the body so that the body's innate healing abilities will be adequate, while other modalities aim to revitalize the defensive processes that have been depleted.

SUBCLINICAL CONDITIONS AND FUNCTIONAL ILLNESS

Another important aspect of the holistic or complementary health model is that sometimes conditions are best treated when they are quite small or subtle, perhaps even below the awareness level of the patient. According to Werbach, allopathic medicine defines disease as "stemming from a recognized etiologic agent or agents, having an identifiable group of signs and symptoms, and resulting in consistent anatomical alterations." But sometimes people experience symptoms for which no disease can be identified. For example, if a person has a marginal vitamin deficiency, such symptoms as fatigue, depression, headaches, impaired concentration, and aches and pains can result. However, the deficiency may not be discovered by the allopathic physician upon physical examination or blood tests. Moreover, the medical view of the test result may not take into consideration the fact that individuals vary with respect to the stress load under which their bodies are laboring. They instead compare an individual's result to a standardized reference range based on "average" levels of the pathogen. For example, analysis of a stool sample may reveal "normal" levels of pathogenic organisms, such as fungi, parasites, or bacteria, leading the physician to rule out several possible causal agents. However, a given patient's body, if too busy coping with other stressors, may succumb to the effects of the "acceptable" level of pathogenic organism. Often, such a patient will then be referred to a psychiatrist, based on the assumption that if no disease can be found then the person must be suffering from a psychosomatic ailment for which psychotherapy or psychotropic medication is the appropriate treatment.

Many of the holistic healing modalities include techniques for assessing imbalances in the body that are too subtle to show up on standard blood tests, x-rays, or biopsies. These techniques allow imbalances to be detected and corrected before they become disease states. For example, some people have thyroid glands that function well enough to yield blood test results in the normal range, yet the holistic practitioner can use a muscle test, pulse analysis, body temperature tracking, detailed constitutional history taking, or other methods to discover the presence of an otherwise insignificant imbalance in that gland. Furthermore, he or she might become aware that this minor imbalance is due not to any overt disease in that gland, but to functional disturbance of other endocrine components such as the adrenal gland, which can, in turn, be traced to certain aspects of the person's lifestyle, such as caffeine intake or lack of exercise. Steps can then be taken to balance out the problem in the endocrine system. So, using these and other highly sensitive assessment techniques, a holistic healer can detect dysfunction before it becomes severe, and understand its root causes to restore it to normal functioning, all well before the allopathic physician would be aware of any difficulty.

With knowledge of these basic concepts used by practitioners of holistic healing arts, you are now prepared to read on and to begin your process of deciding how to maximize your emotional wellness.

HOW TO LEARN MORE

Selye, H. *The Stress of Life*. New York: McGraw-Hill, 1956.

Werbach, M. *Third Line Medicine*. New York: Arkana, 1986.

J. Jamison Starbuck, J.D., N.D.

2 An Introduction to the Politics of Health Care

The politics of medicine are in many ways similar to politics of any sort: Power and money are the motivating factors, the forces underlying a multiplicity of decisions and governmental law-making. However, medical politics in America have involved another factor during the past century, a component whose influence have been critical in shaping both the delivery of health care in the United States, and our collective view of medical and scientific reality. While deeply significant throughout the past 100 years, this third factor is currently being challenged by a renaissance of contemplation about health care, and we might find its influence shrinking as we proceed into the twenty-first century.

This third factor is medical dogma. Medical dogma is defined as that system of thought which declares that there is one, and only one, system of medicine and science. Medical dogma says that the medical system is composed of, and limited to, medical doctors, their support staff and related institutions, pharmaceutical drugs, surgical procedures, highly technical equipment, certain portions of the insurance industry, and some Ph.D.'s. For decades, medical dogma had convinced the American public that its system and medicine were synonymous. When people heard the word "doctor," they thought of medical doctors. When people thought about "medicines," they pictured pharmaceutical drugs. "Treatments" brought to mind surgery, radiation, and chemotherapy. "Medical research" meant work being done by medical doctors or Ph.D.'s at medical schools, universities, or government facilities, on subjects related to pharmaceuticals, surgical techniques, or technological advances in the understanding of pathology.

Medical dogma, and its impact on our consciousness, is responsible for the fact that many Americans, until recently, had never heard of, much less seriously considered, medical options other than those espoused by the dominant medical system. Treatment options such as Ayurvedic medicine, Chinese medicine, naturopathic medicine, homeopathy, medicinal plant therapies, body-work and nutrition, if discussed at all, were relegated to the category of "alternative," and dismissed as "other than," "less than," "faith healing," "snake oil," "worthless," and sometimes even "criminal." Patients who chose to utilize these different modalities were considered daring, foolish, or strange.

The medical-political forces of money and power also affected our lack of awareness of, and access to, a variety of medical options. For all of the nineteenth and most of the twentieth century, no government funds were available for schools which trained naturopathic physicians, acupuncturists, massage therapists, and the like. These institutions had to survive on private funds and tuition fees. Their students were not able to obtain government loans and were not able to participate in government training, research, or employment programs after graduation. No government research dollars were available to explore "alternative" treatment modalities; no pharmaceutical companies offered research grants, nor endorsed academic chairs at institutions of "alternative" medicine.

During the late nineteenth through the late twentieth century, the politics of medicine had established the dominance of a monochromatic, hierarchical, and closed system of medicine. For patients with mental health complaints, as well as for patients with physical ailments, acceptable medical options were allopathic physicians, drugs, and surgery.

Now, as we approach the year 2000, there are signs that we are in the midst of an important intellectual, medical revolution. While for the past century unconventional individuals, perhaps the brilliant, the brave, and the prescient among us, kept alive a wide variety of "alternative" medicines, they are now joined by a multitude of more conventional, middle-of-the-road Americans. Medical dogma is under attack from a variety of sources, and there is an emerging schism in our collective definition of "medicine." This schism is the certain result of our increasing awareness of the world around us. Mass media, worldwide communication, and our inescapable movement toward a global community has broadened our horizons and excited our imaginations. We have learned that medicine is defined differently in other cultures. In the living rooms of our homes, on our computer screens, we see color films of yoga postures from India, of psychic surgery in the Philippines, of acupuncture instead of anesthesia, of the miracles of the mind-body connection.

Our understanding of reality has changed significantly in the past fifty years. As physicists now speak of particles smaller than the atom, and of waves and patterns of energy, intertwined, interdependent, and infinite, the concept of homeopathic medicine healing through infinitesimal doses seems more plausible. With our sharpened awareness of the dwindling rain forests and fragile ecosystems worldwide comes the knowledge that these environments contain plants with an ability to heal disease, that soil content influences food content, which, in turn, affects our health. As we hear scientists, religious teachers, economists, and health care practitioners suggest that we are one with all life and with all matter, the concepts of ecopsychology, self-generated healing, and biofeedback begin to make sense even to the skeptical among us.

We are well aware that technology and modern medicine have not solved all our health care problems. Concurrently, we understand that many new advancements carry with them new health threats. As we face our changing realities, we become aware that the reality of medicine has changed as well. From the holistic side of the schism, we see that medicine is not one method, not one system. It is as multifaceted as life itself, and we, the consumers of health care, have the right, and the obligation, to choose that method which works best for us.

As we look to the future of medicine, we must remember that changing human consciousness is rarely swift; Columbus was ridiculed for his theory of a world which was not flat; physicians resisted the notion of washing their hands because no invading organism was visible to them. Medical doctors have long dominated the medical scene, and they are not likely to easily relinquish the power and control they have so enjoyed. Many in the conventional medical system are loathe to accept what their current science cannot prove, and their scientific methods, double-blind, randomized, single element, placebo-controlled studies are not well-suited for exploring the effects of a holistic, individualized approach to healing.

It is up to us, patients, practitioners, and interested participants, to involve ourselves in the current revolution in medicine and in medical politics. What is required is not rhetoric, but action — positive personal and political action resulting in long-term changes to our medical system. One of the major challenges facing the "alternative" health care movement is eliminating the words "alternative medicine." As we embrace diversity in ourselves and in our world, so, too, should we embrace diversity in medicine. If medicine was a broad spectrum of equally respected possibilities for healing, instead of a hierarchy of "better thans" piled on top of one another with allopathic medicine on top, would not our culture be healthier, wiser, and more amply served?

The revolution in medical politics also requires changes in legislation, at the local, state, and federal levels. Among the needed legislative changes is the recognition of a wider array of health care practitioners through state licensing and insurance equity laws. These changes would allow consumers to freely choose the practitioner they want. Additionally, legislative efforts are required to ensure access to holistic practitioners for citizens dependent on the public health care system. King County, Washington (which encompasses Seattle), recently made national headlines by being the first to have an on-staff naturopathic physician and an acupuncturist in their county public health facility. More public health options like this are needed across the United States if we wish to preserve the health and integrity of all of our citizens. Challenges also exist in Medicare and Social Security, as these programs currently do not pay for the services of even licensed holistic health care providers.

We also face challenges in our education and research arenas, both public and private. In January 1993, the *New England Journal of Medicine* published an article (Eisenberg et al., 1993) stating that approximately one-third of the American people used some form of "alternative" medicine each year. Shortly thereafter, the National Institutes of Health (NIH) established the Office of Alternative Medicine (OAM), ostensibly to objectively study this area of great interest to the American public. While philosophically an exciting step, so far the OAM has been disappointing, receiving a tiny, tiny fraction of the overall NIH budget. The OAM has had little impact on the delivery of health care in America, and sadly, some of the OAM's own scientists have been quoted as labeling homeopathy as "silly."

The final challenge is a personal one, a challenge which asks each of us to explore options other than those offered by mainstream medicine, and to educate ourselves about the wide variety of health care options we indeed have. Such a challenge should be undertaken safely and wisely, but it is a journey which offers much and is well worth pursuing.

The Whole Mind: The Definitive Guide to Complementary Treatments for Mind, Mood, and Emotion is a great source to use when facing the challenges of exploring medical options. *The Whole Mind* represents a fine step in the necessary process of freeing individuals from the limitations of medical dogma and shining clear light on other effective health care options. Individuals with mental health problems will be especially grateful for this book, as they are often more vulnerable to the medical system, and because few reliable resource books on mental health and holistic medicine exist today. It is exciting to see the abundant possibilities for care and treatment of mental health disorders. May each reader take something from, and give something back to, this delightful process of redefining medicine.

HOW TO LEARN MORE

Coulter, H. L. *Divided Legacy: A History of the Schism in Medical Thought. The Patterns Emerge: Hippocrates to Paracelsus.* Vol. I. Washington, DC: Center for Empirical Medicine, 1994.

Coulter, H. L. *Divided Legacy: A History of the Schism in Medical Thought. The Origins of Modern Western Medicine: J. B. Van Helmont to Claude Bernard.* Vol. II. Washington, DC: Wehawken Book Company and Berkeley, CA: North Atlantic Books, 1988.

Coulter, H. L. *Divided Legacy: A History of the Schism in Medical Thought. Volume III. The Conflict Between Homeopathy and the American Medical Association,* Second Edition. Berkeley, CA: North Atlantic Books and Homeopathic Education Services, 1982.

Coulter, H. L. *Divided Legacy: A History of the Schism in Medical Thought. Volume IV. Twentieth-Century Medicine: The Bacteriological Era.* Berkeley, CA: North Atlantic Books, 1994.

Eisenberg, D. M.; R. C. Kessler; C. Foster; F. E. Norlock; D. R. Calkins; and T. L. Delbanco, "Unconventional Medicine in the United States: Prevalence, Costs, and Patterns of Use." *New England Journal of Medicine* (1993): 328, 246–52.

Kuhn, T. S. *The Structure of Scientific Revolutions,* Second Edition. Chicago: University of Chicago Press, 1970.

ABOUT THE AUTHOR

J. Jamison Starbuck, J.D., N.D., has a practice in family medicine in Missoula, Montana. At least 30 percent of her practice is devoted to the treatment of mental health issues, including Attention Deficit Disorder (ADD), depression, anxiety, and eating disorders. She also teaches homeopathy and botanical medicine, is a consulting editor for Time-Life Books, and writes and consults for various publications nationwide. She is a 1989 graduate of National College of Naturopathic Medicine. She is also a graduate of Middlebury College and Willamette University College of Law, and is a member of the state bars of Montana and Oregon.

John L. Stegmaier

3 A Parent's Perspective on the Politics of Mental Health Care

When Dr. Bassman invited me to write this chapter, my wife and I thought long and hard about it because we knew that I would have to talk frankly and personally about our daughter. We were concerned, particularly because inevitably the chapter would tend to stress the bizarre, out of control aspects of psychosis. In a variety of ways, however, the insights brought by my daughter's experiences have already benefited many people who are beset by problems like hers and this has been a source of satisfaction to her. On that basis, we decided to go ahead with the chapter and we hope very much that it will prove useful to patients and parents alike.

JAPAN AND HAWAII

Twenty-five years ago, an abrupt personality shift in our youngest daughter plunged my wife and me into a search for solutions to a severe mental illness that has dominated our lives ever since. When the problem arose, we were living in Japan, where I had long worked in government and business. After careful thought, and despite a high regard for Japanese medicine, we finally decided to take our daughter back to the U.S., confident that "a good American psychiatrist" could make her well in no time. Looking back, we are amazed at the simple-mindedness of that assumption.

Our daughter was 14 years old when she first displayed behaviors sharply at odds with her normally confident, outgoing, achieving ways. Within barely a year, she dropped out of two schools, stopped communicating with us and her many friends, and retreated into a sullen, hostile withdrawal. At first we interpreted this as just a difficult adjustment to adolescence. When she began to suspect that we and others were plotting to harm her, however, we realized that the situation demanded professional help.

We took our daughter directly from Japan to Hawaii, hoping that the mild climate and relaxed social environment might prove therapeutic. (Before going there, we had ascertained that the psychiatric talent compared favorably with what was available on the mainland.) She did do fairly well in Hawaii at the start — was admitted to a leading girls' school and got reasonably good grades. Nonetheless, she was unable to make friends and, instead, repeatedly rebuffed the many schoolmates who tried to make contact with her. She was also increasingly unfriendly toward us and her siblings, and her angry outbursts often disturbed the peace and quiet of our home.

One unforgettable night, she went out of control so badly that my middle daughter's muscular boyfriend and I were unable to restrain her, and she hurled a bottle into a large wall mirror across the living room. Six years later, we began to see that this kind of aberrant behavior stemmed from a wide variety of physiological problems of which we had not been aware — disordered sugar metabolism, food and chemical sensitivities, nutritional deficiencies and imbalances, malabsorption, etc. At the time, we simply thought she was acting outrageously, although our attitude was tempered by nagging doubts, nurtured by the comments of her counselors and by books on psychiatric subjects, that really the fault somehow was ours for having been "bad parents."

We learned a lot about the horrors of mental illness during our three years in Hawaii, how devastating it is for the sick person and how bewildering, frightening, and fraught with helplessness it is for the parents. At one point, our daughter took to stealing away from the house at night and making a beeline to a busy highway not far from our home, where she would dance wildly along the side of the road. More and more delusional, she became convinced that she was the Virgin Mary, and when we came home one day, she was up on the roof acting out the role, much to the fascination of the neighborhood. About this time she decided to become a nun, and several times I drove her to a Catholic church for instruction by a young priest. This brief flirtation with the spiritual life ended when she stalked out of a session shouting curses at him for opposing abortion.

In the meantime, she came to be regarded as hopelessly antisocial at school, and her grades plummeted even in subjects in which she used to shine. For instance, she had been so good at reading that a previous school had chosen her to read aloud before a meeting of the PTA. However, in Hawaii, her ability fell so drastically that the school phoned us and suggested that she receive instruction in remedial reading. Conscious that "problems" were at the root of our daughter's weird behavior, one young teacher suggested that they have lunch together to discuss how she might improve her grades. She accepted the invitation but specified that she could tolerate only "health foods." The teacher came laden with various goodies of unimpeachable purity. True to form, our daughter arrived late, bearing several chocolate-covered icecream bars, which we gathered had long been her standard fare for lunch at school. (Much later we learned that milk, sugar, and chocolate were high on the list of foods to which she was severely allergic and that could precipitate psychotic symptoms whenever she ate them.)

Hazards of Life in Paradise

Despite its impressive charms, Hawaii proved to hold many dangers for a beautiful young lady struggling with serious mental problems. Although she could not bring herself to reciprocate the overtures of her schoolmates, our daughter felt comfortable with drifters, beachcombers, and others on the fringe of society in the fiftieth state. One of our scariest moments came one afternoon when the three of us went swimming at a crowded beach on the north side of Oahu. Before we could find a place to settle down, our daughter raced away and was immediately lost in the crowd. We went searching for her at top speed and spotted her in a parked car talking eagerly to the owner, a swarthy gentleman who spoke English poorly but who was radiating delight that this attractive, amiable young lady had popped into his front seat.

We squelched that budding friendship on the spot but were less successful with the "forever young" smalltime drug dealer and all-around bum whom I'll call Ronald. A member of Hawaii's large contingent of ne'er-do-well Californians, Ronald noticed our daughter one day as she was waiting for a bus and within minutes asked her for a date that night. She came home terribly excited and begged us to drive her to the shopping mall where they had agreed to meet.

Both of us were strongly opposed to letting our daughter go out with a man whom she barely knew and we had never met. At the same time, we were keenly aware of her profound loneliness; we were constantly trying to bring her into contact with other people. Perplexed, we phoned her counselor and asked him what he thought we should do. Without hesitation, he replied, "As things stand, you overprotect your daughter and this is very bad for her feelings of independence and self-worth. You have to let her 'hurt and be hurt' in order to adjust to life. By all means, let her go out on this date. To do less would be unfair to her." That friendship flourished until, mercifully, they parted.

Our daughter's most perilous pass in Hawaii came when she was 18 and her counselor kept stressing that she was much too dependent on us (under prevailing psychiatric doctrine, parents are always basically suspect) and that she must start living independently. Still awed by psychiatric "experts," we arranged for her to move into the YWCA, an easy bus ride from her school and, again at the counselor's urging, we left for a short business trip to the mainland. When we returned, we pieced together a chilling story from our daughter's disjointed account of what happened during our absence.

In conscientious assertion of her independence, she set off one day on a hike up one of the wooded hills overlooking Honolulu. Suddenly, a young Asian man pulled her into the bushes, raped her, and then threatened to kill her. Something, perhaps a subtle compatibility born of our long years in Japan, enabled her to dissuade him from this and she escaped. The very next day, the same man raped and murdered another girl in the same area. Our daughter watched with horror as the police brought him in handcuffs to the police station near the YWCA. She was doubly troubled because in her confused state of mind, she felt that somehow she had helped to bring about the young man's arrest.

A PREEMINENT MENTAL INSTITUTION

When she was just 19, our daughter suddenly begged us to take her some place where there were "other people like me." Delighted at this unexpected change of attitude (previously she had resisted any idea of hospitalization), we immediately arranged for her admission to a Midwestern mental institution with outstanding credentials, feeling that surely here she would stand the best possible chance of putting her mental problems behind her.

As part of the registration process, we had an appointment with the business manager who was visibly elated to find that our insurance would provide full coverage for our daughter for an almost unlimited period to come. Because we were new to the game, the significance of his reaction was lost on us. In our ignorance, we also attached little importance to the fact that the patients, all of whom were fed in the cafeteria, were under absolutely no restrictions as to their choice of foods and could eat nothing but apple pie and ice cream if they chose to do so. Similarly, they could smoke cigarettes to their hearts' delight, and coffee, cream, and sugar were available to them 24 hours a day. (Later we learned that caffeine and tobacco are treacherous "no-no's" in mental illness and that diet is critically related to psychosis.) Looking back, we find it difficult to believe that the organization's top people were unaware of these elementary facts.

Despite its beautifully manicured lawns, luxurious buildings, and large staff, the hospital proved totally incapable of helping our daughter. After nine months she was sicker than when she entered, and we informed her group psychiatrist that we were taking her out. Discomfited by our decision, he said, "But Mr. and Mrs. Stegmaier, many of our patients don't begin to respond to our therapy for five years." We didn't doubt the accuracy of his statement, having observed several patients who appeared extremely ill after protracted stays.

This first major hospitalization proved to be only the start of a quest that involved five major hospitals and individual treatment by well over twenty different psychiatrists and other specialists in thirteen states and the District of Columbia over the next few years. In time, we stopped expecting them to solve our daughter's mental problems but continued to hope that someone, somewhere, could explain persuasively why she was ill. (Typical was the comment of a hospital spokesman whom we encountered along the way: "We think that psychosis stems from disorders of brain chemistry but that's all we know about it.") It was monstrous that this purported psychiatric expert, speaking for a very well known mental institution, could make such a statement when the momentous discoveries of pioneers like Theron Randolph, Abram Hoffer, Carl Pfeiffer, and others were common knowledge to anyone truly interested in finding answers to serious mental illness.

THE COLORADO INTERLUDE

To be near our daughter, my wife and I decided to move to Colorado as soon as she was ensconced in that high-status mental hospital. (In those days we had enough extra money to afford adjustments of this kind; eventually, inevitably,

the illness ate it all up, and more.) We settled in the town of Georgetown, population about 800, at 8,500 feet above sea level and 45 miles west of Denver.
We chose it partly because we felt that it might prove hospitable to our daughter. My wife had roots in the town: her grandfather had owned mines in the
area and her mother was brought up there.

We were right. Thanks to a wonderful principal, our daughter was admitted to the junior class of the high school very late in the year, finished with
passing grades, and graduated the next year. She went on school outings, sang
in the church choir, and even had a few friends for the first time in years. In
short, she was functioning better in that environment than she had for a long
time. In light of what we know now, it's clear that the beautiful mountain air,
cleaner than any that she had breathed for a long time, had a lot to do with
this. Even so, her condition remained constantly vulnerable to the slightest
provocation.

For instance, despite doing well at school a lot of the time, she would get
derailed and behave atrociously at home, particularly on weekends when she
often stayed indoors all day. We later learned information that suggested a
major reason for this was that the building materials and wall-to-wall carpeting
in our new house were still off-gassing formaldehyde and other allergenic chemicals. Similarly, she did well at school in the fall until cold weather came and
the maintenance crew turned on the oil burner. Almost immediately, she reacted so strongly to the minuscule leaks of spent gas that it looked for a while as
though she would have to drop out.

There were other signs that our daughter's condition remained precarious.
After that first major hospitalization, we had taken her to a psychotherapist in
Berkeley, CA, where she was hospitalized for several weeks while receiving his
treatments. (At one point, he had us fly in two of our other three children to
participate with the rest of us in his group sessions, in hope of resolving family
conflicts that he felt were at the root of her mental problems.) He was good at
his specialty, but in the end his "talk therapy" alone proved inadequate and he
was forced to put her on a low dosage of Haldol (haldoperidol, the widely used
antipsychotic medication). When we left for home she was on five mg per day,
but she kept pressing us to reduce the dose and we did so very gradually. (For
most patients, antipsychotic medications have extremely negative connota-
tions.) Eventually, we got it down to one mg per day and she remained quite
stable at this level. (Accustomed to prescribing massive dosages of antipsychotic

medications, psychiatrists whom we later told about this simply refused to believe it.) She then insisted that we drop it entirely and we finally agreed to try this. Within one day, she remarked on the plant growing out of her mother's head and we knew she must go back on the Haldol. Miraculously, she agreed without a major blowup.

During the two years that we spent in Colorado, our daughter was treated by a variety of practitioners, including an offbeat psychiatrist who prescribed a moderate dosage of Mellaril (another major antipsychotic). Probably because she was chemically sensitive, as we discovered much later, she collapsed soon after taking it. We immediately phoned to ask him what to do next and he replied, "Double the dose." We ignored this outrageous advice and never saw him again.

She was also treated by a chiropractor who claimed to know a lot about disorders of sugar metabolism. At the first appointment, he administered a glucose tolerance test to her and informed us that the results showed that she was suffering from chronic, "functional" low blood sugar (hypoglycemia). This was new to us but we soon learned that the problem is common and is often associated with psychiatric symptoms including severe fatigue, mood changes, and even, in some cases, mental confusion. To deal with the condition, he recommended that she go on a low-sugar, high-protein diet featuring items like beef steak for breakfast. (Later testing showed that she could not eat beef without risking psychotic reactions.) Until we learned better, we held her to this regimen while struggling to deal with the upsets that it constantly provoked.

OTHER SETTINGS, OTHER HORRORS

After two years in Colorado, we decided audaciously to take a trip around the world with our daughter, then 21, still assuming that her problems were basically psychosocial and that the stimulations of travel — including a return visit to Japan — might help to cure her mental problems. We proceeded wildly through the U.K., France, Spain, Italy, and Greece with our daughter still on that terribly provocative high-protein diet. Athens turned out to be the end of the line partly, no doubt, because the air was so heavy with pollution that you could cut it with a knife. After a couple of days, our daughter began to manifest suicidal impulses, and a local psychiatrist whom we contacted by phone urged that we immediately return to the U.S. We were on the morning plane for New York.

Upon arrival, our daughter was in such a disturbed state that we had to admit her to a hospital on Long Island, where she remained for two months while we stayed in a Manhattan apartment so that we could go out to see her often. To our great surprise, we found her virtually normal one day, better than she had been for years. Not only was she cheerful and sociable, she invited us to play Ping-Pong with her and beat both of us decisively. Her doctor's personality was basically unfathomable to us, but her dramatic recovery convinced us that he must be a genius, so when he instructed that we not come to see our daughter again for three weeks, we agreed without a whimper. The next time we went to visit her, however, she was "exquisitely psychotic," so desperately ill that she was actually banging her head against the wall. Deeply concerned, we queried the nursing staff about this and one of them commented, "It's funny — she did so well on the water fast." Inquiring further, we learned that her doctor had quietly taken her off everything but spring water for a few days and that an unexpected interval of great clarity had followed. Inexplicably, he had then decreed that she could eat anything she wanted, whereupon she devoured five or six lamb chops and rapidly become extremely psychotic again.

Next we flew our daughter to an ostensibly "orthomolecular" hospital in Florida, where she spent nine months and where we detected few signs of progress during several visits. (On one occasion we arrived unannounced and found her in Intensive Care, literally in rags.) During her stay we were allowed to phone the psychiatrist once weekly to discuss her condition, but he proved to be a poor communicator. For some reason, his speech was often noticeably slurred. Only a day or two after returning from one of our visits, we were dismayed to receive a phone call asking that we come down again to discuss what our daughter would be doing following her discharge. The psychiatrist and two assistants sat us down and informed us gravely that she had decided to go to New York to "make it on her own." (She was barely managing to function on 40 mg of Valium per day at the time.) We suspected that the three of them had cooked up this appalling scheme and were immensely relieved when she joined the meeting and breezily announced that she would be accompanying us to our new home just outside Washington, where we had moved during her stay. (We decided to do this partly because, still incredibly naive, we assumed that the National Institutes of Health surely would have answers to her illness.)

A REMARKABLE PSYCHIATRIST

When our daughter was 23, we heard about Thomas L. Stone, M.D., an Illinois psychiatrist reputed to have marked success treating chronically ill mental patients by addressing their physiological disorders. Ever-hopeful, we immediately arranged for her admission to his special nine-bed unit in one of the wards at a large mental hospital not far from Chicago. While waiting in the lobby, we talked with a man and wife who had brought their daughter from Florida to enter the program a few days before. They beamed, "You're going to be amazed. This doctor is really on the right track." It didn't take us long to agree; the day-to-day occurrences in that unit gave us our first clear evidence that psychotic illness results primarily from myriad disorders of the body.

Dr. Stone had originally been a psychoanalyst but turned away from it when he began to notice that in many cases, his patients' psychotic symptoms resulted from physical ailments, or from exposure to foods and other substances to which they reacted allergically. Treatment of such conditions almost invariably led to a reduction in mental symptoms and in many cases, to full recovery. Exploring further, he perceived that psychosis is multifactorial in nature and that full success in dealing with it demands aggressive treatment of all physiological disorders at the root of the condition. Upon admission to his program, patients went through a battery of tests involving every major organ system and physiological function of the body so that the doctor could develop treatments targeted at their individual needs. In many cases, additional tests were done later as he learned more about the strengths and weaknesses of each patient's physical being.

An important aspect of Dr. Stone's diagnostic approach was to identify any food sensitivities that might be causing or exacerbating the individual's mental problems. He began by putting each new patient on a spring water fast for several days, a procedure that provoked withdrawal symptoms in a few patients, although most of them recovered rapidly in response to countermeasures such as intravenous infusions of vitamin C. (Fasting experts report that in most patients, food deprivation does not begin to produce actual starvation for at least 25 days.)

The majority of patients did well on the spring water fast as the toxins that had caused them pain gradually left their bodies. Many of them were in better shape by the third or fourth day than they had been for years. However, some of them, including our daughter, never fully cleared because, as we discovered later, they were chemically sensitive and were constantly reacting to the polluted hospital air.

As soon as patients had cleared as much as possible, Dr. Stone and his staff began testing them one food at a time, while constantly monitoring them for pulse rate, skin temperature, blood sugar level, and other indicators of physiological function plus, of course, behavior. Whenever patients proved not to be allergic to a particular food, nothing would happen — all indicators, including behavior, remained steady. In contrast, a patient would often be in the grips of a horrendous psychotic episode within minutes after eating a food to which he or she was intolerant. Not infrequently, these reactions were so serious that patients would have to be clapped into restraints and kept in isolation for up to two full days while they were being detoxified to the offending substance.

Avoidance and neutralization offer the best immediate means of dealing with food and chemical allergies, and in many cases, they bring a rapid reduction or elimination of physical and mental dysfunction. When our daughter first entered the program, she tested allergic to all but seven foods. She was then compelled to eat only those foods and do so rotationally — once every four days.

Our daughter was under Dr. Stone's care for 13 months, eight in the hospital and five in his out-patient clinic, after mainline psychiatric interests compelled the administration to close his unit. We were with her every day and many nights. One cardinal lesson that we learned was that virtually everyone is sensitive to one or more foods and/or chemicals. However, "target organs" for such sensitivities run a gamut that includes the stomach and intestines, cardiovascular system, muscles and joints, and, notably, the central nervous system. As we eat a variety of foods and experience chemical exposures, our allergic sensitivities are "masked" and are often imperceptible. Once a person has been on a spring water fast for a few days, however, the allergies become "unmasked" and his or her reactions may become far more extreme.

One day shortly after our arrival, our daughter was scheduled to test Brussels sprouts at lunch. All patients ate in the same large room, cafeteria style. Our daughter received her test serving of Brussels sprouts as she went through the line, joined some other patients at one of the tables, and began to eat. Expecting no problems with such an innocuous-seeming food, my wife and I went to another part of the dining room to have lunch. After a few minutes, our daughter emitted a blood-curdling shriek, let go a string of profanity, and had just time enough to slam her tray against the wall when two or three burly male staff seized her and led her, still screaming, to the "quiet room." It took two days before she stabilized enough to come out and resume testing. She proved totally insensitive to pears, which went on the list of items that she could eat rotationally without reacting. Incidentally, after several months during which she ate no Brussels sprouts, her sensitivity to them dropped enough so that she was able to eat them rotationally without reacting.

During our 13 months in Illinois, we saw massive, overwhelming proof that mental illness is rooted in physiological problems: disorders of sugar metabolism, weakened pancreatic function, nutritional deficiencies, impaired liver, gastrointestinal breakdown, hormonal insufficiencies, and dozens of other purely medical conditions.

GETTING THE COLD SHOULDER AT NIMH

After returning home from Illinois, my wife and I could hardly wait to report our eye-opening observations to the National Institute of Mental Health (NIMH). We rushed over there like two bumpkins, buttonholed a couple of men who we later learned were high in the scientific hierarchy, and regaled them for 10 minutes or so about the wondrous things we had seen and learned. We fully expected them to call an impromptu meeting of colleagues to hear our story. Far from this, they registered complete boredom, made it clear that we were interfering with matters of high importance, and politely but firmly showed us the door.

It took us a long time to understand that the NIMH, its scientists, and the vast number of others whom it funds in laboratories across the country spend little or no time devising solutions to complex pathologies. Instead, the scientists pursue a severely reductionist, *basic science* approach under which they examine small, individual parts of the whole by means of double-blind crossover studies, and rarely look at the big picture or feel compelled to do so. This means that NIMH and its scientific family, individually and institutionally, are poorly equipped to holistically examine a phenomenon like psychotic illness and to develop realistic, effective ways of dealing with it. To do so would be beyond them, partly because this would involve myriad components, many of them not susceptible to double-blind techniques, but also because the main focus of their interest and effort is to "do science" (with a Nobel Prize always in mind) rather than to cure disease.

Someday NIMH may begin to come to grips with multifactorial illnesses by stressing "outcomes studies," an alternative technique in medical research that downplays double-blind crossover investigations and concentrates on therapeutic results. In the meantime, the laborious, time-consuming double-blind approach holds up medical progress outrageously, because most practicing physicians do not dare to deviate from "the medical mainline" until NIMH (and the FDA) have given the green light. Thus, U.S. research scientists, many of them without the slightest knowledge of or interest in clinical activities, have immense power to determine if and when the American public can have the benefit of medical advances, including alternative techniques that have been tested exhaustively and proven safe and sound in other advanced nations.

PLAYING GAMES WITH OTHER PEOPLE'S LIVES

In our peregrinations, my wife and I have encountered more than a few psychiatrists and other professionals who viewed patients with undisguised indifference, even disdain, particularly those with parents who did not hesitate to make clinical suggestions. One of the worst examples was the top psychiatrist and his team at a high-powered hospital in the Washington area who gave our daughter 23 mg of Haldol, despite our urgent warning (or perhaps because of it) that she could not tolerate more than five mg. We arrived shortly after and found that she could not talk, could barely breathe, had great difficulty swallowing, and kept writhing uncontrollably and falling off the bed. When we demanded to see the psychiatrist and asked what he thought was wrong, he answered, "Catatonia." And when we asked what he thought was the source of the catatonia, he said, "Anxiety." (Based on our experience with psychiatrists, we believed this to mean "anxiety reflecting tensions in the home caused by bad parenting.")

Another consequence of the Haldol overdose was that unknown to us, our daughter became ultrasensitive to it. Several months later we arranged an appointment for her at the Pfeiffer Treatment Center in Naperville, IL, headed by former U.S. government research scientist William Walsh, Ph.D., where she was scheduled to receive highly sophisticated testing and clinical recommendations. Our plan was to go by car but she balked at leaving. Our family doctor came to the house and gave her a five mg injection of Haldol, which had always made her cooperative and compliant in the past. Twenty minutes later we were well up the highway at rush hour when she went into an extremely psychotic state, didn't know where she was or who we were, and kept trying to open the back door of the car. Somehow I managed to reach back and hold down the door lock while easing the car over to the shoulder so my wife could get into the back seat and keep her from jumping out. When we reached a motel, I went to phone the police for help, whereupon she broke away, raced across a busy highway, and headed for the rim of a deep abandoned quarry. Fortunately, a young man saw what was happening, caught up with her, and was able to hold her until the police arrived. (We have called on the police for help countless times and they have never failed us.)

PROBABLE ROOT CAUSE AND TANTALIZING POSSIBILITIES

It took years of study and thought before it dawned on my wife and me that our daughter's mental problems may have begun in the garden of the house that we occupied while I was consul general for the Kobe–Osaka area of Japan. Our daughter was fond of the gardener and often followed him around, conversing in Japanese while he worked. A key item of his stock-in-trade was a variety of pesticides sent by the American Embassy. One day termites invaded the house and my wife asked him what could be done about it. With great aplomb, he replied that he would spray the affected areas with an American termite killer called Chlordane. (Years later it was revealed that Chlordane is extremely toxic to humans.) Only a few days afterward, our daughter, who normally enjoyed robust health, came down with a raging fever. She was rushed to the hospital, where she was diagnosed with pneumonia. The American doctor who treated her was baffled as to why she had fallen ill and told my wife there was something mysteriously wrong with her immune system. That bout with pneumonia proved to be the starting point for a long decline in our daughter's physical and mental health that culminated in the psychosis that has bedeviled her for a quarter century.

If we had known then what we know now, we would have declared the house off-limits to Chlordane and all other pesticides not certified as harmless to human beings. It's staggering that simple preventive measures like these might well have spared our daughter the terrible suffering that she has had to endure because of psychotic illness.

The most painful aspect of our daughter's illness has been to watch the years inexorably slip by while the life of this beautiful, intelligent, talented, extremely decent young lady goes down the drain. (Now 39, her greatest desire is to marry and have children.) It has been all the more difficult for us to bear her situation, and those of other patients whom we have followed over the years, as we have come to realize that already existing modalities, expertly combined, could greatly improve patients' prospects of recovery and cure some completely.

HOW IS SHE DOING NOW?

For several years our daughter did quite well on Clozaril, one of the antipsychotic medications developed in Europe and now widely used in the U.S. (We got ahead of the parade by ordering it from Switzerland long before the FDA approved it.) At first Clozaril seemed ideal because it dramatically diminished the extreme paranoia that had severely reduced the scope of our daughter's activities for several years by keeping her in a state of social paralysis. Everything that anyone did or said triggered deep-seated fears as to his or her intentions; my wife and I were constant objects of her suspicion. After a few years on Clozaril, however, she began to show pronounced signs of obsessive-compulsive disorder (OCD). Upon consulting the latest clinical data, we found that this was one of the side effects now mentioned by the manufacturer. When a severe psychotic episode sent our daughter into a brief hospitalization, a cooperative psychiatrist put her on a different antipsychotic medication. (It is extremely hazardous to make such a shift except under controlled conditions because the outcomes are unpredictable.) The change helped somewhat, but a fairly serious OCD persisted.

We read that scientists in Israel were treating OCD effectively with large amounts of inositol, a member of the B-vitamin family available in any good health food store. After checking with Dr. William Walsh, mentioned previously, we began giving inositol to our daughter, gradually building it up to the levels reported from Israel. The OCD visibly began to abate and her overall mental health improved.

We are not so naive as to expect a single natural substance such as inositol to prove the solution to our daughter's psychosis. In dealing with such a vexing problem, however, one has no choice but to keep exploring all possibilities. Our great hope now is that inositol, combined with other remedies, will keep her manageable until a program becomes available that addresses the clinical, social, vocational, and other deficits that now make it impossible for her to live a normal life.

LISTEN TO THE EXPERTS

Everything that my wife and I know about mental illness has been learned by living under the same roof for a quarter century with a psychotic child whom we love dearly, and by studying and listening carefully to concerned professionals and nonprofessionals, including countless parents with whom we have exchanged information over the years. We are fairly well-informed nonprofessionals, but we are just that: deeply interested lay persons lacking in professional credentials. In the interest of credibility, we would urge readers to check out the basic points raised in this chapter by consulting what highly qualified experts have written on the subject.

One of the most authoritative, informative books available is *A Dose of Sanity* by Sydney Walker III, M.D. (1997), a highly experienced practicing psychiatrist who heads the Southern California Psychiatric Institute. Dr. Walker sternly rebukes his colleagues for deserting their medical roots and lazily following the dictates of the *DSM* (*Diagnostic and Statistical Manual*) a psychiatrist's operating bible, instead of using their professional knowledge to dig in and find out what is wrong medically with mental patients and treating them on that basis. To make his case, Dr. Walker cites countless individuals diagnosed as "schizophrenic," "manic depressive," etc., who recovered completely once the physiological problems underlying their mental disorders were diagnosed and treated. In his view, the failure of psychiatrists to conduct themselves in this fashion amounts to participating in a vast system of misdiagnosis with the most tragic consequences for patients. In his words, "psychiatric patients whose disorders are caused by tumors, infections, toxic exposure, hormonal imbalances, or other physical ailments will suffer needlessly, or even die, if they are simply labeled, drugged, and psychoanalyzed."

Another excellent book of this general character is *Ill Not Insane* by Bonnie Sigren Busick, R.N., Ph.D. (1986). Drawing heavily on the professional literature, Dr. Busick makes a strong case for broad acceptance of a medical model in mental illness that "carefully searches for physiological problems which could cause the behavior in question before assuming the problem is of psychological origin." The book identifies more than 200 physical illnesses and conditions that can cause or exacerbate mental problems.

Other medical professionals who have written in this vein include Erwin Koranyi, Robert Hall, and Lorrin Koran, all three of whom report countless instances in which practitioners have misdiagnosed mental patients, often disastrously, by failing to examine the physiological factors at the root of their symptoms.

HOW TO LEARN MORE

Busick, B. *Ill Not Insane.* Louisville, CO: New Idea Press, 1986.

Walker, S. *A Dose of Sanity.* New York: John Wiley and Sons, 1997.

ABOUT THE AUTHOR AND THE NEW HOPE PROJECT

Mr. Stegmaier received his bachelor's degree from Harvard University and was a secondary school teacher for several years. He served as a military pilot/instructor in World War II and as a foreign service officer of the Department of State from 1946 to 1968. From 1968 to 1971 he was president of Encyclopedia Britannica Japan, Inc. and was president of the Well Mind Association of Greater Washington, a not-for-profit, all-volunteer educational and public service organization, during 1984–1996. He and his wife have four children — a son and three daughters — all but the youngest of whom have always enjoyed sound mental health.

Mr. Stegmaier is cofounder and president of the New Hope Foundation, Inc. He and his wife have spent more than a decade working to establish a realistic, effective new model, incorporating techniques that work in diagnosing and treating psychotic illness and scrupulously avoiding those that do not. The project has an excellent site and has attracted intense interest from dozens of families across the country whose mentally ill children have failed to benefit from other programs. One of New Hope's most distinctive features will be a lifelong follow-up program that includes chemically clean, low-rent housing for graduates working gainfully in the general area. Parents will be encouraged to play an active role in the New Hope program, particularly at the graduate level.

New Hope is tentatively scheduled to begin operating in 1998. For details, contact the New Hope Foundation, Inc., Box 201, 3205 Wake Drive, Kensington, MD 20895, (301) 946-6395.

Stanislav Grof, M.D.

4 Rethinking Basic Assumptions about Psychology and Psychiatry:
The Role of Spirituality and Nonordinary States of Consciousness

WHAT ARE NONORDINARY STATES OF CONSCIOUSNESS?

Nonordinary states of consciousness (NOSC) are characterized by dramatic perceptual changes, intense and often unusual emotions, profound alterations in thought processes and behavior, and by a variety of psychosomatic manifestations. This chapter will focus on research findings in a large and important subgroup of NOSC that I call "holotropic" (literally "oriented toward wholeness" from the Greek *holos*, "whole" and *trepein*, "moving toward"). In these states, consciousness is changed, but is not grossly impaired. All intellectual functions are intact and the person remains fully oriented. The content of holotropic experiences is often spiritual or mystical. This state involves sequences of psychological death and rebirth and a broad spectrum of transpersonal phenomena, including feelings of oneness with other people, nature, and the universe, past life experiences, and visions of archetypal beings and mythological landscapes as described by C. G. Jung (1960).

Holotropic experiences can be triggered by various forms of systematic spiritual practice involving meditation, concentration, breathing, and movement exercises that are used in different systems of yoga, Vipassana or Zen Buddhism, Tibetan Vajrayana, Taoism, Christian mysticism, Sufism, or Cabala. Ancient cultures have brought on these states of mind through chanting, drumming, breathing, dancing, fasting, enduring extreme pain, and social and sensory isolation, and ingesting psychedelic plants. Such processes were important parts of shamanic practices, healing ceremonies, and rites of passage.

Among the modern means of inducing holotropic states of consciousness are psychedelic substances isolated from plants or synthesized in the laboratory, and powerful experiential forms of psychotherapy, such as hypnosis, primal therapy, rebirthing, or holotropic breathwork. There are also very effective laboratory techniques for altering consciousness including sensory isolation and brainwave biofeedback.

Episodes of NOSC can also occur spontaneously, without any specific identifiable cause, and often against the will of the person involved. Since modern psychiatry does not differentiate between mystical or spiritual states and mental diseases, people experiencing these states are often labeled psychotic, are hospitalized, and receive medication to suppress the symptoms. My wife and I refer to these states as spiritual emergencies or psychospiritual crises. We believe that when properly supported and treated, they can result in a patient's emotional and psychosomatic healing, positive personality transformation, and consciousness evolution (Grof and Grof, 1989, 1990).

It is useful and important to study nonordinary states of consciousness because of their great therapeutic potential and because they are a rich source of revolutionary new information about the psyche, human nature, and the nature of reality.

HOW IT BEGAN

The therapeutic use of nonordinary states of consciousness is the most recent development in Western psychotherapy. Paradoxically, it is also the oldest form of healing and can be traced back to the dawn of human history. Shamanism is the most ancient religion and healing art of humanity, the roots of which reach far back into the Paleolithic era. Shamanism is not only ancient, it is also universal; it can be found in North and South America, Europe, Africa, Asia, Australia, and Polynesia.

The fact that so many different cultures throughout human history have found shamanic techniques useful and relevant suggests that they address the "primal mind" — a basic and primordial aspect of the human psyche that transcends race, culture, and time. All the cultures, with the exception of the

Western industrial civilization, have held NOSC in great esteem and have spent much time and effort to develop various ways of inducing them. Societies used them to connect with their deities, with other dimensions of reality, and with the forces of nature; for healing, for cultivation of extrasensory perception, and for artistic inspiration. For preindustrial cultures, healing always involves nonordinary states of consciousness — either for the client, for the healer, or for both of them at the same time.

The history of psychotherapy is deeply connected with the study of NOSC. Examples include Franz Mesmer's experiments with "animal magnetism," hypnotic sessions with hysterical patients conducted in Paris by Jean Martin Charcot, and the research in hypnosis carried out in Nancy by Hippolyte Bernheim and Ambroise Auguste Liebault. Sigmund Freud's early work was inspired by his sessions with a client (Miss Anna O.), who experienced spontaneous episodes of nonordinary states of consciousness. Freud also initially used hypnosis to access his patients' unconscious before he radically changed his strategies.

As a result of this shift, Western psychiatry and psychology do not see NOSC (with the exception of dreams) as potential sources of healing or of valuable information about the human psyche, but basically as pathological phenomena. Michael Harner (1980), an anthropologist and a practicing shaman initiated during field work in the Amazonian jungle, suggests that Western psychiatry is seriously biased in at least two significant ways. It is ethnocentric, which means that it considers its own view of the human psyche and of reality to be the only correct one and superior to all others. It is "cognicentric" (a more accurate word might be "pragmacentric"), meaning that it takes into consideration only experiences and observations in the ordinary state of consciousness. Psychiatry's disinterest in holotropic states, and disregard for them, has resulted in a culturally insensitive approach and a tendency to pathologize in its own narrow context all activities that cannot be understood. This includes the ritual and spiritual life of ancient and preindustrial cultures and the entire spiritual history of humanity.

In the 1950s, psychiatrists and psychologists developed LSD therapy and other psychotherapies that emphasize experience rather than talk. This was the start of a movement to reintroduce the therapeutic use of nonordinary states of consciousness.

IMPLICATIONS OF MODERN CONSCIOUSNESS RESEARCH

If we systematically study the experiences and observations associated with NOSC or more specifically, holotropic states, this leads inevitably to a radical revision of our basic ideas about consciousness and the human psyche, and to entirely new forms of psychiatry, psychology, and psychotherapy. The changes we would have to make in our thinking fall into the following categories:

The Nature of the Human Psyche

Traditional academic psychiatry and psychology use a model that is limited to biology, postnatal biography, and the Freudian individual unconscious. This model has to be vastly expanded and a new map of the psyche has to be created to describe all the phenomena occurring in NOSC. Specifically, this new model of the psyche must address two main areas: The first is the perinatal domain related to the trauma of birth. Traditional medicine denies that the child can consciously experience and recall birth. However, many people do relive various aspects of the biological birth process, including photographic details of aspects of the event of which they have no intellectual knowledge. It appears that experiential confrontation with birth and death results automatically in a spiritual opening and discovery of the mystical dimensions of the psyche and of existence.

The second major domain that has to be added to the map of the human psyche is now known under the name "transpersonal," meaning "beyond the personal" or "transcending the personal." These are experiences that have been described through the ages in the religious, mystical, and occult literature. These experiences involve going beyond the usual boundaries of the individual (his or her body and ego) and beyond three-dimensional space and linear time that restrict perception of the world in the ordinary state of consciousness. The American writer and philosopher Alan Watts referred to this restricted range of perception as the "skin-encapsulated ego."

In the ordinary state of consciousness, we cannot see objects from which we are separated by a solid wall, ships beyond the horizon, or the other side of the moon. If we are in Paris, we cannot hear what our friends are talking about in San Francisco. We cannot feel the softness of a lambskin unless the surface of our body is in direct contact with it. In addition, we can experience vividly and with all our senses only the events that are happening in the present moment. We can recall the past and anticipate future events or fantasize about them; however, these are very different experiences from an immediate and direct experience of the present moment. We are all familiar with these limitations from our everyday existence and they are undoubtedly pragmatically relevant. According to the Newtonian–Cartesian paradigm of traditional Western science, these restrictions and limitations are absolutely mandatory and definitive, since they result from the material nature of the world and are determined by physiological laws of perception. However, modern consciousness research has clearly demonstrated that in *transpersonal* experiences these limitations do not apply and can be transcended. This represents a critical challenge not only for psychiatry and psychology, but for the entire philosophy of Western science.

The Cause of Emotional and Psychosomatic Disorders

Emotional and psychosomatic symptoms that are not organic in nature are seen by traditional psychiatry as resulting from traumatic things that happen to us in infancy and childhood. Therapeutic work using NOSC reveals that these symptoms may have additional roots on the perinatal and transpersonal levels. Thus, for example, somebody suffering from psychogenic asthma can discover that the underlying biographical material consists of memories of suffocation during a near drowning accident in childhood and an episode of diphtheria in infancy. On a deeper level, the same problem is also connected with choking in the birth canal, and its deepest root can be a past life experience of being strangled or hanged. To resolve this symptom, it is necessary to allow oneself to experience all the layers of problems associated with it. When properly understood and supported, this process can be conducive to healing, spiritual opening, personality transformation, and consciousness evolution. The emergence of symptoms represents not only a problem, but also a therapeutic opportunity; this insight is the basis of most experiential psychotherapies.

The study of NOSC has revealed that emotional and psychosomatic problems are much more complex than is usually assumed and that their roots reach incomparably deeper into the psyche. Freud once likened the human psyche to an iceberg, of which only the one-tenth visible above the water surface represents the conscious mind, while the submerged nine-tenths are the unconscious realms studied by psychoanalysis. In light of modern consciousness research (and ancient wisdom of perennial philosophy), we can correct this simile and say that all that Freudian psychoanalysis has discovered about the human psyche represents, at best, the exposed part of the iceberg, while vast additional domains remain hidden under water. In the words of Joseph Campbell, Freud was fishing while sitting on a whale.

The Process of Healing

The goal in traditional psychotherapies is to reach an intellectual understanding as to how the psyche functions and why symptoms develop and then to derive a strategy to "fix" the patients from this understanding. A serious problem with this strategy is the amazing lack of agreement among psychologists and psychiatrists about these fundamental issues, resulting in an astonishing number of competing schools of psychotherapy. Work with NOSC suggests a very radical alternative: If the experts can not reach agreement, why not trust one's own healing intelligence, one's own inner healer. This approach was first suggested by C. G. Jung. Jung saw the task of the therapist as helping to establish a dynamic interaction between the client's conscious ego and what he called the Self. The healing then comes from the collective unconscious and it is guided by an inner intelligence that surpasses that of any individual therapist or therapeutic school. The task of the therapist is simply to offer a method that induces a NOSC (e.g., a psychedelic substance or faster breathing and evocative music), that creates a safe environment, and that supports unconditionally and with full trust, the spontaneous unfolding of the process. This trust has to extend even to situations in which the therapist does not understand intellectually what is happening. Healing and resolution can often occur in ways that transcend rational understanding. In this form of therapy, the therapist is not the doer, the agent who is instrumental in the healing process, but a sympathetic supporter and coadventurer. This attitude corresponds with the original meaning of the Greek word *therapeutes*: "attendant or assistant in the healing process."

It seems appropriate to emphasize a very important and amazing characteristic of NOSC that is invaluable for psychotherapy. These states tend to engage something like an "inner radar," automatically bringing into consciousness the contents from the unconscious that have the strongest emotional charge and that are most psychodynamically relevant at the time. This represents a great advantage in comparison with verbal psychotherapy, where the client presents a broad array of information of various kinds and the therapist has to decide what is important, what is irrelevant, where the client is blocking, etc. This automatic selection of relevant topics spontaneously leads the process to the perinatal and transpersonal levels of the psyche, domains not recognized and acknowledged in academic psychiatry and psychology.

The Role of Spirituality in Human Life

From the point of view of traditional psychiatry and psychology, the material world represents the only reality, and any form of spiritual belief is seen as reflecting a lack of education, primitive superstition, magical thinking, or a regression to infantile patterns of functioning. People who have direct experiences of spiritual realities are seen as ill. Western psychiatry makes no distinction between a mystical experience and a psychotic experience, and sees both as manifestations of mental disease. In its rejection of religion, it does not differentiate primitive folk beliefs or fundamentalists' literal interpretations of scriptures from sophisticated mystical traditions and Eastern spiritual philosophies based on centuries of systematic, introspective exploration of the psyche.

In contrast with the Western attitude that pathologizes the entire spiritual history of humanity, transpersonal psychology seriously studies and respects the entire range of human experience, including perinatal and transpersonal phenomena. It is more culturally sensitive and offers a way of understanding the psyche that is universal and applicable to any human group and historical period. It also honors the spiritual dimensions of existence and acknowledges the deep human need for transcendental experiences. In this context, spiritual search appears to be an understandable and legitimate human activity.

People who have experiences of this kind are more open to spirituality found in the mystical branches of the great religions or in their monastic orders, not necessarily in their mainstream organizations. It is spirituality that is universal, all-embracing, and based on personal experience rather than on dogma or religious scripture.

To prevent confusion and misunderstandings that in the past have compromised many similar discussions, it is critical to make a clear distinction between spirituality and religion. Spirituality is based on direct experiences of other realities. It does not necessarily require a special place or a special person mediating contact with the Divine, although mystics can certainly benefit from spiritual guidance and a community of fellow seekers. Spirituality involves a special relationship between the individual and the cosmos and is in its essence a personal and private affair. At the cradle of all great religions are visionary (perinatal and/or transpersonal) experiences of their founders, prophets, saints, and even ordinary followers. All major spiritual scriptures — the Vedas, the Buddhist Pali Canon, the Bible, the Koran, the Book of Mormon, and many others are based on revelations in holotropic states of consciousness.

CONCLUSION

As we have seen, the observations from NOSC research represent a serious challenge to contemporary science. The results also cause us to question some of the more fundamental assumptions about the nature of reality. The observation I would like to use here comes from thanatology, a young scientific discipline studying death and dying. There are many well-documented cases of people who experienced clinical death as a result of cardiac arrest during an operation. At this time, they experienced their consciousness detaching from the body, floating freely above it, and observing it from above with detached interest. They were able to witness efforts of the medical team and to give detailed, retrospective accounts of these activities after they were revived and returned to consciousness. They also could accurately describe how many people were involved, who came through which door, what gadgets were brought in and out, and how they were used.

Michael Sabom (1982), a cardiosurgeon who conducted an intensive study of the near-death experiences of his patients, wrote a book summarizing his observations, *Recollections of Death*. His patients, lying on the operating table with their eyes closed and in a state of deep coma, were able afterward to describe in minuscule details the events in the operating room, including the movements of the little hands on the gauges of the medical instruments during various stages of the resuscitation procedure. In other studies, many patients could describe accurately what was happening in other rooms of the building, or even in remote locations. And there are even observations of persons who were medically blind as a result of organic damage to their optical system. At the time of their clinical death, they were able to perceive the environment visually and in full color. They lost their sight again when they regained consciousness, but could give accurate reports about what they had seen. There are many other types of transpersonal experiences that present similar critical challenges to traditional science. However, I hope that the preceding example from the study of near-death experiences is sufficient to demonstrate the nature and seriousness of the problems involved. Many illustrative case histories can be found in my books (Grof, 1985, 1988, 1992).

When confronted with such challenging observations, we have only two choices. The first is to reject the new observations simply because they are incompatible with the traditional scientific belief system. This involves an arrogant assumption that we already know what the universe is like and can tell with certainty what is possible and what is not. With this kind of approach, there cannot be any surprises, but there is also very little real progress. In this context, anyone who brings critically challenging data is accused of being a bad scientist, a fraud, or a mentally deranged person. This is an approach that characterizes pseudoscience or scientistic fundamentalism and has very little to do with genuine science. There are many historical examples of such an approach: people who refused to look into Galileo Galilei's telescope because they "knew" there could not be craters on the moon; those who fought against the atomic theory of chemistry; those who called Einstein a psychotic when he proposed his special theory of relativity.

The second reaction to such observations is characteristic of true science. It is excitement about and intense interest in such anomalies combined with healthy critical skepticism. Major scientific progress has always occurred when the leading paradigm was seriously challenged and failed to account for some significant findings. In the history of science, paradigms arrive, dominate the field for some time, and are replaced by new ones. If instead of rejecting and ridiculing the new observations, we would consider them an interesting opportunity and conduct our own study to test them, we might very likely find that the reports were accurate. At that point, we would realize that we are something very different from what we were taught and from what the Western industrial culture believes. It would also become clear that materialistic science has an incomplete and inadequate image of reality, and that its ideas about the nature of consciousness and the relationship between consciousness and matter (particularly the brain) must be radically revised. We would literally find ourselves in a different universe.

It is hard to imagine that Western academic science will continue indefinitely to ignore all the challenging evidence that has already been accumulated in the study of various forms of holotropic states, as well as the influx of new data. Sooner or later it will be necessary to face this new evidence and accept its far-reaching theoretical and practical consequences. It is my firm belief that we are rapidly approaching a point when transpersonal psychology and the work with nonordinary states of consciousness will become integral parts of a new scientific paradigm of the future.

HOW TO LEARN MORE

Alexander, F. "Buddhist Training as Artificial Catatonia." *Psychoanalyst* 18 (1931): 129.

Grof, C. and S. Grof. *The Stormy Search for the Self.* Los Angeles: J. P. Tarcher, 1990.

Grof, S. *The Adventure of Self-Discovery.* Albany, NY: SUNY Press, 1988.

Grof, S. *Beyond the Brain.* Albany, NY: SUNY Press, 1985.

Grof, S. and H. Z. Bennett. *The Holotropic Mind.* San Francisco: Harper San Francisco, 1992.

Grof, S. and C. Grof., eds. *Spiritual Emergencies.* Los Angeles: J. P. Tarcher, 1989.

Grof, S. *Realms of the Human Unconscious.* New York: Viking Press, 1975.

Harner, M. *The Way of the Shaman.* New York: Harper and Row, 1980.

Jung, C. G. "The Archetypes and the Collective Unconscious." *Collected Works, Bollingen Series XX.* vol. 9.1. Princeton, NJ: Princeton University Press, 1960.

Perls, F. *The Gestalt Approach and Eye-Witness to Therapy.* New York: Bantam Books, 1976.

Ring, K. *Heading Toward Omega.* New York: William Morrow and Co., 1984.

Sabom, M. *Recollections of Death.* New York: Simon and Schuster, 1982.

Talbot, M. *The Holographic Universe.* San Francisco: HarperCollins, 1991.

Wasson, G., A. Hofmann, and C.A.P. Ruck. *The Road to Eleusis: Unveiling the Secret of the Mysteries.* New York: Harcourt Brace & Co., 1978.

Wilber, K. *A Sociable God.* New York: McGraw-Hill, 1982.

ABOUT THE AUTHOR

Stanislav Grof, M.D., is a psychiatrist and professor of psychology at the California Institute of Integral Studies with more than 40 years of research experience in nonordinary states of consciousness. He was born and educated in Prague, Czechoslovakia, and received an M.D. from Prague's Charles University of Medicine and a Ph.D. from the Czechoslovak Academy of Sciences. He has served as a clinical and research fellow at Johns Hopkins University, and has conducted research on psychedelics at Spring Grove State Hospital in Baltimore, MD. In 1969 he became chief of psychiatric research at the Maryland Psychiatric Research Center and assistant professor of psychiatry at Henry Phipps Clinic, where he continued his research with psychedelic therapy for neurotics, terminal cancer patients, and substance abusers. In 1973 he moved to California and became a scholar in residence at the Esalen Institute in Big Sur. Since that time, he has focused on exploring the potential of experiential psychotherapy without drugs, in addition to writing and conducting seminars worldwide. He was the founding president of the International Transpersonal Association. He has published more than ninety papers in professional journals and is the author of numerous books.

PART 2

The Complementary
Healing Modalities

Joan Arnold

5   The Alexander Technique

WHAT IS THE ALEXANDER TECHNIQUE?

The Alexander Technique® is a mental practice that focuses on improving movement to achieve optimal health for body and mind. Our movement expresses who we are, how we feel about ourselves, and how we relate to others. Each of us has an individual movement pattern. Posture, like a still photograph of the way we move, reflects much about our emotional state, how we expect to be treated, and how comfortably we approach a new challenge.

On a purely physical level, the technique's basic tenet is that, when the neck is not overworked, the head can poise lightly at the top of the spine. That delicate poise sparks the body's antigravity response, a postural reflex that invites the spine to lengthen, rather than compress, as we move. We can use the technique to capitalize on the body's inherent support system, enhancing our sense of ease and pleasure in movement.

Though the technique does not address the psyche directly, the process of peeling away habitual tensions often reveals their underlying emotional logic. One of my clients described his Alexander work as the physical equivalent of psychotherapy: examining his own outdated assumptions about his body. Alexander teachers are not psychotherapists, but the work deeply affects attitudes and emotional states. For example, it can help people with a wide range of problems, including anxiety, depression, performance anxiety, addiction to food, alcohol or drugs, sexual abuse, and the despair associated with chronic pain.

You can use the Alexander Technique to complement a physician's mainstream treatment. If you are taking medication for a psychiatric disorder, the technique will not counteract its positive effects, and its calming influence may enable you to reduce your dosage. It is also a particularly good complement to psychotherapy.

The Alexander Technique is similar to approaches such as massage or reiki, in that you have a private session with a skilled practitioner who, through the hands, elicits your body's capacity to integrate and heal. Like acupuncture and therapeutic touch, the technique can help resolve a wide range of symptoms by bringing your whole system into better balance. But it is different in that you are an active participant, learning to notice and undo unconscious habits that get in your way. Learning the technique can also improve your receptivity to other forms of bodywork.

Like biofeedback, the technique helps you change your inner state, replacing a mechanical beep with the teacher's verbal and tactile cues. Both aim to train your internal monitoring system, making your senses more reliable so that you can modulate your own stress level. The technique echoes the effects of yoga, T'ai Chi, meditation, or prayer in that it is something you learn to do on your own that aligns you with universal forces, inducing a feeling of harmony and aliveness. But it is not a set of exercises or postures. Rather, it is an approach to movement, a set of guiding thoughts that you keep in mind as you do something else.

HOW IT BEGAN

Frederic Mathias Alexander (1869–1955) was an 18-year-old Shakespearean actor when he was plagued by chronic hoarseness. While on stage before an audience, he sometimes lost his voice completely. A doctor's treatment failed to correct the problem, and he began to look at what he was doing to provoke his vocal troubles. He set up a three-way mirror to observe himself, and he noticed that every time he began to speak, he tightened the muscles in the back of his neck, lifted his chin, and tilted his head back and down. The resulting pressure on the spine restricted his breathing and shortened his stature.

Changing this habit proved surprisingly difficult. Many hours of experimentation revealed that "inhibiting" — stopping the habit — was far more useful than trying to correct the habit. His whole concept of correctness was untrustworthy, based on years of faulty habits. Alexander discovered that deliberate muscular work was not as effective as envisioning an activity, what he called "directing." He also found that if he was too concerned with his goal, his overanxiety to perform well interfered with his ability to do so. He was trying too hard. When he focused on the process rather than the goal, his overactivity lessened. His voice and body worked much more easily, becoming the expressive tools he yearned for. He could do more, he found, by doing less.

By the end of Alexander's nine-year odyssey of self-observation, he had discovered how to restore his voice and enrich his stage presence. He became known for his mellifluous voice. As he taught his method to those who sought him out, he found that it resolved a wide range of symptoms. His students' overall health improved. Polio victims regained their balance, recovered more of their movement range, and felt far less disabled. People who suffered from awkwardness, stuttering, or stage fright overcame their difficulties. He continued to teach his technique in England and the United States until his death in 1955 at the age of 86.

Among those who have studied the technique are Jacqueline Kennedy Onassis, Paul McCartney, Marlo Thomas, Kevin Kline, James Earl Jones, Sting, Mary Steenburgen, Paul Newman, and Joanne Woodward. Today there are 2,500 Alexander Technique teachers throughout the world and 700 in the United States. They offer their students a way to apply the important principle that Alexander articulated: When we stop the fear reaction that drives our holding patterns, a harmonious organism is beneath, waiting to unfold.

HOW IT WORKS

We begin life with a body exquisitely designed to meet life's challenges. You can see this in young children. They have naturally erect spines and can effortlessly balance their large heads on little necks. They walk and play, often with regal posture. They are also spontaneously expressive. They know how they feel. When they are hurt, they cry. When they want something, they grab it. They become enraged, and then suddenly, it's over. Barring birth defects, we all began that way.

Over the years, we lose some of that poise and immediacy, that freedom to explore. We spend more time in shoes and chairs. The expectations of others loom larger, and the voices of parents, teachers, or peers may drown out our internal cues. We learn which behaviors and emotions are unacceptable to those around us, and learn to control them. But suppressing a genuine response takes effort. Unspoken feelings may lodge in a tight jaw, injured sexuality in a tight pelvis. Since muscular tension also serves as an anesthetic, we hold back tears or rage when a trauma or loss is too painful to bear. Whether from a single incident or the cumulative assaults so common in all our lives, the body's tissues continue to register unresolved conflicts and childhood fears. They can become limiting habits that infiltrate our thoughts and actions. The Alexander Technique assumes that by stripping away harmful habits, we can restore the accuracy of our responses and much of our original poise.

When one feels threatened, the body goes into the startle pattern — a fear reflex marked by a tight neck and contracted body. If while reading this book, you heard a deafening crack, you would automatically react like a cat with the startle pattern. Vigilant for danger, your body would compress, ready to fight or flee. But once the danger is past, you should return to a neutral state.

Chronic stress occurs when muscles stay contracted and the body does not restabilize. We continue to respond with life or death alarm to a threat that may be long gone. If we are braced in a perpetual state of anxiety and fear, what began as an adaptive instinct becomes a prison. An external shell of tension makes it impossible to give in to gravity and benefit from the natural oppositional force that makes flowing, graceful coordination possible. Real strength lies in a strong, connected center. Paradoxically, we must let go to be better supported.

We do not live in an ideal world. Irrevocable change, pain, and loss are part of existence. But by restoring resiliency in body and mind, we can awaken the resources sleeping within us, and find satisfaction in going through life with the fullness of our own experience intact.

WHAT THE RESEARCH SHOWS

Like many alternative approaches, the Alexander Technique's beneficial effects are primarily shown by anecdotal evidence — people's stories of their own recovery. However, a growing number of studies attest to the beneficial impact of touch, meditation, energy exchange, and stress reduction — all of which are part of the Alexander Technique.

Research increasingly shows that most diseases and chronic conditions are stress-induced. Kenneth Pelletier, M.D., of the Stanford Center for Research in Disease Prevention, wrote in *Mind/Body Medicine: How to Use Your Mind for Better Health*: Goleman and Gurin (1993) "A 1992 review of stress and disease from two physicians, researchers at the National Institutes of Health, noted the role of stress in a wide array of psychiatric disorders, autoimmune diseases, coronary heart disease, functional disorders of the intestinal tract, chronic pain, and a range of other medical and psychological disorders."

Studies of stress reduction techniques have verified their value many times over. The Alexander Technique helps to reduce stress by inhibiting the body's fear response — the startle pattern — thus raising the baseline of physical and mental health.

In the 1950s, Dr. Wilfred Barlow, a British physician who studied with F. M. Alexander and became a teacher of his technique, conducted studies that demonstrated its effects (Barlow, 1952). He photographed participants, analyzed their posture with a scale of postural faults, and measured their progress. The control group of forty-four students at London's Central School of Speech and Drama did not receive Alexander lessons, but were given exercises to improve their posture. Their number of postural faults actually rose, from an average of nine before the exercises to ten afterward. The forty students at the Royal College of Music in London who did receive Alexander lessons increased their height and shoulder width and reduced their number of postural faults from ten to five. Their teachers noticed that the students became easier to teach, improved their singing and acting ability, and became more psychologically balanced.

Performance anxiety is something we all contend with at times. It can block effectiveness whether we face an audience, a classroom, a business meeting, a social occasion, or an empty page. To modulate performance anxiety, professional musicians increasingly take drugs, especially beta-blockers. Chris Stevens, a physiologist and Alexander teacher, collaborated with two Danish physicians on a study of thirty-nine members of the Aarhus Symphony Orchestra in Denmark (Stevens, 1994). For eight weeks, three groups of performers each used a different stress-reducing alternative: beta-blockers, exercise, or the Alexander Technique. To determine stress level in a test concert, changes in heart rate and blood pressure were measured. Results showed that the Alexander Technique was more effective than exercise and as effective as beta-blockers in reducing performance anxiety.

In a 1988 study published in *Holistic Medicine* (Fisher, 1988), participants in a multidisciplinary pain management program were interviewed about their preferred approach. Patients rated the technique as the most highly valued method of managing their pain.

REAL PEOPLE AND THE ALEXANDER TECHNIQUE

When Linda came for her first Alexander lesson, her feet hurt so much that she was reluctant to walk barefoot a few steps across the studio's carpeted floor. Several months before, she had bruised her feet on a long walk on pavement in a thin pair of boots. Though her physician said they had healed, the tenderness continued and she could no longer distinguish between the original injury and her own reaction to it. Mystified and frightened by the pain, she was concerned that her range of function was narrowing. She longed to dance and exercise again. At age 38, Linda was recuperating from a miscarriage six months before. Since taking Prozac for chronic depression, she had gained 25 pounds. She was plagued by frequent bouts of despair as she juggled career demands with the needs of her husband and energetic six-year-old daughter. As a successful attorney, direct confrontation is part of her job. But when I met her in January 1996, her movement had a fragile, tentative look.

In her first few lessons, Linda thought that she first had to step up onto a stool to reach the bodywork table. At my suggestion, she leaned against the table's edge to swing her legs up. When she did so easily, she realized the stool was superfluous. Many students have irrational fears about their bodies, and say things like, "I'm afraid if I let my neck go, my head will fall off," or "If I don't grip my legs, I'll lose my balance." Our patterns are based on beliefs established sometime in the past. Linda traced her fearfulness to her mother's dramatic reaction to any physical problem, whether mild or severe. She seemed afraid to trust the ground beneath her feet — literally.

When she was on the table, her feet felt tight, as if she customarily pulled them up from the floor. As she learned to notice and release that pull, she saw that her foot pain was not a condition from a mysterious source, but linked to her pattern. Her hands had a similar taut quality, and she complained of pain in her arms and wrists. When I encouraged her, with words and touch, to let her palms open, she felt her own resistance. "I don't want to open my hands," she mused, making tight fists.

She told me then that when she was seven years old, she washed her hands so often that they bled. Though this behavior was diagnosed later as obsessive-compulsive disorder, at the time her mother told her, "That's just a phase that children go through." While a splinter in Linda's foot provoked high drama, her compulsive hand-washing caused barely a ripple. Her hands became scaly and ragged, "like alligator skin," she said. "I was ashamed and tried to hide them."

To this extraordinary story, I said, "You've been through a lot."

"I guess so," Linda said softly. And then, in a surge of emotion, "It makes me feel strange when you say that. I guess it makes it concrete for me. If I don't talk about it, it's not that real, not that bad."

Linda had been in psychotherapy for 15 years with a woman who, she felt, saved her life. Yet the Alexander lesson — which addressed the pattern, not its origins — provided something unique. As she let her hands uncurl, the childhood feeling of withdrawn shame resurfaced. As children, we muffle some of our genuine responses to survive in our families, but the original feelings endure within us. My empathy sharpened her sense of the sadness, shame, and loneliness of those years. In therapy she had learned the value of allowing, not denying, such feelings, and brought the insight gleaned from her Alexander work to her psychotherapist. The reciprocity of the two approaches continues to enrich her explorations.

After 5 months, Linda's foot pain dissolved almost completely. She wears cushioned shoes, but easily walks barefoot across the floor. After 10 months of Alexander study, this basically healthy, energetic woman works out several times a week. Her increased sense of control over her body has quieted her lifelong fear of illness. She has taught her daughter some of the breathing practices she has learned. She still takes an antidepressant and wrestles with her personal demons. Her life is just as stressful, but she enjoys it more. With less fear and more confidence, she is freer to move.

∾

In 1993, Frank woke up one morning unable to lift his head. Getting out of bed became a complicated, excruciating procedure to avoid the stabbing pain in his neck. He consulted with a family practitioner, who asked what event might have triggered this attack. That question made Frank reflect on the deteriorating atmosphere in his office, where he had worked as an administrator for 12 years. "Things were just horrid," he recalled. "You couldn't turn your back because you could never tell who might plunge a knife into it." Several days after his physician pressed hard into the offending muscles, Frank experienced some relief. But later the problem returned. Anti-inflammatory medication was helpful, but there were side effects. Still, he always carried his bottle of pills, "just in case. If it really got bad, I would take them." A fit, active 61-year-old, he couldn't jog because of the pain.

When Frank came for Alexander lessons beginning in July 1996, he began to see how "the tension and the way I carried myself were causing this terrible pain." After six lessons, he eliminated the tension almost completely. "I still have achiness, but it's a lot better," he said. "If I can learn how to reduce the tension in my muscles, then the pain doesn't progress. Now that it's under my control, I'm not afraid of it anymore." He is off the anti-inflammatories, and many times during a day, he uses his new method of sensing his inner state and readjusting. "I notice I'm a little tight and remember to loosen up, stand erect, let my shoulders go, and walk bending my knees more. Every time I get up to move, I'm more conscious."

There was also a shift in his body image. Many people suffer one kind of self-loathing or another: "I'm too fat . . . too thin . . . too old . . . too lazy to stand up straight . . . I walk like a duck." But such judgments don't encourage progress. Offering a more generous, constructive internal voice, an Alexander teacher creates an environment of support, while recognizing the student's full responsibility for change.

After Frank's 4 months of study, he said of our lessons: "Often when I'd stand up, you'd put one hand on my stomach — an area I'm very self-conscious about. But it didn't seem to bother you at all, in the service of doing your work. I got the feeling of your complete acceptance of my body."

∞

Rachel, an athletic 35-year-old corporate training coordinator, came to the technique to relieve the pain in her right shoulder. But the work led to something deeper. Early on, my touch elicited muscular tremors in her, one evidence of tension release. Rachel found herself crying often and writing in her journal, returning to emotional issues she had examined in her 10 years of psychotherapy.

When she was 11 years old, Rachel was already a talented tennis player, winning tournaments and relishing the game's challenge. But her parents discouraged her from becoming a professional. She now believes that her father's unfulfilled desire to become a musician engendered his dark response to her success. Though she pursued her passion, her confidence was shaken beginning at age 13. Sometimes, when the pressure was on during a game, "my whole body would tighten with this intense fear. I'd choke and lose the point." As if her life were in danger, she froze. "The worst was the finals of a major mixed doubles event when I was 29. A big crowd was watching. I was playing well, but suddenly a wave of panic came over me. I started crying and could barely hit the ball. It was absolutely horrible. I stopped playing for a while after that. I thought, 'I'm outta here.' "

I knew nothing of Rachel's performance anxiety when we began our work together. Noting her awkwardness — surprising in an accomplished athlete — I encouraged her to decompress her spine and expand in movement. I helped her relearn how to improve her swing, distributing its force through her whole body, not just the shoulder. After 3 months, her shoulder pain vanished. Her muscular tremors lasted for more than 6 months and gradually stopped. Now Rachel continues to refine her movement skills both on and off the court, and has radically altered her playing style.

When she recently won a doubles match and excitedly told me the story, it was the first time I heard the history of her anxiety episodes. "During a panic attack," she said, "I used to think, 'Uh oh. I made a mistake. Now it'll only get worse. I'm about to embarrass myself.' " In this downward spiral, her mistake became an indictment. Rather than staying in the present with all its inherent possibilities, she imagined catastrophe in the future. But as Rachel learned the technique, she used her new way of thinking in activity to still her fear response. Then she could be in the moment, free of paralyzing judgments. "In this last game," she said, "instead of freaking out about a mistake, I stayed calm and focused, reminding myself that my body really knows what to do." Learning to inhibit her body's fear reaction restored the relaxed focus that encourages success. Though panic still occasionally troubles her, her love of challenge now supersedes her fear of losing. "I could always give up playing tournaments," she said, "but then I'd be bored. It's the competition that makes me stretch and play my best game. That's what keeps it interesting."

Though the Alexander Technique works through simple, accessible principles, its applications are as varied as human experience. Whether the resulting changes are quick and direct, or slow and subtle, the technique's rich ideas continue to resonate through all our efforts, informing our understanding of ourselves and each other. With all the complexity and difficulty of being human, we can use the technique on the path to integration, each in our own way.

WHAT TO EXPECT

Though the Alexander Technique has therapeutic benefits, it is primarily an educational method. The practitioner is called a teacher; the private session, a lesson; and the client, a student. Students can be at any functional level, from elite athletes to the wheelchair-bound. Most teachers work in an office, but some go to a home or hospital to work with the dying or those recuperating from injury or surgery.

An Alexander lesson is an opportunity to unwind and observe how your mind and body work. From the teacher you get focused, sympathetic coaching on how to use your increased awareness to calm your system and raise your level of functioning. A teaching studio is usually a low-tech environment with a chair, bodywork table, and mirror. You wear loose, comfortable clothing that allows free movement of the arms and legs. The teacher may ask what problem or goal brings you there and what you would like to achieve through your

Alexander work. You also might discuss other relevant information, such as your medical history, how active or sedentary you are, and what your life demands of you.

Though every lesson reiterates the same principles, each one is a bit different. Similarly, all practitioners teach the same principles, but with varying styles. The teacher will observe you doing simple actions — like sitting, standing, and walking — and help you learn to notice your movement pattern. Some students hold themselves up in a rigid posture; others pull themselves down into a slump. Some say, "I hate the way I walk," or "I'm always uncomfortable and anxious," or "I have a bad back." The teacher can explain how your pattern connects with your concerns and helps you see yourself in a new way by guiding you to watch your own movement in the mirror. To demystify the workings of the body, you might look at a muscle chart and miniature skeleton. Appreciating the elements of your neuromuscular design helps you understand how to attain more ease and effortless support. Part of the session is an opportunity to release accumulated tension. While you lie clothed on the table and settle into a restful state, the teacher gently moves your limbs to encourage expansion, helping you to breathe more fully.

Movement becomes the vehicle to improve your functioning. As you walk, for example, the teacher may use touch to give you the feeling of a lighter, more fluid stride, while encouraging you to direct and engender that fluidity in yourself. As you get up from a chair, the teacher might ask you to notice compression in your neck, release it, and envision your spine lengthening. Ordinary activities — writing, speaking, washing dishes — then become imbued with a spirit of observation as you explore your tendencies and discover your own capacity for efficient movement.

Alexander teachers practice a unique touch. Placing their hands gently on the head, torso, or limbs, they can sense your body's imbalances and tense areas. This light touch does not intrude or manipulate, but invites your muscles to lengthen, suggesting a freer way to move. Such a release may be the first time you sense how much you have been holding. This touch is also a conduit for the teacher's thought, informing you how to direct, and inviting you to participate. Such experiences then become reference points, memories to call on once you have left the studio. The next day, you might catch yourself hunched over your computer or unnecessarily gripping a coffee cup, and remember that you can breathe, lengthen, and streamline your efforts. As time goes on, you improve your ability to recall an idea or a sensation from your lesson and to replicate it.

The Alexander touch often evokes a feeling of relaxation. But unraveling tensions can also expose held emotions. When a student suddenly recalls a suppressed painful memory or bursts into tears, the teacher can offer a sympathetic presence and may invite you to talk about your experience. Though this can open a door to further insight, it is best to have the support of a psychotherapist who can address the issues involved more fully. Still, the technique offers one way to unwind the body's emotional holding patterns.

The Alexander Technique is a skill — like speaking French, playing tennis, or playing the piano. If you are intrigued by your first lesson and decide to try it, it is best to give your initial study three to six months, attending regularly once or twice a week. Lessons are generally 45 minutes long, with initial sessions up to an hour. Many students begin applying their new understanding after their first lesson. It can be liberating to find that you have more choice than you realized about how you look and feel. Some experience pain relief and greater ease immediately; others may take six months to a year to reverse the adverse effects of lifelong habits. Some students take lessons for several years, continuing to deepen their understanding. Your choice will depend on how serious your problem is, your available time and resources, and your interest. Many students solve the problem that first drove them to study, and then continue, fascinated by the process of removing inner obstructions and refining their skills.

The success of the work depends on how you use what you learn. The goal is not to make you depend on the teacher, but to train you to find greater comfort, confidence, and peace in all your interactions. Given time, the Alexander Technique offers a gentle mindfulness, a way to work on yourself each day, throughout your life.

HOW TO FIND A PRACTITIONER

NASTAT — The North American Society of Teachers of the Alexander Technique. All members have completed a three-year, 1,600-hour course of training. To find a teacher in your area, call (800) 473-0620.

Personal referral — Ask acquaintances who have studied the technique about their experiences and their teacher's style and emphasis. Verify the teacher's qualifications.

Professional referral — If your physician or mental health professional is not familiar with the Alexander Technique, consult an alternative practitioner or a directory of holistic health services.

Institutions — Continuing education programs, college performing arts departments, wellness programs, or pain clinics are potential referral sources. Some sponsor introductory Alexander Technique group classes.

Find an instructor whose personality is right for you. Alexander teachers come from a variety of backgrounds that will be reflected in their work. Though the technique's principles are consistent and the practitioners are exceptionally well-trained, individuals have different styles and degrees of interest in the work's psychological aspects. Lessons will vary from a half hour to a full hour, and cost from $30 to $100. When speaking to prospective teachers, you might inquire:

- Where they studied and the number of years they have been teaching.

- About other areas of expertise, such as physical therapy or psychotherapy.

- Whether they have experience in dealing with a problem similar to yours.

- About fee, location, schedule, and appropriate attire.

HOW TO LEARN MORE

For a free catalog of books and videos available through NASTAT Books, call (800) 473-0620.

Austin, J. and P. Ausubel. "Enhanced Respiratory Muscular Function in Normal Adults After Lessons in Proprioceptive Musculoskeletal Education with Exercises." *Chest,* 102 (1992): 486–490.

Barlow, W. "Postural Homeostasis." *Annals of Physical Medicine* 1 (1952): 77–89.

Caplan, D. *Back Trouble.* Gainesville, FL: Triad Publishing, 1987.

Fisher, K. "Early Experiences of a Multi-Disciplinary Pain Management Programme." *Holistic Medicine* 3 (1988): 47–56.

Gelb, M. *Body Learning.* New York: Henry Holt and Co., 1987.

Goleman, D. and J. Gurin, eds. *Mind/Body Medicine: How to Use Your Mind for Better Health.* Yonkers, NY: Consumer Reports Books, 1993.

Stevens, C. *The F. M. Alexander Technique: Medical & Physiological Aspects.* London: STAT Books, 1994.

ABOUT THE AUTHOR

Joan Arnold, a certified teacher of the Alexander Technique, has performed and taught dance, yoga, and exercise for more than 25 years. Since her 1988 graduation from the American Center for the Alexander Technique, she served on its faculty for three years and maintains a private practice in Brooklyn and Manhattan. She has taught at Equinox Fitness Clubs, New Age Health Spa, Hunter College, and the American Academy of Dramatic Arts and has demonstrated the technique on *CBS Good Morning* and Fox Cable's *FX/MD*. Her articles on dance, alternative health, psychology, and bodywork have appeared in *New York Woman, Self, Family Therapy Networker, Living Fit, Shape,* and *New Woman,* where she is a contributing editor.

Walter H. Schmitt, Jr., D.C., D.I.B.A.K., D.A.B.C.N.

6 Applied Kinesiology:
Individualized Assessment Using Applied Kinesiology Procedures

WHAT IS APPLIED KINESIOLOGY?

Applied kinesiology (AK) is a simple way to measure how well messages are carried by the nerves in your brain and central nervous system, and to find out which nerve circuits are working normally and which ones are "short circuiting." The AK doctor does not evaluate for destruction or pathology of nerve pathways, which is the traditional realm of the medical neurologist, but for dysfunctional states that readily may be restored to normal function.

How we feel and how we act depend, to a great extent, on our body's ability to receive and send unimpaired messages through our complex nerve pathways. If we wish to listen to a radio or transmit a radio signal, we want to do so with as little static and background noise as possible so the signal gets through as clearly as possible. Likewise, we would like to eliminate as much static as possible in the body and mind for optimum clarity of our thoughts and actions, and to maximize the potential with which each of us was born.

AK doctors approach the patient from a comprehensive, holistic framework. Starting with an open mind, the AK doctor interacts with the patient directly, using feedback from the patient's nervous system to guide the work. AK researchers have shown the well-known body-mind connections to be reflected in the function of the muscles. Therefore, AK doctors employ manual muscle testing to measure patients' responses to various stimuli. Nowhere in the Western healing traditions are the principles of touching and healing and body-mind relationships more elegantly or completely exemplified than in the application of the techniques of AK.

AK doctors blend a multitude of natural and alternative therapies, based on the individual assessment of each patient. AK doctors can design individualized treatment programs for people with most mental health problems including anxieties, phobias, decreased motivation, learning disabilities, depression, and schizophrenia. In people without named mental health problems, AK has been equally effective in the quest for maximizing human potential and improving quality of life.

HOW IT BEGAN

In 1964, an original observation by Detroit chiropractor Dr. George Goodheart gave birth to AK. While working with a patient who had a long-standing shoulder disability, he noticed a muscle weakness in an important muscle in that shoulder. A simple manipulation immediately restored the strength of the muscle and normal function of the shoulder. Goodheart realized that what was commonly referred to as muscle "spasm" or muscle "tightness" is not usually the primary problem, but a secondary consequence of another muscle being weak due to underfunctioning. Visualize two guy wires attached to the mast of a sailboat. Loosening one wire allows the mast to shift to the other side and gives the appearance that the other wire is tighter when there is no more pull in that wire than previously. To straighten the mast, the loose wire must be tightened. The same is true for muscles and muscle balance, except it is the nerve pathways to the muscles that control their function.

By applying simple AK procedures to strengthen weak muscles, immediate return of muscle strength is observed. The tightness or spasm in opposite muscles is reduced just as quickly. Muscle balance is achieved, along with a return to normal nerve function.

The clinical ramifications of this simple principle have expanded to include all healing professions in many parts of the world. The International College of Applied Kinesiology (ICAK) was formed in 1974 and has now evolved into an international organization. Meetings of ICAK chapters gather numerous practitioners from varied backgrounds to share their observations and experiences with other professionals. Dentists may use AK to improve their approach to jaw and bite problems. Medical doctors may use AK to identify which medication is most compatible with an individual patient. Psychologists may use AK to aid in understanding the interplay of various stressors for their clients. As more practitioners become involved with AK, the applications of AK principles continue to penetrate new frontiers of the various healing arts.

HOW IT WORKS

The function inside our bodies is reflected in the function of our muscles. The network of nerve connections begins in the sensory nerve endings throughout the body, goes to the central nervous system (brain and spinal cord), and ends in the nerves to our muscles. Our muscles are hooked to all other functions of our bodies and minds.

An AK muscle test is an interaction between the doctor and the patient. The doctor places the patient's arm or leg in a position to isolate a specific muscle with specific neurological connections. The patient is then asked to resist the doctor's force as the doctor pushes against the arm or leg in a direction that measures the strength response of the specific muscle. The strength of the muscle testing response depends on the nerves going to the muscle. The nerve pathways that affect the muscle test response can originate virtually anywhere in the brain or nervous system.

The ability of the patient to resist the doctor's pressure is further evaluated while a variety of sensory nerve endings are stimulated. For example, the muscle testing response may be measured with the patient's body in a certain position, with various nutrients placed in the mouth to stimulate taste bud nerve endings, or while the patient mentally focuses on stressful events.

TRIAD OF HEALTH

Applied kinesiologists symbolize their view of the body as an equilateral triangle (see Fig. 1), with structure as the base and chemical and mental factors as the sides. A change in any of the three factors in this "triad of health" will have an impact on each of the other two factors. Likewise, therapies directed toward any one factor will affect the other two factors whether or not the therapy was designed with this purpose.

This triangle is more than a convenient representation of a philosophy. It has been the basis for the open-ended investigation of anything that affects the nervous system and may result in muscular imbalance. Any factor monitored by the nervous system can be evaluated by muscle testing procedures. AK procedures identify the source(s) of static in our nervous systems and employ treatments to remove the static and restore a clear signal. Following are examples of techniques based on these principles.

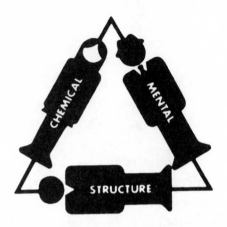

Figure 1. The Triad of Health.
© Systems DC, Pueblo, CO
(from David Walther, with permission)

The Mental Side of the Triangle: Emotional Recall Technique

The emotional recall technique is used to identify a neurological short-circuiting based on mental or emotional stress patterns. The patient is asked to think of a stressful situation, past or present. In many instances, there will be an immediate, temporary weakening of muscle strength, often all over the body, while the thought is maintained. This is a perfect example of identifying interference or static in the nervous system from a mental source.

Treatment is based on identifying sensory receptors and nutritional factors that negate the weakening effect of the emotional recall. When this pattern is corrected, the person can recall the emotionally stressful event or thought without any resulting muscle weakness. Further, confrontation with the previously distressful thought or situation is usually met with remarkable calm and tolerance by the patient. Thoughts or memories that previously caused butterflies, cold palms, or other uncomfortable symptoms can now be tolerated with none of these symptoms.

A number of AK doctors have refined the emotional recall technique to deal with specific problems such as addictions, phobias, grief, post-traumatic stress syndrome, and even overcoming academic, sales, and sports barriers.

Many of the techniques employed to reset emotional or mental circuit breakers can be taught to the patient so that therapy may be performed at home or whenever needed. The simplicity of these techniques is out of proportion to the often dramatic changes they make in people's abilities to cope.

The Chemical Side of the Triangle: Neurotransmitter Chemicals and Their Nutritional Precursors

Why is it that some people seem to be clear-headed and some people never seem to think clearly? Why is it that some people easily fall into depression while others stoically accept fate? There are obviously many reasons why people react differently, but one of the reasons is the chemical makeup of the person, particularly the availability of neurotransmitters. Neurotransmitters are the chemical substances our nerves use to communicate with each other.

All messages carried in the nervous system depend on the presence of these chemical neurotransmitters. Whether the nerve message is a thought, a reflex reaction such as removing your hand from a hot object, or an intentional movement such as walking, turning your head, or reading this page, the message relies on a fascinating system involving the release of chemical neurotransmitters at the end of one nerve that stimulates the next nerve to carry the message.

How we think and how we feel, our sleepiness and our wakefulness, our ability to sense our surroundings, and how we react to various stimuli from our environment depend on the presence of neurotransmitters in our brains. These neurotransmitters are constantly being used up and must be replenished.

Neurotransmitters are derived directly from substances in our diets. What we eat and how completely we digest and absorb it can significantly affect how our nervous systems function. The foods we eat can have a fairly rapid (within a few hours at most) effect on our entire sense of well-being.

But what if a person's nutritional status is compromised in such a way as to affect the adequate production of neurotransmitters? Such is the case in many people who have mental symptoms.

Medical practice uses drugs to enhance or block neurotransmitter activity. Applied kinesiologists and other nutritionally minded practitioners try to stimulate production of neurotransmitters through natural means. If we can identify what nutrients are needed for the production of neurotransmitters, we can supply those nutrients, which allow the body to make the needed chemicals. Of course, there are many cases where medications are necessary, especially in the short term. But with our growing experience in how to manipulate the body chemistry, we find that there is less frequently a long-term need for anti-depressants and tranquilizers.

Just as there is a need for adequate availability of nutritional substances for nerve and brain function, an excess of certain chemicals will also interfere with the ability of our brains to function optimally. Poor diet, food allergies, or exposure to certain chemicals from the environment can have a major impact on mental (and physical) functioning. Allergies to foods are rampant in our society and have a huge effect on the function of the brain. So does toxicity arising from the person's digestive system. These critical chemical factors are rarely considered by many doctors. AK individual assessment procedures identify which patients have too little of some nutrient or too much of some toxic substance.

The Structural Side of the Triangle: Chiropractic Manipulation and Other Sensory Stimulation

We are all conditioned to believe that everything in our bodies is okay as long as there is no pain. This is far from the truth. One does not go from optimal health to disease without a period of time when function first declines without symptoms. Deviations from normal, balanced posture are often among the first signs of dysfunction, whether structural, chemical, or mental. Optimal muscle balance is rarely found among even the strongest athletes and the healthiest fitness enthusiasts. If you look closely at a person's relaxed, standing posture, you will almost always observe at least slight alterations of the levels of the hips, shoulders, and head. Muscle imbalances allow misalignment of the spine and other joints in our bodies. Muscle imbalances and bony misalignments cause abnormal sensory nerve stimulation and make normal daily activity more difficult, which adds considerably to a person's stress. These postural patterns are most easily corrected by chiropractic and other manipulative therapies. Following manipulation, the mechanical sensory nerve endings will once again send normal messages to the brain and central nervous system. Muscle, organ, and brain function will operate closer to their optimum levels as a result of the restoration of normal sensory input from the vertebra and other joints. Many people report that they feel like "someone just turned on the lights" as their mental clarity immediately improves following chiropractic manipulation.

With AK treatment, mechanical sensory nerves are normalized from the muscles and the joints. By stimulation of sensory nerve endings at strategic locations all over the body, changes can be made in our structural, chemical, and mental factors. Normalizing all three sides of the triangle affects how our brains function. It is these structural aspects that are overlooked by many other approaches. Yet it is by normalization of sensory input to the brain that some of the most dramatic influences are made to help people achieve their human potential.

WHAT THE RESEARCH SHOWS

Since 1976, ICAK has published *Proceedings*, which include hundreds of articles and papers by its members. Most of these papers are designed to share ideas rather than meet strict scientific criteria. Until recently, all AK doctors were trained as clinicians and not researchers. The scarcity of AK doctors trained in research methodology, combined with the extremely limited money available for natural health care research, has resulted in almost no clinical papers appearing in peer-reviewed research journals.

The Foundation for Applied Conservative Therapies Research (FACTR) has recently been created by ICAK as a research foundation with the purpose of generating and publishing scientific research on AK. To date, studies published have dealt only with the neurophysiological mechanisms of AK. So far, no clinical outcome studies of the effectiveness of AK have been completed, although several have been started. Two clinical papers have recently been published based on the relationship of muscle testing responses to emotional stress. Both used concepts developed by Scott Walker, D.C., which he calls "Neuro Emotional Technique." The first was a preliminary study that found that induced emotional arousal (threatening stimuli in phobic patients) showed weakening responses during muscle testing in a high percentage of people, if a number of previously unidentified variables were controlled (Peterson, 1996). The other paper reviewed two patients with elevated cholesterol levels who had spinal adjustments performed while pondering stressful events (Peterson, 1996). Both had significant reductions in their cholesterol levels (27.8 percent and 22.5 percent) following the procedures. Follow-up studies are being performed but have been not been published at this time.

REAL PEOPLE AND AK

∞

Sarah's brother had died in a tragic automobile accident when he was 17 and she was 15. Now in her late twenties, Sarah still thought of her brother daily, but her memories were mainly of the hours and days surrounding the tragedy. She could not enjoy any fond memories of her brother without being shunted into thoughts of his death. For the past 10 years, any thoughts of her brother would make her tearful and unable to function.

In the AK doctor's office, when Sarah was asked to recall her brother's death, she immediately broke into tears. Any muscle test performed by the doctor tested as weak. The doctor evaluated acupuncture points by tapping them until he found one that negated Sarah's muscle weakness. He continued to tap this point while Sarah continued her emotional recall. After a few seconds, Sarah's tears stopped. After 30 seconds of tapping, her recall of her brother's death caused no muscle weakness. Sarah remarked that for the first time since his death, she didn't feel like crying when thinking about her brother.

Now Sarah can recall her brother's life fondly, and she can recall her brother's death with sadness, but without tears and without being incapacitated. On followup visits with her AK doctor, the recall of her brother's death did not result in any muscle weakness.

∞

Many AK practitioners work with mental health care professionals. When combined with traditional mental health approaches, the AK techniques often help patients past blocks in therapy, as the following case history demonstrates.

Ted had a tumultuous relationship with his father throughout his early life and into his college career. Ted felt that the only way to earn his father's love was to excel at whatever he did. Yet none of his achievements seemed to please his father. He was extremely successful in college, but in the middle of his junior year, his father died. Ted became depressed, lost his motivation, dropped out of school, and worked at odd jobs to support himself. He sought therapy, and after years of professional help, he understood his problem logically, but he felt no better and still had no motivation to pursue his potential as a human being.

Ted was seen by an AK chiropractor for chronic back pain that had been present for many years, even before his father's death. The effects of the treatment were good, but they would last no longer than a day or two. The doctor asked Ted to think about the major stressors in his life, one at a time. This recall pattern caused a weakening response to muscle testing for four of the six stressors Ted identified, including several related to always being unable to please his father. The doctor tapped a different acupuncture "circuit breaker" each time Ted recalled a new emotional stressor. He also identified that tasting folic acid, an important nutrient for brain neurotransmitter function, negated the weakening effects of the emotional recall. The weakening pattern of emotional recall never recurred in Ted. In the next 6 weeks, he made remarkable progress in his therapy and was able to decrease sessions to twice a month and eventually once a month. He returned to school, finished his degree, found a job based on his training, made new friends, and felt the return of his life, which had been put on hold for many years.

Nancy is a middle-aged, full-time clinical psychologist whose practice includes many depressed and anxious patients. Prolonged stress arising from family illnesses, combined with her stressful lifestyle, resulted in exhaustion and depression. She tried psychotherapy and antidepressant medication, which helped somewhat with her daily levels of depression, but she was still tired and would occasionally have such severe depressive episodes that she was unable to function.

Nancy consulted an AK doctor who found that her adrenal glands (the body's antistress glands) were near total exhaustion. The doctor used AK treatment methods and placed Nancy on supplements of folic acid, vitamin C, B_6, and pantothenic acid (B complex). Nancy improved greatly. Her energy returned and her daily depression lifted, but she still had occasional, unexplainable, transient bouts of uncontrollable crying and hopelessness. By her next visit, Nancy had not experienced a depressive episode in 3 weeks, and her AK doctor found very little wrong. In the subsequent visit, though, she burst into tears the minute she entered the treatment room and wondered out loud if she would ever be better. The AK exam showed multiple problems, almost as if all the previous problems had recurred at once. AK assessment showed that these factors were associated with an acute allergic reaction. Questioning revealed that Nancy had eaten at a Chinese restaurant the night before and that she usually ate this type of food about once a month. The doctor found food allergy reactions to soy and the food additive monosodium glutamate (MSG). These were later confirmed by laboratory tests. The AK doctor treated Nancy for the acute allergic reaction and immediately Nancy stopped crying. Further treatment that day left her feeling tired but otherwise close to normal. She was instructed to avoid soy and MSG as if they were poisons, which, for her, they are. She returned to normal functioning with the exception of occasional recurrence of short-term depression if she accidentally ingested soy or MSG.

WHAT TO EXPECT

Since AK crosses many interdisciplinary lines, your experience with an AK practitioner will vary. If you see an AK chiropractor, osteopath, or medical doctor, most likely you will receive a physical examination and possibly a laboratory workup. If you see an AK-trained psychologist, dentist, or other practitioner, a different approach will be taken, depending on the person's discipline.

One of the most unique things about AK is that as the patient you are not passive but directly involved in each step of the office procedure. This is because most procedures involve before-and-after muscle testing to evaluate the effectiveness of the therapy. We call this interactive assessment of the patient's problem.

All AK practitioners perform manual muscle testing procedures. This involves you resisting the practitioner's force as it is directed against one of your limbs. Sometimes you will be able to resist the examiner's pressure and other times your muscle strength will easily be overcome by the force of the tester. Factors from each side of the triad of health will be evaluated with muscle testing before and after each step.

You may be asked to place your hands on specific areas of the body or the examiner may push or tap various important "circuits" to determine if these circuits are involved or not. You may be asked to taste various substances such as vitamins or minerals or other remedies. As mentioned earlier in the case histories, you may be asked to mentally focus on stressful events in your life. In each case, the examiner will observe changes in muscle strength that will guide you both to the proper treatment and lifestyle recommendations.

Most people are fascinated by the process. You may or may not be able to feel the difference in muscle strength changes during your exam. Remember that the outcome of any one muscle test is only a part of the larger picture that your practitioner is trying to develop. Your professionally trained practitioner will be able to describe the significance of the findings and outline further recommendations for treatment and lifestyle which are unique for your case.

HOW TO FIND AN AK PRACTITIONER

AK, by definition of ICAK, is performed by licensed health professionals and is used with professional training and appropriate examination and diagnosis of the patient. There are a number of people, both professional and nonprofessional, who have adopted some of the concepts of muscle testing to suit their own purposes. The ICAK maintains a list of members in the United States, Australia, Europe, and other areas of the world who practice according to the ICAK's professional standards.

Certification is available to AK doctors at various levels. The highest level of certification is D.I.B.A.K. (Diplomate of the International Board of Applied Kinesiology). For referral to an ICAK member in the U.S. or abroad, contact ICAK, 6405 Metcalf Ave., Suite 503, Shawnee Mission, KS 66202-4080. Phone: (913) 384-5336. Fax: (913) 384-5112.

HOW TO LEARN MORE

Callahan, R. J. *How Executives Overcome Their Fear of Public Speaking and Other Phobias.* Wilmington, DE: Enterprise Publishing, Inc., 1987.

Durlacher, J. V. *Freedom From Fear Forever.* Tempe, AZ: Van Ness Publishing Co., 1994.

Goodheart, G. *You'll Be Better — The Story of Applied Kinesiology.* Privately published and available from Dr. George J. Goodheart, 20567 Mack Ave., Grosse Pointe Woods, MI. (313) 881-0662. Fax: (313) 881-8691, 1985.

Maffetone, P. *Everyone Is an Athlete.* Mahopac, NY: David Barmore Productions, 1994.

Maffetone, P. *The Health Capsules Book II.* Shawnee Mission, KS: ICAK, 1994. (6405 Metcalf Ave., Suite 503, Shawnee Mission, KS 66202-4080 (913) 384-5336. Fax: (913) 384-5112).

Peterson, K. B. "A Preliminary Inquiry into Manual Muscle Testing Response in Phobic and Control Subjects Exposed to Threatening Stimuli." *Journal of Manipulative and Physiological Therapeutics* 19 (1996): 310–316.

Thie, J. F. *Touch for Health.* Marina Del Rey, CA: DeVorss and Co., 1985.

Valentine, T. and C. Valentine. *Applied Kinesiology.* New York: Thorson Publishing Group, 1985.

ABOUT THE AUTHOR

Dr. Walter H. Schmitt, Jr., is a chiropractic physician practicing in Chapel Hill, NC. He is a graduate of Duke University and the National College of Chiropractic. He served on the board of directors of the International College of Applied Kinesiology for 19 years and is a charter diplomate of the organization. In 1991, he received a diplomate in chiropractic neurology from the American College of Chiropractic Neurology. He was the first doctor to hold diplomate status in both applied kinesiology and neurology. His memberships also include the American Chiropractic Association and the North Carolina Chiropractic Association. He is an adjunct member of the postgraduate faculty of Logan College of Chiropractic and serves on the editorial review boards of the journals *Chiropractic Technique* and *Alternative Medicine Review.* Dr. Schmitt is a trustee for the Foundation for Allied Conservative Therapies Research (FACTR).

Dr. Schmitt is the author of *Common Glandular Dysfunction in the General Practice* (1981) and *Compiled Notes on Clinical Nutritional Products* (Second ed., 1990). He has authored numerous papers and frequently lectures to professional groups, both nationally and internationally. His lectures and papers include such subjects as pain and pain relief, functional endocrine problems, the relationships between body chemistry imbalances and structural faults, and applied kinesiology, particularly the use of muscle testing in enhancing neurological diagnosis of functional problems. In 1983, he served on a special Chiropractic Research Protocol Committee formed by the United States Olympic Committee Sports Medicine Modalities Commission.

Christa Obuchowski

7 Aromatherapy

WHAT IS AROMATHERAPY?

"Aromatherapy" is a term recently coined to describe the healing and medicinal properties found in the essential oils of various plants and herbs. These properties have been familiar to people throughout recorded history. Aromatherapy is a powerful, effective, natural healing therapy that has a profound effect on body, mind, and soul. It has been found to be an effective tool when used with other healing practices.

Aromatherapy uses distilled extracts, also called essential oils, refined from plants and herbs. This therapy can relieve pain, kill bacteria, cleanse the body of toxins, treat immune deficiencies and stress, and support the health of the body, mind, and spirit. Essential oils are extremely concentrated. For example, it takes thirty large roses to harvest one drop of essential oil. Essential oils are found in the barks, stems, flowers, branches, roots, and leaves of plants and are extracted through a process of steam distillation or cold-pressing.

The essential oil gives a plant its fragrance. But the term "aromatherapy" is somewhat misleading. It suggests that the value of essential oils is found only in the aroma of the oil. Aromas are powerful in and of themselves, as is evidenced by the stimulation of pleasant memories and associations carried by a specific odor. But essential oils also have specific pharmacological properties that can help with minor everyday ailments such as a sore throat or a winter cold, and even more serious problems like bronchitis, sinusitis, and rheumatism. Bacterial infections found at the root of many lung ailments, as well as diseases of the immune system, are being addressed by aromatherapy. In the area of mental health care, aromatherapy can be an invaluable tool, not only to improve and uplift a patient's mind, but also to address many underlying physiological problems that may go hand and hand with depression, insomnia, anxiety, grief, learning disorders, and the myriad of other overt symptoms of an unbalanced system.

HOW IT BEGAN

The use of essential oils appears to have been practiced since the earliest recorded history of humankind. In almost every country, we have discovered the remains of incense burners, pots that held cosmetic potions, and oil lamps that indicate the use of infusions of herbs high in essential oils. Frankincense and other resins were used in the temples of Egypt. Essential oils were used for mummification. Hindu texts refer to countless aromatic products used for both liturgical and therapeutic practices. Ancient Semitic people used essential oils in religious practices, to expand consciousness, and to improve meditation. In Europe, plagues and epidemics were combated by fumigation with powerful essential oils. The Greeks perceived that aromatics were useful in the treatment of anxiety, hysteria, grief, and depression. Many cultures sent prayers to the gods through fragrance.

The cosmetic use of essential oils dates back more than 5,000 years. Egyptians, Greeks, Romans, and Europeans designed personal perfumes to elicit various emotions. Unlike modern synthetic perfumes, an essential oil does not merely mask foul odors of the atmosphere or the body, but actually suppresses them by a physiochemical action that destroys, hinders, or neutralizes germs.

In 1920, Rene-Maurice Gottefosse, a French chemist, coined the term "aromatherapy." In his work in the perfume industry, he had discovered that many of the essential oils used were superior to chemical antiseptics. He tells the story of burning his hand and plunging it into pure lavender oil. To his surprise, his hand was healed within a short time without infection or scarring. This amazing discovery led him to explore the uses of essential oils in the cosmetic and dermatological industry. Gottefosse's work inspired other medical and commercial researchers to continue the work of exploration into the myriad of healing and restorative properties of essential oils.

In England, lavender is used in hospitals to aid cancer patients with pain and insomnia. With the invention of penicillin by Alexander Fleming in 1928, chemical antibiotics were viewed as a scientific wonder, and the interest in research focusing on essential oils dwindled. It was not until 1982, with the publication of *The Practice of Aromatherapy* by Jean Valnet, M.D., and then *L'Aromatherapie Exactement* by Franchomme and Penoel (1992), that the remarkable properties of essential oils once again came to the attention of the healing community and to the public.

Aromatherapy is an ancient science with a new name. We are just beginning to understand the depth of benefit available to us even though our relationship with it is an ancient one.

HOW IT WORKS

Aromatherapy can be practiced as self-care or with the aid of a health care professional. Aromatherapy has been incorporated into the practices of many different healing and aesthetic professions. Those interested in simple and practical self-care can find workshops and books that give an introduction to the different methods of using essential oils. Many oils can be used for personal enjoyment. It is fine to experiment at home with diffusers, baths, and inhalation.

Discuss the use of essential oils with a certified aromatherapist when your health issues necessitate the help of a professional. Seek help from a certified aromatherapist if you have any questions or concerns regarding the use of oils, especially if you have asthma, high or low blood pressure, are on chemotherapy, or have eczema or hypersensitive skin. If you are pregnant, consult an aromatherapist about which oils you may use safely during your pregnancy. Do not use essential oils on children under three months.

Following are some of the ways the oils can be applied. There is some overlap between the techniques listed under each of the following categories:

Aromatherapy Massage

A hands-on method using essential oils and massage. It addresses a variety of body and mind ailments. Massage with essential oils can address problems ranging from those that stem from lymph congestion to stress management and insomnia. Therapeutic massage is often considered to be the most effective use of essential oils. Whether through the work of a trained massage therapist, or at home with a friend or loved one, the senses are stimulated as the essential oil penetrates the body. If a full massage is not possible, massaging the hands and feet is an excellent way to stay in good health. The reflex or zone points for the body are stimulated by this method. This helps to balance the body's energy flow.

Medical (Clinical) Aromatherapy

In France and Germany, doctors and naturopaths are using essential oils given through prescriptions and taken orally to treat infectious diseases. Diffusers are being used in hospitals in England to promote states of relaxation and deep rest after surgery. At homes in Europe and the United States, mothers of small children are learning to use diffusers with essential oils to combat airborne infection during childhood illness. A trained aromatherapist can create personalized formulas for use in a diffuser.

Steam inhalation is an excellent treatment for direct absorption of essential oils. In the home, one to two drops of an essential oil can easily be added to hot, steaming water. Cover your head with a towel and breathe in through your nose for quick relief. Whether using essential oils in a steaming bowl of hot water, a cold or hot humidifier, or a sauna, inhalation can easily address both chronic and immediate problems.

Aesthetic Aromatherapy

Essential oils are used by beauty therapists to treat skin problems, for regeneration, and to uplift the spirit. Treatments may include facials, herbal wraps, herbal masks, personalized perfumes, moisturizers, body oils, and skin cleansers. The spa industry is in the process of expanding its use of aromatherapy into every area of body care.

A hot bath at the end of a busy day helps keep body and soul in harmony. It is one of the most wonderful ways of using aromatherapy at home. Choose essential oils that will provide the desired stimulus; mix them with an emulsifier like honey, liquid soap, Epsom or sea salt; add them to your bath water; and relax.

Environmental Aromatherapy

The use of essential oils to modify and enhance our living spaces is increasing. Diffusers are being used at home for personal mind-body care, in large office buildings to stimulate mental concentration, and in hotels and casinos to subtly create environments of luxury and well-being.

Essential oils do not mask unwanted smells; instead, they cleanse the air by altering the structure of the molecules. Diffusers or aroma lamps disperse essential oil molecules into the air. Diffusers come in many different forms and are usually made of ceramic, glass, or marble, with a small container for water that is heated by a candle or electricity. Drops of essential oil are added to the water; the number of drops of essential oil is determined by the size of the room and the intensity of fragrance desired. Heat releases the volatile essential oil molecules into the atmosphere. The influence of the scent is very subtle but can have a profound effect. You can begin using a diffuser at home simply for the pleasure it can create aesthetically. The formulas designed for use in a diffuser can disinfect a room, increase concentration, bring a sense of calm and peacefulness, and stimulate and strengthen the immune system.

A SELECTION OF ESSENTIAL OILS AND THEIR APPLICATIONS

It is crucial that only pure essential oils be used in aromatherapy. These are natural plant essences extracted by steam distillation or expression. Plants grown in the wild or grown organically yield essential oils of optimal quality. In choosing essential oils, choose the best. Reconstituted products or chemical copies of natural essences simply do not work.

Chamomile Roman (Anthemis noblis)

Action: Soothing antispasmodic. Chamomile is one of the most useful essential oils. It is anti-inflammatory and carries extreme soothing action. It eases anxiety, tension, anger, and fear. It is a wonderful oil for children.

Indications: Overactive mind, impulsive behavior, fear, tension, anger, insomnia, stress-related complaints, stomach conditions, inflamed skin, menstrual problems.

Clary Sage (Salvia sclarea)

Action: Calming and euphoric. Clary sage is used to relieve nervous tension, a racing mind, and panicky states. It encourages feelings of well-being and the capacity to see life in perspective.

Indications: Migraine headaches, hormonal imbalance, menstrual cramps, panic attacks, exhaustion, depression, hysteria, insomnia, anxiety, obsession.

Frankincense (Boswellia carteri/thurifera)

Action: Sedative. Frankincense has a calming effect on the nervous system.

Indications: Shortness of breath, anxiety, obsession, hopelessness.

Helichrysum (Immortelle/Helichrysum angustefolium)

Action: Rejuvenates and promotes cell growth. Helichrysum has a strong psychological effect. It helps to ground the mind and foster acceptance of changes in life. It is often used for pain relief.

Indications: Lethargy, nervous exhaustion, neuralgia, stress, shortness of breath, menstrual cramps.

Lavender (Lavandula officinalis)

Action: Balancing, calming. Lavender is known for cleansing and soothing the spirit, relieving exhaustion and anxiety. It has a balancing action on the nervous system, resulting in a calmer approach to life.

Indications: Insomnia, fear, mood swings, nervous conditions, worry, depression, shock, hypertension, headaches, exhaustion.

Marjoram (Origanum marjorana)

Action: Calming. Marjoram is well-known for its warming, relaxing qualities. It is extremely helpful for nervous muscle spasms, aches, and insomnia.

Indications: Menstrual disorders, high blood pressure, grief, hyperactivity, insomnia, nervousness, muscle cramps.

Peppermint (Mentha piperita)

Action: Cooling stimulant. Peppermint is an excellent oil for a tired mind. It has historically been used for nausea. It is cooling and refreshing and is used for nervous exhaustion and fatigue.

Indications: Hysteria, fatigue, depression, shock, indigestion, nausea, dizziness, lymph congestion.

Rose (Rosa damascena)

Action: Soothes the emotions and lifts the heart. It is used traditionally in times of grief and sadness.

Indications: Grief, nervous tension, poor self-image, frigidity, impotence, sorrow, cardiac congestion, emotional exhaustion, disappointment.

Rosemary (Rosmarinus officinalis)

Action: Stimulant. Rosemary is a stimulating, uplifting essential oil that can be used effectively for both mental and physical problems. It clears the mind and aids memory. It is good for mental fatigue, general dullness, and lethargy.

Indications: Depression, lethargy, exhaustion, poor memory, headaches, water retention.

Sandalwood (Santalum album)

Action: Calming. Sandalwood aids in the relief of underlying anxiety and, for that reason, has often been used as an aphrodisiac. It helps with obsessional attitudes. It encourages relaxation and a sense of well-being. It can stimulate the immune system and keep infection at bay.

Indications: High blood pressure, muscle spasms, frigidity, impotence, depression, anxiety, grief, insomnia.

Tangerine (Citrus reticulata)

Action: Emotionally uplifting. Tangerine is refreshing to the mind and helps to release anxiety and depression.

Indications: Indigestion, depression, anxiety in adults and children, sadness.

Ylang Ylang (Cananga odorata)

Action: Aphrodisiac. The exotic aroma of ylang ylang has a sedating effect on the nerves, but at the same time, it uplifts the spirit and mind. It has traditionally been used as an aphrodisiac. It calms overly excited systems. It regulates adrenaline flow. It balances hormones.

Indications: High blood pressure, impotence, frigidity, nervous tension, anxiety, hormonal imbalance.

WHAT THE RESEARCH SHOWS

Today, scientists are studying the effect of aromatherapy on every aspect of health, from the aging process to the treatment of cancers and the stabilization of the immune system. Essential oils vary in chemical makeup and carry with them specific properties that act upon the thyroid, adrenals, and ovaries — the regulators of the body. Essential oils are capable of stimulating the drainage of the lymph glands and detoxifying the body. They invigorate or calm the system and assist in the digestive process. Many essential oils hold antiviral properties and are effective in treating infection.

The science of aromatherapy addresses the tie between fragrance and memory triggers in the brain. With each breath, fragrance molecules reach the brain. The olfactory membrane, located in the nasal cavity, consists of millions of olfactory nerve cells. These are brain cells capable of carrying tremendous amounts of information. The olfactory membrane is the only place in the body where the central nervous system is in direct connection with the environment. Odor molecules are carried by nerve cells in the form of electrical impulses into the brain. These impulses of information reach the oldest and innermost control centers in our brain. Neurotransmitters are released by the odor stimuli. For example, encephaline, a neurotransmitter, that can be released by a scent, reduces pain and creates a sense of personal well-being. Endorphin, another neurotransmitter, stimulates the feeling center and reduces pain. In reality, we are deeply touched by scent.

Giovanni Gatti and Renato Cayola (1923, cited in Lawless, 1994) found that sedative and stimulating plant essences were useful in relieving anxiety and depression. Paolo Rovesti, a chemist and pharmacologist, conducted many clinical experimental studies on patients suffering from "hysteria or psychic depression" that showed aromatherapy to be very effective (1975). The research of Gatti, Cayola, and Rovesti has given us documented evidence of the psychotherapeutic effects of specific essential oils that are sedatives, relieve anxiety, and treat psychological ills.

Today, research with essential oils is continuing in the field of brain wave technology. Essential oils are introduced to a patient and the impact of the fragrance is traced through neurological activity. The research of Dr. John Steele (1984) and Robert Tisserand (1978) has found that certain essential oils, when inhaled or smelled, have a tranquilizing or stimulating effect because they alter the brain waves. In clinical studies conducted by Alan Hirsch (1991, 1993), a Chicago neurologist and head of the Smell and Taste Treatment and Research Foundation, essential oils from lavender, chamomile, lemon, and sandalwood calmed brain activity more effectively than Valium. Hirsch has also documented certain oils that can stimulate the brain and heighten the sense of expansion and energy. In Japan, scientists have studied the effect that lemon's essential oil has on mental concentration. They found that in office environments, typing mistakes were reduced by 54 percent when the essential oil from the lemon was diffused in the room (Fischer-Rizzi, 1989).

REAL PEOPLE AND AROMATHERAPY

Richard is a 42-year-old man who sought help with lower back pain that had persisted for four years and for exhaustion. He had tried both a chiropractor and an osteopath and both had agreed that the source of his pain was not structural. He was using aspirin and cortisone shots to relieve the back pain.

In my first consultation with Richard, it became clear to me that his problem was a result of mental and physical stress. Richard's job was very demanding. He was the manager of a large and successful business, and his sense of responsibility was driven and compulsive. He was aware that he needed time out for himself and he had taken up tennis. He played twice a week with the same compulsive drive that characterized his attitude at work. He described skin problems that occurred during particularly demanding times and didn't seem to know the difference between extending and overextending himself. His body awareness was not strong in any area of his life, and he often found himself exhausted and drained and still feeling that he should do more.

Richard made a commitment to see me weekly for aromatherapy massages. He also agreed to work with me to make some lifestyle changes that would support the treatments. My first consideration in Richard's treatment was to address the physical manifestations of his stress and relieve the pain he suffered. In long-term treatment, our goal was to change his mental attitude toward life from one of competition, fear, and worry to one of harmony. His program included personal time spent in relaxation. He began to take hot baths three times a week with an essential oil formula designed to relax and balance the mind-body connection. We developed a massage oil that his wife agreed to apply after his weekly tennis matches or a particularly hard day at work. These formulas included essential oils of lavender, frankincense, rosemary, immortelle, roman chamomile, marjoram, and ginger.

Richard began to feel more comfortable spending downtime in quiet personal activity. After the first month he reported that his sleep patterns had greatly changed. He was sleeping more deeply and for longer periods of time. His attitude toward his job began to shift. Although his job remained as demanding as before, Richard was beginning to recognize the limits of his body. After two years of treatment, Richard now feels that his commitment to his work has grown deeper, as he has learned to approach it with harmony and cooperation. His back problems have disappeared, he has no more problems with skin rashes, and his general quality of life seems to be much more satisfying. He looks forward to a massage with aromatherapy once a month and continues with his personal formulas at home. He no longer feels the need for either aspirin or cortisone and feels that the essential oils have had profound effects in many other areas of his life as well.

Judy is a 53-year-old woman who had been in a successful marriage since her early twenties. Her appearance was youthful and vibrant. When she entered menopause, however, she began to feel a deep loss of her identity and female sexuality. She was haunted by the fear that she would no longer be attractive to her husband and that her life was over. Her nights were sleepless, with mental visions of the regrets of her life. Although still young and healthy, Judy felt that time was running out for her. On a physical level, she suffered from hot flashes, poor digestion, and frequent headaches. She kept her fears and obsessive thoughts of failure to herself. She felt that menopause was simply a process she had to suffer through alone. As her depression increased, she attracted the very thing she feared. She began to gain weight and, with the loss of self-confidence she experienced, she also began to avoid intimacy with her husband.

Judy came to me weekly for body work and aromatherapy. During her first massage session, I began to discuss the opportunities and problems that come with menopause. I recommended several books that could open the process for her in a more positive way. I also recommended that she begin to discuss her personal experience of this profound life change with her women friends and with her husband.

From a selection of essential oils specifically chosen for their hormonal balancing qualities (sandlewood, ylang ylang, rose geranium, rose, lavender, roman chamomile, jasmine, clary sage, and peppermint), I asked Judy to choose fragrances that most attracted her. Using those oils, I blended a special massage oil for her to use at home on her legs to help reduce the hot flashes. I was also interested in helping her regain a sense of her deep feminine nature. It is true that menopause changes the way a woman looks at herself sexually. I chose a selection of essential oils that not only addresses the hormonal system but also the emotional body — oils that stimulate natural sensuality. It was important for Judy to relax and feel her desirability in her new phase of life.

From the oils Judy was most attracted to, I blended a bath oil and personal perfume. I added relaxing formulas to the bath oil to improve her sleep patterns. In her personal perfume I concentrated on deep sensuality to increase her personal attractiveness. I created a formula based on jasmine, which is especially effective in psychosomatic disorders. Jasmine is a natural analgesic that brings deep relaxation and euphoria to darkness.

After several sessions, Judy's creativity began to blossom. She was enjoying her sensuality again in a new way. She began to feel her connection to nature, which led her into new activities like hiking. She began to paint the landscapes through which she hiked. The additional weight dropped away and she felt herself to be reborn.

WHAT TO EXPECT

If you choose to go to an aromatherapist for aromatherapy massage, an office visit will usually take one to two hours. Commonly, a patient will be asked to give a personal health history. From the history, the therapist will choose a selected group of essential oils. The patient will participate by sampling the fragrances and choosing ones that are pleasing. A patient's preference for a certain essential oil may tell us much about that person's mental, emotional, or physical state. The therapist will then prepare a face oil and a body oil. The patient is asked to undress and lie on the massage table. The comfort and warmth of the client is always paramount. Pillows may be placed under the knees when the client is on his or her back, or a special face cradle used when lying face down.

Many styles of massage may be used with the application of the essential oil, from deep tissue to the light touch of lymph stimulation. A deep bond is created between the therapist and the patient during the treatment and is always characterized by the personal respect shown for the body's communication of its needs. Special techniques such as foot reflexology or sacro-cranial work may be used as well. Often, music, which is chosen to aid in relaxation and enhance a sense of well-being, is an integral part of the treatment. The therapist may also choose to work on specific organs of the body to enhance the effect of the essential oil. A major focus of the massage is the establishment of an olfactory reference to specific states of being. In other words, the therapist wants the patient to associate warmth, relaxation, and well-being with specific scents so that when those essential oils are used at home, the patient unconsciously recalls the experience of his or her treatment.

At the end of the treatment, the therapist might make a personal blend of oils for the patient. The client might be directed to use the oil blend in the bath, a diffuser, or when massaging the feet, hands, legs, or face. Often weekly massages will be recommended for a period of time. A patient should notice immediate shifts in his or her well-being and can discuss with the therapist what length of time will pass before more profound changes appear.

HOW TO CHOOSE A PRACTITIONER

As of 1998, there is no licensing agency in the U.S. for aromatherapists. There are, however, a variety of schools that offer classes in aromatherapy and can supply the names and addresses of certified practitioners. There is no national standard for certification, so each school establishes its curriculum. In discussing certification of aromatherapists, Michael Scholes, president of Aromatherapy Seminars, says, "I consider a health practitioner a fully certified aromatherapist when they have participated in a minimum of 300 hours of class work and hands-on work, and have been active in the field of aromatherapy for at least three years."

Fees for these services may fluctuate from $55 to $150, depending on the length of the session and the therapy used. If the therapist recommends an oil or an oil blend for home use, the cost may range from $15 to $50, depending on the essential oils chosen.

Many health practitioners incorporate essential oils into their work. Massage therapists, naturopaths, psychologists, estheticians, home health care specialists, nurse practitioners, and others are adding the use of essential oils to their healing methods. If you are interested in discussing your health needs with an aromatherapist trained in blending formulas for home or personal use, it would be best to contact one of the following aromatherapy schools and ask for referrals in your area. These organizations also offer aromatherapy products, seminars, and workshops.

AMERICAN ALLIANCE OF AROMATHERAPY
P.O. Box 309
Depot Bay, OR 97341
Tel: (800) 809-9850
Aromatherapy newsletter, information center, and referral service.

AROMA BOTANICA INSTITUTE
Christa Obuchowski, owner and lecturer
Tel: (505) 984-1879
Practicing aromatherapist and therapeutic blender, aromatherapy workshops, seminars and trainings for private individuals and the spa industry.

AROMATHERAPY SEMINARS
Michael Scholes, president and head lecturer
1830 South Robertson Blvd., Suite 203
Los Angeles, CA 90035
Tel: (800) 677-2368, (310) 838-6122

ARTEMIS INSTITUTE OF NATURAL THERAPIES
Peter Holmes, L.Ac, M.H., director
P.O. Box 1824
Boulder, CO 80306
Tel: (303) 443-9289
Offering classes, aromatherapy training, and high-quality essential oils.

LIFE TREE AROMATICS
John Steele, owner and master blender
3949 Longridge Ave.
Sherman Oaks, CA 91423 (please send $2.50 for information packet)
Tel: (818) 986-0594
Offering classes and high-quality essential oils.

NEW MEXICO ACADEMY OF HEALING ARTS
Christa Obuchowski, teacher, applied aromatherapy
501 Franklin Ave.
Santa Fe, NM 87501
Tel: (505) 982-6271
Offering classes in aromatherapy training.

PACIFIC INSTITUTE OF AROMATHERAPY
Kurt and Monica Schnaulbelt, facilitators
P.O. Box 6723
San Rafael, CA 94903
Tel: (415) 479-9121
Specializing in scientific and medical aromatherapy and high-quality essential oils.

HOW TO LEARN MORE

Balacs, T. "Essential Oils in the Body." *Aroma '93: Harmony from Within* Brighton, UK: Aromatherapy Publications, 1994. (P.O. Box 746, Hove, E. Sussex BN3 3XA, UK. Phone: 0273-772-479).

Damian, P. and K. Damian. *Aromatherapy: Scent and Psyche*. Rochester, VT: Healing Arts Press, 1995.

Fischer-Rizzi, S. *Complete Aromatherapy Handbook*. New York: Sterling Publishing Co., Inc., 1989.

Franchomme, P. and D. Penoel. *L'aromatherapie Exactement*. Limoges: Roger Jollois Editeur, 1990.

Gattefosse, R. *Aromatherapy*. Saffron Walden, UK: C.W. Daniel, 1993.

Gumbel, D. *Principles of Holistic Therapy with Herbal Essences*. Heidelberg, Germany: Karl F. Haug, 1986.

Hirsch, A. R. "Olfaction and Anxiety." *Clinical Psychiatry*, 16 (1993): 4.

Hirsch, A. R. "Olfaction and Psychiatry." 144th Annual Meeting, American Psychiatric Association, New Orleans, LA, May 16, 1991.

Kirk-Smith, M. "Human Olfactory Communication." *Aroma '93: Harmony from Within*. Brighton, UK: Aromatherapy Publications, 1994. (P.O. Box 746, Hove, E. Sussex BN3 3XA, UK. Phone: 0273-772-479).

Lawless, J. *Aromatherapy and the Mind*. London: HarperCollins, 1994.

Rovesti, P. *Alla Ricerca dei Cosmetici Perdutti*. Venedig, France: Publisher unknown, 1975.

Steele, J. "Brain Research and Essential Oils." *Aromatherapy Quarterly* 1 (1984): 5.

Stoddart, D. M. *The Scented Ape*. Cambridge, England: Cambridge University Press, 1993.

Tisserand, R. *Aromatherapy to Heal and Tend the Body*. Santa Fe, NM: Lotus, 1988.

Tisserand, R. *The Art of Aromatherapy*. Rochester, VT: Healing Arts Press, 1978.

Valnet, J. *The Practice of Aromatherapy*. Rochester, VT: Healing Arts Press, 1982.

Worwood, V. A. *The Fragrant Mind*. Novato, CA: New World Library, 1996.

ABOUT THE AUTHOR

Christa Obuchowski is a certified aromatherapist who received her training in Europe and the United States. She began her work by studying massage therapy and related fields. For the last seven years, she has devoted more and more of her practice to working with essential oils. She has worked extensively with some of the foremost aromatherapists, conducting and participating in seminars with Dietrich Gumbel, Ph.D, Kurt Schnaubelt, Marcel Larbre, and Michael Scholes. Her goal is to design a personalized, client-oriented experience that will stimulate the natural healing potentials inherent in the body. Obuchowski is on the staff of the New Mexico Academy of Healing Arts, where she teaches aromatherapy and hydrotherapy.

Jim Brooks, M.D.

8 Ayurveda:
Maharishi Ayurveda and Mental Health

WHAT IS AYURVEDA?

Ayurveda is the system of traditional medicine from India. Maharishi Ayurveda is a more comprehensive and complete version of Ayurveda developed by Maharishi Mahesh Yogi. The term "Maharishi Ayurveda" has recently been expanded upon, and is referred to as "Maharishi's Vedic approach to health," or "Maharishi's Vedic medicine." These terms refer to the application of all forty branches of Vedic literature to the field of health. For a more in-depth description of Vedic literature and how it relates to health look at the book *Human Physiology: Expression of Veda and the Vedic Literature*. Maharishi Ayurveda has many practical applications to the fields of mental health and substance abuse treatment. Ayurveda also emphasizes strategies for preventing illness and for promoting mental and physical health; it includes methods such as transcendental meditation (TM) for developing higher states of human consciousness beyond the three most familiar states: waking, dreaming, and sleeping. The theoretical underpinnings are sound and simple to understand, and the clinical application of the principles significantly contributes to current treatment modalities. Techniques of Maharishi Ayurveda, which include meditation, diet, herbal preparations, purification treatments, changes in daily routine, and taste and aroma therapies, all act in a holistic and synergistic way. These treatments serve to enhance the benefits of other mainstream treatments. For instance, psychotherapy and medication can sometimes have the unwanted side effect of promoting dependency and a lack of control over one's healing process. A Western-trained physician who is also trained in Maharishi Ayurveda can use an integrated approach that primarily emphasizes natural treatment methods but, if necessary, add additional approaches. In this way, patients truly get the best of both worlds — East and West.

HOW IT BEGAN

Ayurveda is thought by medical historians to be approximately 6,000 years old. There are textbooks on this system of healing, including the *Charaka Samhitas* by Sharma and the *Sushruta Samhitas* by Bhishagratha, still available today, that were written approximately 3,000 years ago. Due to hundreds of years of foreign rule in India, much of the essential knowledge of ayurveda has been lost. Since India's independence, there has been a resurgence of ayurvedic medicine. There are more than 100 ayurveda colleges in India, a number of which are fully supported by the Indian government. The World Health Organization has formally recognized and given support to the reestablishment of this system of health in India. Over the last eight years in particular, there have been significant strides in bringing the knowledge of ayurveda back to its original status. The individual most responsible for this is Maharishi Mahesh Yogi, a renowned expert in Vedic knowledge, who is the founder of the transcendental meditation program and a number of academic institutions around the world, including the Maharishi Institute for Vedic Science and Technology in India and the Maharishi University of Management in the United States. Maharishi, working with leading ayurveda physicians in India, including Brihaspati Dev Tri Guna and Bal Raj Maharishi, has rediscovered the essential knowledge of ayurveda and has made courses available to physicians around the world so that they can become trained in this system of natural health. Hundreds of medical doctors on five continents have now taken courses in Maharishi Ayurveda and are integrating it with their medical practices.

HOW IT WORKS

The classical textbooks of ayurveda describe four causes of mental illness: psychological, physiological, behavioral, and environmental. The main psychological cause of mental illness, according to Maharishi Ayurveda, involves what is called in Sanskrit "*pragyaparadha*." The English translation means "mistake of the intellect." *Pragyaparadha* is the tendency to misperceive and misunderstand the world around us. It occurs when a person has lost contact with his or her inner self, or "pure consciousness." This loss of contact affects such elements of personality functioning as self-esteem, creativity, capacity for experiencing pleasure, outer versus inner dependence, frustration tolerance, reality testing, and overall ability to achieve one's goals in an effective and life-supporting manner. People can regain contact with their inner selves through the regular practice of meditation or other methods of transcending the usual states of consciousness. According to Maharishi Ayurveda, during meditation, the regular experience of pure consciousness results in a completely new style of psychophysiological functioning and changes the qualitative experience of an individual in a dramatic and significant way. These changes include mental calmness, broadened awareness, and profound inner contentedness, called "*sat-chit-ananda*" in Sanskrit. The calmness of mind that grows with the regular habit of meditating enables the individual to be less anxious and less prone to distraction. A less distracted mind is less likely to be shaken from a sense of inner stability. The individual develops the ability to have a more open mind and to see a situation with a broader perspective. Such a person will not have much need to obtain pleasure from outside one's self. Also, being more alert means having more energy and motivation. Obviously, the significant enhancement of inner well-being is likely to have a positive effect on many psychiatric conditions and addictive behavior. Research has shown that the TM technique helps individuals gain control over their personal habits.

A second factor seen by ayurveda to contribute to the development of psychiatric conditions is an imbalance of the three basic underlying metabolic principles that govern human physiology (as well as the physiology of the animal and plant kingdoms). These three organizational principles are called *Vata*, *Pitta*, and *Kapha* (Chopra, 1990). *Vata* represents the principle of movement in physiology. It is responsible for the functioning of the nervous system and the flow of the circulatory and digestive symptoms. *Pitta* is responsible for the digestion and metabolism, and *Kapha* is responsible for the structure and fluid balance of the body. All of the modern and scientific understandings of the body's composition and function can be placed into one of these three categories.

There are several advantages to categorizing the physiology according to *Vata*, *Pitta*, and *Kapha*. First, every individual can be categorized as one of seven different psychophysiological constitutional types, based on the combination of these three elements, which are called "*doshas*." Once an individual's constitutional type is determined (through a comprehensive history and physical examination, including the examination of the pulse), then it is possible to determine what types of food would promote balance in any given individual. Also, if there is some psychological or physiological imbalance, or disease, present, herbal preparations and recommendations can be prescribed to restore balance for that individual. Patients are taught to understand their psychophysiological constitutional type so that the foods eaten in the future will not contribute to the development of illness. Patients are also given exercise recommendations, because exercise, in the proper amounts, is seen in ayurveda to be very strengthening to the immune system. Ayurvedic physicians also teach appropriate daily routines to maintain proper balance between the patient's biological rhythms and the natural rhythms of the environment.

For example, if an individual has primarily a *Vata* type of constitution, then that individual may be prone to such psychiatric conditions as insomnia and anxiety. For such an individual, certain food types that reduce excess *Vata* in the system will be extremely helpful in reducing the symptoms. Warm and heavy foods with more of a sweet, sour, or salty taste would be appropriate. Also, regular, mild exercise, a daily warm oil massage, regular practice of transcendental meditation, certain herbal preparations that provide a soothing influence to the nervous system, and a variety of other behavioral recommendations will serve to correct the anxiety and insomnia. Ayurvedic treatments often can be administered without having to resort to modern drugs, which may tend to have harmful and unwanted side effects. This system for understanding the human physiology is simple to learn for the physician and for the patient, and it gives the psychiatric patient a tremendous sense of control over his or her recovery.

A third perspective for understanding the etiology of mental imbalance and addiction is Maharishi Ayurveda's principle of the "violation of natural law." This refers to the idea that we create much of our own misery. In medicine, this idea is becoming well-known and scientifically proven. For example, cigarette smoking and alcohol consumption are proven to be related to such disorders as lung and throat cancer, heart disease, strokes, hypertension, auto accidents, homicides, and suicides. Thousands of years ago, ayurveda not only recognized this fact, but more importantly, provided a methodology for reducing and ultimately eliminating the tendency to violate natural law.

If a person is emotionally healthy, with positive self-esteem, he or she has less of a tendency to behave in a manner that creates harm to him or herself, or others. Behaviors that result in harm to one's nature result from an inner feeling of lack. Improper diet, too little or too much exercise, smoking, drinking, drug abuse, etc., will be significantly reduced if a person reduces the feeling of inner lack.

Each of the approaches of Maharishi Ayurveda serves in a natural way to greatly enhance one's sense of self. TM and other techniques of Maharishi Ayurveda promote a natural experience of well-being that, for many, eliminates the need to use drugs or alcohol.

The fourth factor seen to contribute to mental illness is environmental influence. Our environment definitely plays a role in daily life. A loving, nurturing environment does a lot more to foster normal human development than an environment in which one's parents and/or siblings are hostile, judgmental, and stressed. Maharishi Ayurveda maintains that it is possible for us to enhance the quality of our environment from two perspectives.

The first is that it may be difficult to change another person's behavior, but we certainly can change our own. If a person is improving his or her physical and mental well-being through the technologies of Maharishi Ayurveda on a daily basis, then he or she may be able to step out of the vicious cycle often seen in unhealthy relationships. If we can improve ourselves and develop more inner strength and stability, we often can begin to respond to our family and/or peers in a less defensive and more supportive and empathic manner. This can go a long way in reversing negative trends and tendencies that we previously viewed as unchangeable and hopeless aspects of our environment.

Secondly, and more profoundly, Maharishi Ayurveda states that on the deeper levels of our mind we are intimately connected with those around us. Just as two houses may look very different on the outside and yet contain the same atoms and subatomic particles on the inside, ayurveda states that the deeper aspects of personality, especially the underlying pure consciousness of the individual, has the property of infinite correlation. We are all the same at this deepest level of our nature. Consequently, if we can enliven this field of infinite correlation through individual and, especially, through group transcending, it should be possible to significantly influence our environment in the direction of greater peacefulness and positiveness.

WHAT THE RESEARCH SHOWS

A great deal has been written on the physical health benefits of Maharishi Ayurveda, and there are now a number of published papers describing the benefits of Maharishi Ayurveda for mental health. There is also a growing body of clinical experience in applying Maharishi Ayurveda therapies to psychiatric patients.

Scientific research clearly demonstrates improvements from the practice of ayurvedic techniques, both in psychological and physiological health (Barrett and Brooks, 1992). Group practice of the TM and TM Sidhi (advanced meditation techniques) programs results in a reduction of crime, accidents, sickness, and suicides. In addition, numerous published studies indicate that the use of Maharishi Ayurveda in prison has a significant and positive impact on the rehabilitation process (Dillbeck and Landrith, 1981). Repeated findings include decreased recidivism, improvement in inmate-inmate and inmate-guard relationships, and increased participation in educational and recreational activities (Bleick and Abrams, 1987). Research on the transcendental meditation technique indicates that this state of restful alertness has a corresponding style of physiological functioning that includes EEG coherence (Banquet, 1973), marked reduction in metabolic rate (Wallace, 1970), increased skin resistance (Orme-Johnson, 1973), low levels of cortisol (Bevan, 1980), and a constellation of other neurophysiological parameters (Jeuning and Wilson, 1978; *Results of Scientific Research*, 1984).

Major depression is one of the more common conditions, with approximately 20 percent of the population afflicted at some point in their lives. The techniques of Maharishi Ayurveda help to treat this condition to a significant degree. Research has demonstrated that herbal medications, ayurvedic physical therapy procedures (including *Shirodhara*, an ancient treatment for mental conditions involving the pouring of herbalized oil across the forehead), and transcendental meditation are all helpful in treating not only depression but a number of other conditions (Sharma et al., 1990; Hauser et al., 1988). These treatments appear to work by virtue of effecting change in physiological parameters, including changes in EEG, serum cortisol, endogenous endorphin production, and endogenous imipramine receptor binding. Also, factors such as stress reduction, increased inner contentment associated with enhanced self-esteem, and increased energy all contribute to the alleviation of depression.

REAL PEOPLE AND AYURVEDA

Carla is a married nurse with two children. She became severely depressed, which caused her to be unable to function at work or at home. She was extremely suicidal. She was given a trial of antidepressant medication in the hospital but, due to side effects, she was unable to take an effective dose. She was prescribed transcendental meditation and within a few days, she had a significant improvement of her depression to the point where she was able to leave the hospital. This patient previously was stuck in her therapy sessions. She was unable to look at some difficult issues related to early childhood abuse. After learning to meditate, she had more self-confidence and was able to face many difficulties in her life from which she had been emotionally hiding.

Mental health professionals who integrate Maharishi Ayurveda into their practice are finding similar benefits in the treatment of other conditions including anxiety disorders, borderline and narcissistic personality disorders, psychotic disorders, and substance abuse disorders.

Ralph is a 40-year-old attorney. He suffered from a variety of addictions including narcotics, amphetamines, and minor tranquilizers. He had been struggling for years to get off these substances. With a combination of Maharishi Ayurveda therapies including herbal preparations, transcendental meditation, dietary recommendations according to his constitutional type, music therapy, etc., he has been able to stop using drugs. He is also feeling a sense of inner happiness and strength, which he was able to achieve previously only by taking drugs. He described his experience with ayurveda as follows:

> Having been a poly-substance abuser for the last 20 years, I was nearly ready to give up and simply maintain a crippled lifestyle. I had studied TM in the seventies, but my drug use had all but precluded its use in my daily life. After some prompting from my ayurveda-oriented physician, I began twice-daily meditation.

Any attempt at describing the positive effects would be minimizing. It has been the only competing approach to altered consciousness that has been effective against the tremendous anxiety and craving produced by the drug withdrawal I have had to endure. After 20 minutes of meditation, I become relaxed and focused, and feel that my life has meaning. Meditation is so simple yet powerful that it seems almost impossible that its effect can be so valuable. My aftercare plans' foundation is the inclusion of this most useful tool. I would recommend its use unconditionally for those who suffer, as well as for those who are healthy but simply want to greatly improve their lives.

WHAT TO EXPECT

When a person sees a Maharishi Ayurveda trained physician, the individual is given an extensive mind and body assessment, based on physical characteristics and mental and emotional tendencies. Ayurvedic pulse diagnosis is used to determine constitutional type and any imbalance that might be present. Following this, a comprehensive set of recommendations is given to help balance the mind-body system, and also to promote a more perfect state of health and enlightenment. Recommendations may include transcendental meditation for development of higher states of human potential and for stress management, herbal nutritional supplements and dietary advice, a body purification program (called "*panchakarma*"), and daily and seasonal routines. The whole experience is very uplifting and highly educational, with an emphasis on self-empowering each person, so individuals can become self-sufficient in their health care.

HOW TO FIND AN AYURVEDIC PRACTITIONER

It is recommended that you choose a physician (M.D., D.O., or chiropractor) who has been fully trained and qualified in Maharishi Ayurveda. At present there are no states offering licenses to practice ayurvedic medicine in the U.S., although efforts are being made in this direction. To find a practitioner of ayurveda in your area, call (515) 472-9580.

HOW TO LEARN MORE

Banquet, J. P. "Spectral Analysis of the EEG in Meditation." *Electroencephalography and Clinical Neurophysiology* 35 (1973): 143–151.

Barrett, P. and J. S. Brooks. "Transcending Humiliation: An Ancient Perspective." *Journal of Primary Prevention* 12 (1992).

Bevan, A. J. W. "Endocrine Changes in Transcendental Meditation." *Clinical and Experimental Pharmacology and Physiology* 7 (1980): 75–76.

Bhishagratna, K. L. *Sushruta Samhita.* Chowkhamba Sanskrit Series Office, undated.

Bleick, C. R. and A. I. Abrams. "The Transcendental Meditation Program and Criminal Recidivism in California." *Journal of Criminal Justice* 15 (1987): 211–230.

Brooks, J. S. and T. Scarano. "Transcendental Meditation in the Treatment of Post-Vietnam Adjustment." *Journal of Counseling and Development* 64, no. 3 (1986): 212–215.

Chopra, D. *Perfect Health.* New York: Harmony Books, 1990.

Dillbeck, M. C. and G. Landrith. "The Transcendental Meditation Program and Crime Rate Change in a Sample of 48 Cities." *Journal of Crime and Justice* 4 (1981): 25–45.

Hauser, T., K. Walton, J. Glaser, and R. K. Wallace. "Naturally Occurring Ligand Inhibits Binding of (3H)-Imipramine to High Affinity Receptors." *Society of Neuroscience* 14 (1988): 244.

Jeuning, R. and A. F. Wilson. "Adrenocortical Activity During Meditation." *Hormones and Behavior* 10 (1978): 54–60.

Nader, T. *Human Physiology: Expression of Veda and the Vedic Literature.* Available through MAPI at (800) 345-8332. More information can be obtained by calling Maharishi University of Management of Maharishi Vedic Medicine at (515) 472-7000.

Orme-Johnson, D. W. "Autonomic Stability and Transcendental Meditation." *Psychosomatic Medicine* 35 (1973): 341–349.

Results of Scientific Research on the Transcendental Meditation and Transcendental Meditation-Sidhi Program. Jabalpur, India: Age of Enlightenment, 1984.

Sharma, H. M., et al., "Effect of Maharishi Amrit Kalash on Depression and Substance Abuse." Presented at the annual meeting of the American Association of Ayurvedic Medicine, Boston: Spring, 1990.

Sharma, P. V. *Charaka Samhita.* Chaukhamba Orientalia, undated.

Wallace, R. K. "Physiological Effects of Transcendental Meditation." *Psychosomatic Medicine* 167 (1970): 1751–1754.

ABOUT THE AUTHOR

Jim Brooks, M.D., is currently the clinical director of the Mental Health Institute of Iowa at Mount Pleasant. He is a board-certified psychiatrist and has had extensive training in the application of Maharishi Ayurveda to the field of mental health. He has cowritten a book on this subject entitled *Aurvedic Secrets to Longevity and Total Health*, published by Prentice-Hall. He has published research on the benefits of Maharishi Ayurveda in the rehabilitation of victims of post-traumatic stress disorder.

Frank Andrasik, Ph.D.

9 Biofeedback

WHAT IS BIOFEEDBACK?

Imagine primitive man walking about, when suddenly he is confronted by a dangerous animal. Immediately, his body prepares for one of two possible actions: Remain and fight to the end or flee to safety. The bodily reaction is the same for either course: His pulse quickens, heart rate and blood pressure increase, muscles tense, digestion slows, sweating increases, blood volume in his extremities is reduced, pupils dilate, clotting factors are released into the blood stream, etc. All of these bodily changes are part of the fight or flight response. They prepare a person for physical action. For example, blood is diverted from the hands and feet to the belly muscles (to prepare the person for combat or running) and to the brain (to ensure that mental processes are optimal). Reducing blood flow in the extremities also reduces the likelihood of bleeding, because hands and feet deliver and block blows and are more likely to be injured. Clotting factors are increased to promote healing. Increased sweating of the hands makes it more difficult for an aggressor to grab the person. Pupils dilate to sharpen vision. Energy is diverted from digestion. The body senses a need to channel energy to those activities necessary for immediate survival.

The fight or flight response was very adaptive long ago, when our lives required more physical responses to our environment. Carrying out a physical response served to discharge the excess arousal. Today, we rarely face such life-threatening situations, but our bodies continue to react in a very similar manner to the things that create stress and anxiety for us, such as criticism from a spouse or unreasonable deadlines from a boss. Without an effective outlet, these bodily reactions can rage at full force over time. A certain amount of arousal is needed for optimal functioning; it energizes, motivates, and focuses us on the tasks at hand. However, when the fight or flight response is activated frequently enough, it is no longer adaptive and a full-fledged clinical problem can develop. What is needed is a way to restore bodily functioning to a more reasonable level.

Biofeedback teaches people how to prevent this exaggerated bodily reaction from occurring in the first place, or how to tone it down when it does occur. Biofeedback treatment involves monitoring various bodily states and using the information gained to make meaningful changes. In biofeedback, a person learns to sense when bodily response systems are becoming overly aroused and to apply strategies to combat the arousal problem.

Biofeedback shares a close kinship with the diverse approaches that use relaxation as a way to combat life stresses, such as meditation, mindfulness, yoga, autogenic training, progressive muscle relaxation training, paced breathing, and imagery. Biofeedback typically combines one or more of these allied relaxation-based approaches. The goals of biofeedback, in its most common application, are quite complementary to these procedures. The distinguishing characteristic is that biofeedback uses instruments that record information about your body as a way of gauging targets for treatment and evaluating progress. Think of it as instrument-aided relaxation.

Biofeedback can be helpful with anxiety, panic disorder, addictions, attention deficit disorder, self-confidence, self-efficacy, elevated mood, and enhanced problem-solving skills. It can successfully be combined with psychotherapy. Biofeedback therapists typically maintain close working relationships with other health care providers, particularly physicians. Physicians need to rule out medical causes prior to treating certain disorders, and the biofeedback therapist will regularly consult with the physician if physical problems arise during treatment. Also, a favorable response to biofeedback may necessitate medication adjustments. For instance, significant reductions in blood pressure as a result of biofeedback may leave a person over medicated and in need of a lower drug dose.

HOW IT BEGAN

Biofeedback, like so many treatments, owes its beginning to multiple influences. Mark Schwartz, a past president of the Association for Applied Psychophysiology and Biofeedback, traces at least ten separate influences that converged to spur the development of biofeedback (Schwartz, 1995).

One of the pivotal influences resulted from some basic laboratory studies conducted with animals. In a series of experiments, it was shown that these laboratory animals could learn to control bodily responses that previously were assumed to be outside of voluntary control. These bodily responses were labeled "autonomic responses" to reflect "automatic" control (Miller and DiCara, 1967). Imagine the excitement as researchers learned that animals could be taught to alter blood flow, blood pressure, and heart rate. It was just a matter of time before researchers began to see whether the phenomena that emerged from the highly controlled laboratories would translate to the real world with humans. In short, they did and continue to do so. Biofeedback researchers continue to place a strong emphasis on using basic research to pave the way to applying and conducting critical analyses of approaches.

HOW IT WORKS

No single explanation can do justice to how biofeedback works. The mechanisms vary with the type of biofeedback used and the condition treated. Common to all approaches is awareness of how symptoms are expressed, what factors are most likely to trigger symptoms, and the relation between thoughts, emotions, feelings, and bodily reactions. Armed with this awareness and with the aid of the biofeedback therapist, individuals are taught new, more adaptive ways to respond.

For example, with tension-type headaches, a major cause of the pain is overactivity of shoulder, neck, head, and/or facial muscles. These increased contractions typically occur in response to stressors encountered in daily life, as if one is guarding or bracing against the stress. Stressors can be mental, physical, or more likely, both. For example, when faced with a pressing deadline that is mentally taxing, you may end up frantically working at the computer keyboard and holding your body rigid for extended periods of time. Before long, it would not be surprising to find that your muscles ached and your thinking was impaired. How might this problem be approached therapeutically? A physician might prescribe a muscle relaxant, while a physical therapist might use heat, massage, or exercises. If positional problems are involved, instruction in body mechanics might be in order, as well as use of special furniture and keyboards. A biofeedback approach would involve attaching tiny sensors to various muscles suspected to be contributing to the problem. Once the source of muscle tension is identified, the biofeedback therapist would instruct or coach the person in ways to prevent muscle tension levels from increasing, and in how to relax muscle tension levels when they begin to approach dangerously high levels.

Feedback is the critical link and the distinguishing feature of this approach. Feedback and feedback loops are vital to all types of learning. Imagine how difficult it would be to learn to play tennis if you were blindfolded and were not told when a ball would be served your way. If you should happen to hit the ball, you would have little idea where it went. Removing the blindfold establishes a feedback loop that allows learning to take place more quickly. With biofeedback, changes in physical processes in your body, such as muscle tension, hand temperature, and sweat gland activity, are translated into signals that you can see or hear. Feedback can be provided through any of the senses, and it is made to mirror changes in bodily response. For example, learning how to decrease muscle tension in the neck can be done by providing a sound that becomes softer, or a bar on a computer screen that shrinks in height as muscle tension decreases. Computer-based biofeedback systems allow a great deal of variety and the creation of special forms of feedback. When teaching someone how to warm his or her hands, the image of an ice cube can be displayed on the screen and made to melt as temperature goes up, and to expand or harden as temperature goes down. With children, feedback can be provided in a game-like format to enhance interest and motivation. This direct feedback helps you learn what makes your symptoms get worse and what you can do to make them get better.

WHAT THE RESEARCH SHOWS

Biofeedback is a dynamic, evolving field, with new research findings generated on a regular basis. One current source that addresses both efficacy and cost-effectiveness is a document published by the Association for Applied Psychophysiology and Biofeedback (AAPB), "Clinical Efficacy and Cost-Effectiveness of Biofeedback and Therapy: Guidelines for Third Party Reimbursement" (Shellenberger et al., 1994). The authors defined various criteria by which to judge effectiveness and then listed diagnoses that meet these criteria. The list contains the following diagnoses: anxiety disorders, asthma, attention deficit disorder (hyperactivity), cerebral palsy, disorders of intestine motility, enuresis, epilepsy, essential hypertension (high blood pressure), incontinence (urinary and fecal), insomnia, motion sickness, neuromuscular disorders (Bell's palsy, whiplash, muscle-tendon transfers, low back strain, joint repair, torticollis, peripheral nerve problems, spasm, incomplete spinal cord lesion, lower motor neuron lesion, ataxia, dystonia, and paralysis), pain (headache, back, rheumatoid arthritis, and myofascial/temporomandibular), Raynaud's disease, and stroke. AAPB, at various times, has commissioned blue-ribbon panels or task force committees to systematically review available literature for a given disorder and to prepare detailed, critical reports of biofeedback as a treatment. The most recent collection of task force reports may be found in Hatch, Fisher, and Rugh (1987).

Researchers are exploring more cost-efficient ways for administering biofeedback-based therapies, and one of these is what we have termed "minimal-contact" treatment. By giving patients instructional manuals and cassettes, the number of trips to the office can be reduced considerably without a corresponding reduction in effectiveness for some problems (Rowan and Andrasik, 1996). Studies have shown that children are especially good candidates for biofeedback, often responding more quickly and with greater improvement than adults (Attanasio et al., 1985).

REAL PEOPLE AND BIOFEEDBACK

For several years, Tom had been experiencing panic attacks, described as an intense fear or discomfort that would reach a peak within 10 minutes. During an attack, he experienced a rapid heart rate, sweating, trembling, dizziness, and shortness of breath (a smothering feeling). When these symptoms first appeared, Tom feared he was about to die and these worries continued, so much so that they served to further intensify his condition and started a cycle of panic. A psychophysiological stress profile revealed that Tom's panic attacks were accompanied by marked elevations in skin conductance response, which is a measure of sweat gland activity.

It was first explained to Tom that panic attacks are best thought of as harmless false alarms that are compounded by worries about them. The body is preparing to cope with danger, but since the danger is strictly internal, there is nothing to run from or to fight (Gilbert, 1986). Tom gradually came to realize that his worries served only to exacerbate the condition.

Next, Tom was taught various strategies to relax to decrease his skin conductance activity. Treatment then entered the final stage, wherein panic attacks were induced in the clinic so Tom could work on his biofeedback-aided relaxation skills "live." The therapist coached and supported Tom through successive panic episodes, until he reached the point where he was comfortable warding off attacks by himself.

Greco (1994) recently reported on the successful use of a very specialized form of biofeedback, termed "neurotherapy," for treating two individuals who experienced severe eating disorders. Treatment for one individual is summarized here. S. W., 45, began binge eating and purging (self-induced vomiting) more than 25 years ago, and when seen for treatment, she was purging 20 times each day on average. This took considerable time, required a lot of money to purchase food, and led her to become isolated from family and friends. She has previously been treated for depression and suicide attempts, including electroshock therapy, two hospitalizations, various medications, and counseling. She reported a prior addiction to alcohol but stated that she had been sober for three years. She related that "bulimia was a substitution for drinking alcohol in that I experienced a high when I purged."

Treatment was based on an approach that has shown promise with alcohol addiction (Peniston and Kulkosky, 1989), called "alpha-theta brain wave training." Treatment begins with six sessions of temperature feedback to facilitate general relaxation and continues with thirty or more sessions of neurotherapy, during which the person attempts to increase brain wave activity in the alpha-theta range. Learning to control brain wave activity is quite difficult, so multiple sessions are typically held each week (S. W. was seen four times per week). When brain wave activity is increased in the alpha-theta range, people often report experiencing a deep state of relaxation. Remaining in this state for an extended period can unleash images that are very vivid and often traumatic and anxiety producing. Such "abreactive reactions" occurred frequently with S. W., and the content centered on themes of abuse she had experienced as a child. The therapist helped her work through these distressing images.

At the end of treatment, S. W.'s eating patterns had stabilized. Six months later her purging had not returned and now her long-standing depression had cleared as well. Two years later she was maintaining her weight with a normal diet. Greco theorized that changes in brain wave activity produced changes in certain brain chemicals, called endogenous opioids, which were ultimately responsible for the improvement noted, along with S. W. working through certain adverse situations experienced as a child.

WHAT TO EXPECT

Once a detailed clinical history is taken, the biofeedback therapist typically performs an assessment called a "psychophysiological stress profile." It consists of recording bodily responses when the person tries to relax, when attempts are made to place mild stress on the person, and when simulating real world behaviors in an attempt to identify which response systems are the most reactive or sensitive and most likely to be contributing to the target problem. Armed with this knowledge, the biofeedback therapist instructs or coaches the person to respond to stressful situations in more adaptive ways and teaches how to keep bodily responses from becoming too extreme in the future. We like to think of the biofeedback therapist as a coach, or as a teacher when working with children. A coach is someone who has special skills and knowledge and can impart this information to others in a supportive way.

Biofeedback therapists use numerous techniques to augment biofeedback, including diaphragmatic breathing (breathing that is slow, deep, and rhythmic), guided imagery (focusing on pleasant, relaxing scenes), autogenic training (a form of self-suggestion to enhance feelings of deep relaxation), and progressive muscle relaxation training (systematic tensing and relaxing of major muscle groups designed to promote deep relaxation of the entire body).

To be successful at biofeedback, a person must take an active role in treatment and learn to behave and think in new ways. This often leads to important psychological changes, such as a newfound sense of mastery, improved self-confidence and self-efficacy, elevated mood, and enhanced problem-solving skills. Skills acquired for a particular problem may be useful when dealing with other significant problems as well.

It is helpful to distinguish between the general practice (GP) biofeedback clinician and the biofeedback specialist (Andrasik and Blanchard, 1984). The GP biofeedback clinician treats conditions that share certain characteristics: The symptoms are generally related to heightened arousal or excessive sympathetic nervous system activity and are believed to have some association to stress or anxiety, or conditions activated by the fight or flight response. Examples include anxiety disorders, recurrent headaches, elevated blood pressure, and nervous stomach. For these types of problems, many forms of therapy have been attempted with success.

Other types of problems treated by biofeedback require more specialized approaches and training. Examples include modifying brain rhythms (EEG) for deterring epilepsy, for improving cognitive functioning in people who have experienced a stroke, and for enhancing attention and concentration in children who are diagnosed with attention deficit disorder; increasing muscle tone for people experiencing paralysis due to stroke; and enhancing muscle tone and muscle coordination for people having disorders of intestinal motility. Successful treatment within this cluster of disorders requires specialized biofeedback instruments and knowledge above and beyond that of the GP biofeedback clinician. In certain neurotherapy applications, such as treatment of alcohol and drug addictions, for example, therapists need to be especially vigilant for unexpected side effects, and to have skills to deal with these difficulties should they occur. The type of treatment provided by the biofeedback specialist is more involved and time-consuming, taking perhaps forty sessions or more, while conditions treated by the biofeedback GP most commonly require eight to twenty individual sessions.

HOW TO FIND A PRACTITIONER

Biofeedback clinicians can be found in mental health centers, universities, medical schools, hospitals, and private practice. These clinicians hold degrees in psychology, medicine, physical therapy, social work, counseling, or related disciplines. Their training in biofeedback may have been formal (university courses, intensive workshop programs) or informal (self-directed study). They may or may not hold a certificate from the Biofeedback Certification Institute of America (BCIA). BCIA was founded in 1980, and it is the only entity that presently defines and monitors standards for competence in biofeedback. Certification is now available for the GP biofeedback clinician and for stress management. BCIA is just now establishing a third certification, which concerns specialization in EEG biofeedback or neurotherapy.

One approach to locating a practitioner is to contact BCIA, which maintains a geographical registry of therapists meeting minimal standards for competence in administering biofeedback. If a certified provider is not available in your area, a search of the local directory may reveal professionals who list biofeedback among their offerings. Questions to ask potential therapists concern their extent of training in biofeedback, academic pursuits involving biofeedback (does the provider present workshops, teach courses, or conduct research on biofeedback), experience with the problem at hand, and the professional standing in his/her specific field (e.g., licensing). Certification in biofeedback is voluntary at present, and many competent therapists have elected not to pursue this option. While certification ensures a minimum level of competence, the absence of certification does not imply the absence of this level of competence.

RESOURCES

The two best sources for gathering further information are the Biofeedback Certification Institute of America (BCIA), 10200 West 44th Ave., Suite 304, Wheat Ridge, CO 80033-2840; (303) 420-2902; fax: (303) 422-8894; E-mail: bcia@resourcenter.com, and the Association for Applied Psychophysiology and Biofeedback (AAPB), 10200 West 44th Ave., Suite 304, Wheat Ridge, CO 80033-2840; (303) 422-8436 or (800) 477- 8892; fax: (303) 422-8894; E-mail: aapb@resourcenter.com. Both organizations request that you send a stamped, self-addressed envelope to receive information and referrals, rather than calling on the telephone.

AAPB, founded in 1969, is a multidisciplinary professional society. Its members include nurses, educators, social workers, physical and occupational therapists, psychologists, psychiatrists, physicians, dentists, and mental health counselors. This organization conducts an annual scientific meeting, offers periodic workshop programs around the country, publishes and distributes various publications for professional and lay audiences, and sponsors a scientific journal, *Applied Psychophysiology and Biofeedback* (formerly known as *Biofeedback and Self-Regulation*).

The following items published by AAPB may be of particular interest to readers: the brochure "Biofeedback Training: A Client Information Paper" and a series of white papers prepared for consumers that discuss biofeedback approaches to varied disorders. Popular books abound and may be obtained at local bookstores or libraries.

HOW TO LEARN MORE

Andrasik, F. and E. B. Blanchard. "Applications of Biofeedback to Therapy." In *Clinical Psychology: Theory, Research, and Practice* (Vol. II), edited by C. E. Walker, 1123-1164. Homewood, IL: Dow-Jones-Irwin, 1984.

Attanasio, V., F. Andrasik, E. J. Burke, D. D. Blake, E. Kabela, and M. S. McCarran. "Clinical Issues in Utilizing Biofeedback with Children." *Clinical Biofeedback and Health* 8 (1985): 134–141.

Clinical Applications of Biofeedback and Applied Psychophysiology: A Series of White Papers Prepared in the Public Interest by the Association for Applied Psychophysiology and Biofeedback. Wheat Ridge, CO: AAPB, 1995.

Gilbert, C. "Skin Conductance Feedback and Panic Attacks." *Biofeedback and Self-Regulation* 11 (1986): 251–254.

Greco, D. "A Case Study Approach Examining the Effects of Alpha-Theta Brainwave Training upon Bulimia Nervosa." *Advances in Medical Psychotherapy* 7 (1994): 163–174.

Hatch, J. P., J. G. Fisher, and J. D. Rugh, eds. *Biofeedback: Studies in Clinical Efficacy.* New York: Plenum, 1987.

Miller, N. E. and L. DiCara. "Instrumental Learning of Heart Rate Changes in Curarized Rats: Shaping and Specificity to Discriminative Stimulus." *Journal of Comparative and Physiological Psychology* 63 (1967): 12–19.

Peniston, E. G. and P. J. Kulkosky. "Alpha-Theta Brainwave Training and B-endorphin Levels in Alcoholics." *Alcoholism: Clinical and Experimental Research* 13 (1989): 217–279.

Rowan, A. B. and F. Andrasik. "Efficacy and Cost-effectiveness of Minimal Therapist Contact Treatments of Chronic Headaches: A Review." *Behavior Therapy* 27 (1996): 207–234.

Runck, B. *Biofeedback: Issues in Treatment Assessment.* Washington, DC: U.S. Department of Health and Human Services, 1980.

Schwartz, M. S. *Biofeedback: A Practitioner's Guide.* Second Edition. NY: Guilford Press, 1995.

Shellenberger, R., P. Amar, C. Schneider, and J. Turner. *Clinical Efficacy and Cost Effectiveness of Biofeedback Therapy: Guidelines for Third Party Reimbursement.* Second Edition. Wheat Ridge, CO: Association for Applied Psychophysiology and Biofeedback, 1994.

ABOUT THE AUTHOR

Dr. Andrasik received his doctorate in clinical psychology from Ohio University, upon completing an internship at the University of Pittsburgh School of Medicine in 1979. He presently holds the positions of professor, director of the Center for Behavioral Medicine, and director of Graduate Programs in the Department of Psychology at the University of West Florida, Pensacola. He has been the recipient of several federal and foundation grants to conduct research on biofeedback and has published and presented extensively on this topic. In 1992, he received the "Merit Award for Long-Term Research and/or Clinical Achievements" from AAPB. He served as president of this same organization from 1993 to 1994. He currently serves as editor-in-chief for this association's professional journal, *Applied Psychophysiology and Biofeedback*. Dr. Andrasik can be reached at the Center for Behavioral Medicine, University of West Florida, 11000 University Parkway, Pensacola, FL 32514-5751; (904) 474-2041; fax: (904) 474-2042; E-mail: fandrasi@uwf.edu.

Preparation of this chapter was supported in part by a grant from NIH-NINDS, NS-29855.

Carol Bush, M.S.W., L.C.S.W.
Sara Jane Stokes, Ph.D., M.T.-B.C.

10 The Bonny Method of Guided Imagery and Music

WHAT IS THE BONNY METHOD OF GUIDED IMAGERY AND MUSIC?

The Bonny Method of Guided Imagery and Music (GIM) is a music-centered experiential therapy and a method for uncovering deep levels of the mind. This new form of psychotherapy makes use of music, combined with the ability of the mind to access images to communicate feelings and root causes. The GIM experience is much like a waking dream and enables people to connect to their deeper selves. It can illuminate or help to resolve current life issues.

Clients may experience emotional releases, new connections and insights, and often a spiritual unfolding. This work encourages unresolved issues to surface and helps to remove mental, emotional, and spiritual blocks. It also awakens new levels of creativity while encouraging a deep inner connection to what is most meaningful. The music is chosen from the great masterworks, such as compositions by Bach, Beethoven, Strauss, Mozart, and Wagner. GIM makes use of the fine art of great music as a potent healing force that allows people to directly participate in their own health and well-being.

Unlike many visualization and imagery techniques, GIM imagery is not directed from a script but unfolds spontaneously, stimulated and carried by the music and by skilled guidance. Clients are encouraged to find answers by being honest with themselves, since images do not lie and the dream-like nature of the images is hard to manipulate. It differs from some therapies because it directly engages beyond the intellect, at the sensory and feeling levels.

This method is best-suited for people with depression, anxiety, and most stress-related and relationship problems. It is helpful for those who find themselves in life transitions, such as career change, geographical moves, divorce, or even hospice. It is very well-suited to people with addictions, especially those who are in recovery. To enter this type of inner work there must be a motivation to explore, heal, and perhaps get on with life. Whether the motivation is the desire to ease emotional pain or the urge for growth, GIM moves people toward their goals. Additional benefits are the promotion of body awareness, the growth of spontaneity, faster symptom resolution, enhancement of creativity, intuition, and deep appreciation of music.

GIM is not recommended for people with serious mental disorders, because it has the potential for uncovering deep emotional issues and unconscious material. This is not helpful for people who are struggling to maintain balance and coping with the realities of everyday life.

HOW IT BEGAN

In the past several decades, the emergence of holistic thought in health care has led to a renewed appreciation of the way the ancients used music. They knew the potential of music to alter consciousness.

The origins of GIM date back to when a tremendous push to explore outer space spawned a similar push to explore inner space. Man had just walked on the moon. People, especially youth, were restless for change. This was the time of Kent State and the Beatles. Old forms were breaking up; it was a time to seek and stretch. The Menninger Foundation in Kansas and the Maryland Psychiatric Research Center received government grants to explore consciousness using hallucinogenic drugs. Several renowned pioneers in consciousness research gathered at these two research centers.

Helen L. Bonny, Ph.D., R.M.T., a music therapist, brought her special knowledge of music's potential for altering consciousness to the research team in Baltimore. She felt that music was the perfect vehicle for exploring the psyche, because it could carry someone through the heights and depths of an experience. She developed a powerful yet safe therapeutic method for healing called guided imagery and music (GIM). Since then, GIM applications have been pioneered in such diverse areas as individual and group psychotherapy, development of creativity, uniting mind/body in the healing arts, spirituality, and cross-cultural issues. In all areas, this method honors the ancient idea that we can awaken our inner vision and reconnect with our deep source.

The Association for Music and Imagery (AMI), founded in 1980, publishes a professional journal for GIM and credentials GIM practitioners through endorsed training programs worldwide. There is a growing number of skilled practitioners of the Bonny method of GIM, under the title of fellow, who continue to research new applications of the method.

HOW IT WORKS

The guided imagery and music process works without having to think about it. Through the skilled guidance of a specially trained therapist, the appropriate use of music, and the willingness of the client to be spontaneous, the process energizes the psyche's innate ability to heal itself. GIM provides a creative, often dramatic means of tapping into this complex means of healing. While listening to inspired performances, the music provides a projective screen for creatively connecting many levels of mind, body, and spirit. Through the GIM process we connect our conscious mind to our unconscious mind.

The material that emerges is often metaphoric, so it is important to establish trust in this way of communicating with the inner self. Often the experience of being able to release bottled-up emotions enables a client to feel immediate relief and to trust that something significant is happening.

WHAT THE RESEARCH SHOWS

Dr. Kenneth James of the University of Chicago observed in an unpublished presentation at the AMI Conference in 1980 that the brain responds to music quite differently than it does to the spoken word. The brain's right hemisphere is activated by stronger impressions with music than with the spoken word. Such feeling-laden images can be processed by the brain almost simultaneously. The time-space barrier of the logical left brain is circumvented. This allows millions of bits of information to be processed in seconds. Since the human has an enormous capacity to store information, the retrieval of significant impressions and images becomes an effective way of accessing the conscious and the unconscious mind.

Dr. Robert McDonald, a GIM practitioner from Minneapolis, studied the effects of GIM on the body and mind (1990). He studied thirty adults with essential hypertension who were not taking medication. A third of these subjects received GIM once a week for 6 weeks. A third received verbal therapy once a week for six weeks, and the remaining third received no intervention. Blood pressure in the GIM group steadily declined. At a six month follow-up, the blood pressure of that group remained lowest of the three groups studied.

Dr. Cathy McKinney (McKinney, 1994) found that listening to music while imaging has a more intense effect on the body and mind, in terms of accessing emotions and effecting body states, than just listening to music. A synchronization occurred between the music, feelings, images, breath and pulse rate, causing a potent effect. She studied a group of fifty-six adults, half of whom had latent Epstein-Barr virus, and gave them a short series of GIM sessions. She found that the mood states of both groups were significantly and positively altered in terms of anxiety, depression, and confusion. Also the Epstein-Barr group showed significant improvement in terms of fatigue on follow-up. Her results indicate that a short series of GIM sessions (at least six) can positively effect mood.

Dr. Elizabeth M. Jacobi (publication in press) recruited 30 subjects diagnosed with rheumatoid arthritis to participate in a 90-minute individual GIM session per week for 10 weeks. Data were collected on three levels: medical/physical, psychosocial, and behavioral functioning. Results from the study showed statistically significant improvement in the level of psychological distress and subjective experience of pain.

GIM therapy has been applied to a wide range of special populations. Case studies by GIM therapists, published in *The Journal of the Association for Music and Imagery*, include such diverse areas as trauma and abuse (Pickett, 1995; Borling, 1992), collective grief from the World War II Holocaust (Merritt and Schulberg, 1995), post-traumatic stress disorder with Vietnam veterans (Blake, 1994), and addictions and recovery (Stokes, 1992). GIM has also been adapted for a nonverbal man with autism (Clarkson, 1995). Bruscia (1992) reports the use of GIM with several people with AIDS. Clarkson and Geller (1996) and Wrangsjö and Korlin (1995) discuss the effectiveness of GIM from a psychiatric and psychoanalytic perspective.

REAL PEOPLE AND THE BONNY METHOD

Liz came to therapy with relationship problems. She found herself avoiding intimacy with her husband, Rob, and admitted that all her previous relationships had been difficult as well. She couldn't seem to feel close to anyone. She had come from a home in which her parents had frequent fights before they divorced when she was 11. Her brothers teased her constantly and during childhood she frequently suffered from night terrors.

I had been seeing Liz for approximately five months on a once-a-week basis. We had an equal number of GIM and talk sessions. She had learned to trust her inner wisdom and the metaphoric way in which the imagery expressed her feelings. But one day, she felt miserable when she showed up for a session. She and Rob had had a bitter argument. He was fed up with her aloofness. I suggested that we explore the blocks in the relationship as the music of Bach began. She saw herself in a park with her husband approaching. She couldn't face him. She felt too ashamed. When urged to explore that shame, she became aware that she felt wounded in her genitals. She knew that only a pure white light could help her, but she was cut off from the light. As she looked more closely, she saw that connected with, yet separate from, the wound was a pure, innocent child. The child had somehow split off from her and was hiding.

The form of a defender emerged within this scene. This defender looked like a haggard, frazzled form of her adult self. It informed her it was tired of constantly standing between her and anyone who would get close to her. It had been doing this to protect the child.

With my urging, Liz was able to ventilate all the pent-up feelings of the worn-out defender. She raged and cried. Finally, she indicated it was over but now she was seeing the ones who had first wounded her. In her mind's eye she was back at the beach as a five-year-old. She was at an outdoor evening concert with her family. She remembered she had gone to the bathroom alone. Some boys jumped her as she came in the door. Threatening to kill her if she told anybody, each one raped her. By briefly reexperiencing the trauma of this event, she was able to release it. As this occurred, a bright light appeared in her inner world, filling the void and healing the wound. Suddenly the child found herself transforming into Tinkerbell (a child-woman) while her shadow was sewn back on.

Returning to her normal state after this music session, she was amazed at what had occurred. She had never connected the rape with her hesitancy in relationships. She was not aware that she still carried the shame from that long ago event. The fear had lodged deeply in her psyche and had made her overly protective of her emotional attachments. This one session had an enormous effect on the intimacy problem with her husband, and she felt it helped to save her floundering marriage. After 10 years they are still happily married.

Mary was an attractive 35-year-old who was married and had a well-paying job as a computer consultant. Her appearance belied her inner turmoil. Previously, she had tried conventional talk therapy for her feelings of depression but felt frustrated that her insights had not produced any real change. She sang in a community chorus and was intrigued that somehow music could be used for counseling. Because she loved music, she decided to give it a try and committed for twelve GIM therapy sessions.

Her initial imagery revealed that there were two Marys — the competent career woman and dutiful wife, and the woman who was carrying on a secret affair and whose increasingly heavy drinking was getting harder to hide. Her overriding feelings were of loneliness and guilt. In her third session, we began to see the dynamics that contributed to her aloneness.

As Mary lay relaxed on the couch, the music from a Bach fugue evoked a sensation of spiraling downward. Though she felt apprehensive, she reported, "The strings say I need to go down to that cave and go in." There in the hidden recesses of the cave, she encountered her brother, who had committed suicide when she was 8 years old. "How could you have done this to me?" she cried out in anguish, "You were my best friend!" Music selections for grief work encouraged Mary to fully feel the anger and abandonment she had hidden deep inside. Afterward, Mary was amazed that her loss from long ago could be so filled with emotion and so real. She thought she had dealt with her brother's death "long ago." The next few weeks, Mary's frozen feelings began to thaw and she was more ready to face what she referred to as "how my life is a lie."

In her sixth GIM session, she reported that she had been arguing with her husband, Bill, and she just couldn't trust him with her feelings. She felt impelled to keep her secret affair going, though she suffered from guilt pangs. I used the nurturing music of Britten, Vaughan Williams, and Berlioz as she explored her life. Sharing her imagery, Mary said, "The sky is brilliant blue; the scent of fall is in the air. I hear the crowds cheering. I'm 16 in my blue and gold cheerleader outfit at the game. Tommy, my boyfriend, just made a touchdown. I look excited and bubbly on the outside, but on the inside I know something is wrong. As I look at myself, I don't have any face!" I encouraged Mary to continue sharing. "I look happy," she said, "but on the inside I'm hollow and split." I asked her to try to explore her feelings. Mary softly cried, "I want to be whole and stop hurting . . . I have no heart, no soul — I'm just empty."

Later in the session, as her tears subsided, Mary was able to let the lovely voices from Pucinni's "The Humming Chorus" from *Madam Butterfly* caress her, and she felt their gentle harmony as angels of mercy. Mary's face was relaxed now. "They're comforting me," she whispered, "and the darkness is beginning to lift. They are telling me that it's going to be all right." In the weeks afterward, we discussed the significance of the imagery. "It's like the mask I still wear today," she mused, "living a secret life."

Mary had grown up in a family in which her father would often drink and her mother was aloof. Kids were to be seen and not heard. Having friends over was discouraged and Mary remembered excelling at making excuses. The family rule was to look good and Mary's job was to be popular and get good grades. In the imagery sequence, Mary had found a way to face her deep childhood wounds of isolation and feeling split, and was able to begin to allow herself the comfort and caring that she never felt from her parents. Even though she did not consider herself religious, Mary accepted the angel helpers without question.

Gradually, in the weeks that followed, Mary felt like she was more aware of her reactions and behaviors. She wondered if she could trust more, yet still was churning over her affair and all the secrets in her life. She also saw her daily cocktail hours as a way to numb out the hollow feelings of her current life.

In her eighth session, Mary found herself stuck in the middle of a bridge surrounded by a barren landscape, and could not move. "I can't decide whether to go back to Bill or leave him for my lover," she lamented. The music mirrored her ambivalence as the melody and rhythm swayed back and forth. "The affair is over," she admitted quietly, "but I don't know if I want to be with Bill." The feeling of being stuck intensified. "This can't go on," she moaned, "I have got to move!" To the strains of Brahms' Piano Concerto, the scene shifted to an old-fashioned ballroom filled with dancers. To her surprise, she and Bill were dancing, feeling the rhythm of their movements in tune and time to the music. "We used to do this back when we dated," she exclaimed. "I forgot how natural we could be and how much fun it was." Afterward, Mary stated that she felt relieved to say her affair was over but felt scared to really end it for once and for all. "Am I really getting an answer from myself about all this?" Mary wondered.

During the following week, Mary was asked to use the dance image as a metaphor for exploring some risk-taking with Bill. Could things between them really be different? Could she open up more and tell him her real needs? In the weeks that followed, Mary made some critical decisions to end her affair and seek out couples counseling with her husband. She felt she could at least trust her own instincts and give the marriage another chance. In the last session, she found herself once again in the dark cave where she had grieved over her lost brother, and a curious thing happened. She relayed, "I see a pool of water with ripples on the surface . . . it's the kind you want to get into." She fell silent and then continued, "There is a kind of glow coming up from down under. It is sort of a diffused light coming up through me and all around me. It's wonderful!" Later, during Wagner's exquisite masterpiece "Lohengrin," Mary closed the session with a memorable reunion. "Ted, my brother is here," she declared. "We are holding each other. He says he is proud of me. I feel so grateful. There are no words."

Today, Mary regards herself as a different person. She states that she is much more open emotionally and willing to try new things. She feels much more confident and reports that she and Bill are getting along much better. They actually signed up for ballroom dancing classes, something they had always talked of doing. To Mary, GIM therapy was amazing. The images were powerful metaphors that told the story of her life. Her journey contained the wounds of the past and the present, yet also held the treasures and her strengths to be the real person she longed to be. The music was her constant companion, urging her forward, mirroring her pain, giving comfort. Today she is free to grow, to risk, and to love — no longer split or stuck but free to make choices and take chances trusting herself and others.

WHAT TO EXPECT

In GIM therapy, the client and therapist work together as a team. We refer to the client as "traveler" and the trained therapist as "guide." This terminology supports a mutual cooperation to solve problems and empowers clients to trust in their own capacity for healing and insight.

In conventional talk therapy, getting to the core of a presenting issue normally would take months or even years to accomplish. In GIM therapy, the combination of the music, deep relaxation, and a trained guide greatly accelerates the time frame. For instance, during a series of 10 sessions, which may take 3 to 4 months, major shifts usually occur in enhanced self-concept, restoration of more healthy behavior patterns, positive attitudes, and capacity for change.

Sessions are generally 60 to 90 minutes long. The client/traveler usually commits to a series of six to twelve sessions. This may occur weekly or biweekly. In other cases, the number and frequency of sessions may be determined by the guide and client as needed. The client stays fully dressed. The guide may assist with bodywork, to facilitate release of intense emotions or supportive touch during a GIM session, with prior permission from the client.

Each session begins with the traveler and guide exploring significant issues and concerns of the client. A focus or intention is often reached and the guide chooses appropriate music to be used. The client/traveler may sit up or, preferably, lie down on a couch or mat, and is assisted by the guide to relax through breathing or autogenic relaxation suggestions. These suggestions help shift the traveler into a relaxed yet focused mind state. The music starts, and as it evokes images, sensations, and feelings, the traveler and guide talk together. The traveler describes experiences as they occur while the guide supports and encourages the inner action. The active involvement with the music usually lasts approximately 30 to 40 minutes. Afterward, the guide assists the traveler to gain closure and to return to an alert state. The remainder of the session is spent reflecting on the images and experiences that the traveler felt and, if appropriate, their relevance to life issues. Often the art therapy technique of the mandala (a circular drawing that helps to connect the conscious to the unconscious) is used for further nonverbal assessment.

Sometimes the thoughts, feelings, or images accessed during a GIM session indicate a certain course of action that supports the healing process. The guide would encourage the client to trust this information and to follow it. Since GIM therapy is an in-depth process, it requires the expertise of a trained GIM guide. However, people who want to do this work on their own may experience an adaptation of this process in a limited way (see Chapter 17 from Carol Bush's book *Healing Imagery and Music,* 1995).

HOW TO FIND A PRACTITIONER

A listing of certified GIM practitioners is available from the Association for Music and Imagery (AMI) c/o executive secretary James Rankin, 331 Soquel Ave., Ste. 201, Santa Cruz, CA 95062, (408) 426-8937.

GIM practitioners are graduates of approved GIM training programs and credentialed by AMI. A GIM trainee undergoes a basic and advanced training consisting of two to three years of short-term residential courses plus practical applications in the field. The trainee must have a master's degree in a mental health or related field to graduate. Upon completion of the training program, the trainee is granted the title of fellow by AMI. He or she is then qualified to practice the Bonny method of GIM.

Practitioners may work with groups and/or individuals. They may be specialists and have a private practice or work in a clinic or institutional setting.

Charges vary but an individual session may range from $60 to $90 for an hour and a half.

RESOURCES

If you are interested in attending a class or introductory workshop in GIM, you can get a directory of approved GIM training programs and a newsletter with workshop information from AMI. Some workshops offer CEU credit for professionals or may be affiliated with a university for credit. International trainings are held in Germany, Denmark, Mexico, Australia, England, and elsewhere. Membership in AMI is available to anyone, and an annual national conference is held.

The authors are directors and trainers of the Mid-Atlantic GIM Training Program (P.O. Box 4655, Virginia Beach, VA 23454, (757) 498-0452, or for the MD office, (410) 757-9719). They grant CEUs and graduate credit for all three levels of training through Virginia Commonwealth University, Richmond, VA.

Helen Bonny's original monographs and other publications by Lisa Summer may be ordered from The Bonny Foundation, 2020 Simmons St., Salina, Kansas 67401, (913) 827-1497. An excellent source of articles from the field is the *Journal of the AMI* c/o Eugenia Pickett, 500 West University Parkway, Baltimore, MD 21210, (410) 243-7300.

HOW TO LEARN MORE

Achterberg, J. *Imagery in Healing: Shamanism and Modern Medicine.* Boston, MA: New Science Library, 1995.

Beaulieu, J. *Music and Sound in the Healing Arts.* New York: Station Hill Press, 1987.

Blake, R. "Vietnam Veterans with Post-Traumatic Stress Disorder: Findings From a Music and Imagery Project." *Journal of the AMI* 3 (1994): 1–4.

Bonny, H. L. "Music Listening for Intensive Coronary Care Units: A Pilot Project." *Music Therapy* 3, no. 1 (1983): 4–16.

Bonny, H. L. *The Role of Taped Music Programs in the GIM Process.* GIM Monograph #2. Baltimore, MD: ICM Books. 1978.*

Bonny, H. L. and L. M. Savary. *Music and Your Mind.* New York: Harper and Row, 1973.

Borling, J. "Perspectives on Growth with a Victim of Abuse: A Guided Imagery and Music (GIM) Case Study." *Journal of the AMI* 1 (1992): 85–98.

Bruscia, K. E. "Visits from the Other Side: Healing Persons with AIDS Through Guided Imagery and Music." In *Music and Miracles*, edited by D. Campbell. Wheaton, IL: Theosophical Publishing House, 1992.

Bush, C. "Dreams, Mandalas, and Music Imagery: Therapeutic Uses in a Case Study." *Arts in Psychotherapy* 15, no. 3 (1988): 219–226.

Bush, C. *Healing Imagery and Music: Pathways to the Inner Self.* Portland, OR: Rudra Press, 1995.

Campbell, D., ed. *Music and Miracles.* Wheaton, IL: Theosophical Publishing House, 1992.

Clarkson, G. "Adapting a Guided Imagery and Music Series for a Non-verbal Man with Autism." *Journal of the AMI* 4 (1995): 121–127.

Clarkson, G. and J. Geller. "The Bonny Method from a Psychoanalytic Perspective: Working with a Psychoanalytic Psychotherapist in a Guided Imagery and Music Series." *The Arts in Psychotherapy* 23, no. 4 (1996): 311–319.

Copland, A. *Music and Imagination.* New York: Mentor, 1952.

Goldberg, F. S. "Music Psychotherapy in Acute Psychiatric Inpatient and Private Practice Settings." *Music Therapy Perspectives* 6 (1989): 40–43.

Jacobi, E. M. and G. Eisenberg. "The Efficacy of GIM in the Treatment of Rheumatoid Arthritis." *Association for Music and Imagery* (in press).

Leuner, H. "Guided Affective Imagery: A Method of Intensive Psychotherapy." *American Journal of Psychotherapy* 50, no. 1 (1969): 4–22.

McDonald, R. G. "The Efficacy of Guided Imagery in Music as a Strategy of Self-concept and Blood Pressure Change Among Adults with Essential Hypertension." Unpublished doctoral thesis, Walden University, Minneapolis, MN, 1990.

McKinney, C., M. Antoni, A. Kumar, and M. Kumar. "Effects of Guided Imagery and Music on Depression and Beta-Endorphin Levels." *Journal of the AMI* 4 (1995): 67–78.

Merritt, S. *Mind, Music and Imagery.* Santa Rosa, CA: Aslan, 1996.

Merritt, S. and C. Schulberg. "GIM and Collective Grief: Facing the Shadow of the Holocaust." *Journal of the AMI* 4 (1995): 103–120.

Nolan, P. "Insight Therapy: GIM in a Forensic Psychiatric Setting." *Music Therapy* 3, no. 1 (1983): 43–51.

Pickett, E. "Guided Imagery and Music: A Technique for Healing Trauma." *Journal of the AMI* 4 (1995): 93–102.

Stokes, S. "Letting the Sound Depths Arise." *Journal of the AMI* 1 (1992): 69–76.

Stokes, S. "Music Synergy." Unpublished doctoral dissertation, Walden University, Minneapolis, MN, 1985.

Stokes, S. and C. Bush. "Guided Imagery and Music: Ancient Roots, Modern Practice." *Open Ear* Winter (1992): 7–11.

Storr, A. *Music and the Mind.* New York: Macmillan, 1992.

Summer, L. *GIM in the Institutional Setting.* St. Louis, MO: MMB Music, Inc., 1988.

Summer, L. "Imagery and Music." *Journal of Mental Imagery* 9, no. 4 (1985): 83–90.

Tame, D. *The Secret Power of Music.* Rochester, VT: Destiny Books, 1984.

Wrangsjö, B. and D. Korlin. "Guided Imagery and Music as a Psychotherapeutic Method in Psychiatry." *Journal of the AMI* 4 (1995): 79–92.

*Available from the Bonny Foundation (listed in "Resources").

ABOUT THE AUTHORS

Carol Bush, M.S.W., L.C.S.W., is a pioneer in guided imagery and music. Her more than 25 years of clinical experience have included a variety of mental health settings, including private practices in Miami and Virginia Beach. She is the author of *Healing Imagery and Music: Pathways to the Inner Self* (Rudra Press, 1995). In addition, she has authored scholarly articles for professional journals and is a specialist and trainer in the use of mandalas and the Mandala Association and Research Institute (MARI®) Card Test. Currently, she travels widely, conducting workshops and training seminars.

Sara Jane Stokes, Ph.D., M.T.-B.C., is a clinician, educator, and consultant, and received her training in GIM with Dr. Helen L. Bonny in 1973. Her doctoral work pioneered further applications of GIM. She is a past director of music therapy at St. Mary-of-the-Woods College. As a seasoned workshop presenter, her specializations include such diverse areas as recovery, leadership development, and spiritual formation. She has also produced a series of relaxation tapes used in health care settings and is published in the *AMI Journal* and *Music and Miracles* (Quest Books, 1992).

Glenn Doman

11 Child Brain Development in Brain-Injured and Well Children

WHAT IS CHILD BRAIN DEVELOPMENT?

Child brain development is a nonsurgical treatment for brain-injured children, and a series of techniques for making well children intellectually, physically, and socially splendid. These treatments are directed at the brain, the source of the paralysis, speechlessness, blindness, deafness, apparent mental retardation, and other problems that beset the brain-injured child. This is in contrast to the traditional, widely used rehabilitation approaches aimed at symptoms rather than at the source of the problems. An approach aimed at symptoms alone leads to institutionalization or extremely limited goals for the millions of children worldwide with brain injury. The cost of this traditional approach, both in human and economic terms, staggers the imagination.

The half-century of work on the part of the child brain developmentalists who make up the staff of the Institutes for the Achievement of Human Potential has established clearly that brain growth and development are not predestined and unchangeable facts. Brain growth and development can be accelerated by giving the child visual, auditory, and tactile stimulation with increased frequency, intensity, and duration, in recognition of the extremely orderly way in which the brain grows.

This chapter will report that, using these principles, many blind, brain-injured children began to see and read; many deaf children began to hear and speak; many paralyzed children began to walk and run; many speechless children began to talk; and many severely mentally retarded children began to read, write, and think as well as (and sometimes substantially better than) their noninjured peers of the same age. In addition, many well children were able to gain knowledge and skills at levels far above what is usually considered normal for their age. The techniques described here are carried out at home, by the families of the children, rather than by professionals.

HOW IT BEGAN

Discouraged by the lack of results achieved by the traditional symptomatic treatment of brain-injured children, a multidisciplinary team began to form immediately prior to World War II. This team was led by a distinguished neurosurgeon, Temple Fay, who then occupied both the chair of Neurosurgery and the chair of Neurology at Temple University Medical School in Philadelphia, and the team included a young physical therapist: this author.

In the years immediately following World War II, this team grew to include a physiatrist, a nurse, a speech therapist, a psychologist, and an educator. The objective of the team was to find efficient and effective means to treat the brain, rather than the symptoms, thus achieving results that were curative rather than palliative. By 1955, the team had grown to include pediatricians and other appropriate specialists, and a new discipline was formed. The new discipline was called child brain development, and the methods employed complemented and reinforced the results being achieved by the neurosurgical members of the team.

When hundreds of profoundly and severely brain-injured children began to perform as well as or at even higher levels than well children, many perplexing problems arose. What did it mean if children who had suffered profound or severe brain injury performed at higher levels than uninjured children twice their age? It became clear that well kids were not nearly as well as they were capable of being.

By 1963, we turned our attention to making all children intellectually, physically, and socially splendid, and changed our name from the Rehabilitation Center at Philadelphia to the Institutes for the Achievement of Human Potential. There are currently Institutes affiliates in Italy, Brazil, and Japan.

HOW IT WORKS

To be successful, treatment of brain dysfunction must take place on the brain's own terms. In short, we must deal with the principles upon which the brain functions. The brain is the most sophisticated system known to humans. The brain, like the biceps, grows by use. This fact has been well-known to neurophysiologists for half a century. They have also known that the opposite is true. Both of these points have been proven repeatedly by animal experimentation that gives sensory deprivation to one group of laboratory animals while providing sensory enrichment to their matched litter mates. David Krech summarized the findings of his research group at the University of California at Berkeley, "After a lifetime spent in giving environmental enrichment to one group of rats and environmental deprivation to their matched litter mates, it is clear that the rats raised in environmental enrichment have large, highly developed, highly intelligent brains, while their litter mate brothers and sisters, raised in environmental deprivation have small, stupid, underdeveloped brains. . . . It would be scientifically unjustifiable to assume that, because this is true in rats, that it is also true in people. . . . And it would be socially criminal to assume that it were not true in people." These vital studies have been continued and expanded by Marian Diamond at UCLA.

Tragically, there are indications that the same is true in people. Infrequently, but all too often, we discover a child whose insane parents kept the child prisoner by chaining them to a bedpost in a darkened attic, or confined to the darkness and silence of a locked closet. Such children, depending on the duration, depth, and age at which the child suffered this epitome of child abuse, have consequences ranging intellectually from severe retardation to absolute idiocy, and ranging physically from paralysis to profound arrest of growth. This treatment is the exact opposite of a program of child brain development.

Neuroscience research has also shown over the past two decades that the brain is very capable of recovering from certain kinds of injury. This research has shown that the brain responds to stimulation of the senses and to movement by growing and developing. There is also compelling evidence that at any age, and in both normal and pathological states, behavioral events alter the functioning of brain chemicals and that this can change behavior (Institutes, unpublished).

Brain pathways can be divided into two broad categories: sensory (afferent) pathways, which bring information into the brain, and motor (efferent) pathways, through which the brain reacts by commanding motor responses to the information it has received. All incoming sensory, or afferent, pathways are a one-way road into the brain and incapable of carrying an outgoing message. All outgoing, or efferent, pathways are incapable of carrying a message into the brain. This is a long-recognized and well-known fact of neurology that seems to have been completely overlooked in conventional rehabilitation of brain-injured patients. The normal functioning of the brain is completely dependent on the integrity of these pathways. The destruction of motor or sensory pathways will result in a lack of functional performance of the human being. Such a lack will continue until the specific pathways are restored to function, or until new pathways are established that are capable of completing the total cybernetic loop from the environment to the brain and back again to the environment. All efforts in treatment of the brain-injured patient must be directed at locating the break and closing the circuit.

Following is a summary of some of the techniques used at the Institutes which make use of the above principles.

Procedures That Supply Discrete Bits of Information to the Brain for Storage

It is not possible to extract either function or information from a brain that has none. Such a brain is in a zero state and will remain so until information is supplied. Brain injury creates a barrier between the brain and the environment that, in the case of the patient in a coma, cannot be penetrated by sensory stimuli at normal levels of frequency, intensity, or duration. To penetrate the barrier, it is necessary to increase the frequency, intensity, and duration of stimuli by multiples of five, ten, and even more. The principles of child brain development demand that such a child be provided with the greatest, rather than the least, impingement from his environment.

When a child has been traumatically brain-injured and has been in a coma for an extended period of time, he or she has traditionally been provided with life-sustaining medical and nursing care, in a room kept as quiet and free from stimulating environmental impingement as possible. His bed is in a private room with curtains drawn, with silence enforced as far as possible. He is handled only when necessary. Exactly the opposite is required if such a child is to have a chance for recovery.

For example, at the Institutes, such a child's bedside table might contain a flashlight, two blocks of wood, a tuning fork, pins, brushes, sniff jars containing various strong smelling but harmless substances, and a variety of other stimulus-producing tools, as well as jars containing strong-tasting substances such as horseradish, garlic, mustard, and so on. In addition to regularly and frequently scheduled periods during which the following procedures are used, each professional person who passes the child's room is directed to stop long enough to open the child's eyes and shine the flashlight into them, to strike the blocks of wood together sharply near his ear, to pinch his skin, to stick him gently with the pin, to place the vibrating tuning fork on various joints, to brush his skin briskly with textured brushes, to pass various aromas under his nose briefly, and to place on his tongue very small amounts of strong-tasting foods, insufficient in quantity for him to choke or aspirate.

All of these procedures are entirely sensory in nature and do not anticipate a motor response. They are intended purely to supply the brain with bits of random intelligence. These procedures provide basic sensory stimuli that range from such simple information as the presence of light, sound, or feeling to such much more sophisticated bits of information as reading a word, hearing a word, or feeling a specific object. When such stimulation is introduced, one frequently sees a patient respond by seeing, hearing, feeling, tasting, and smelling in a matter of days or a very few weeks, even though the individual may have been in a comatose state for months or even years. Much less spectacular, but much more common, is the child whose injury is at a level just below the level required to produce coma. The child's problem is often identical and simply varies in degree. The same procedure can be applied with success.

The techniques for supplying basic, discrete bits of information to the brain are geared precisely to the patient's developmental stage in the area of sensory competence being treated. Levels of competence in different sensory areas may differ greatly. The patient's levels of competence are determined, and he or she is supplied with input normal to those levels. The patient is then supplied with all the sensory input normal to the next higher level, which he or she is unable to accomplish due to brain injury or due to environmental deprivation. However, in supplying the next higher level, a carefully planned program of greatly intensified and enriched auditory, visual, tactile, gustatory, and olfactory stimuli is made an integral part of the environment. Treatment begins to supply the brain with sensory stimulation with increased frequency, intensity, and duration, in recognition of the orderly way in which the human brain develops and grows.

Procedures That Demand an Immediate Response from the Brain to a Basic Discrete Bit of Information That Has Just Been Supplied to the Brain

Procedures under this principle might range from tapping the patellar tendon with a hammer, demanding a patellar reflex response from the spinal cord (if extension of the knee is a desired developmental response), to visually presenting a card upon which the word "Mommy" has been written in very large red letters, demanding the cortical response of the spoken word "Mommy."

Procedures That Program the Brain

These procedures range from those that are life-saving to those which add the final level of sophistication to human communication. Very basic programs of sensory input are supplied to the lower and more primitive levels of the brain, such as the tactile programming of how it feels to breathe rhythmically, or simple crawling movements. To the higher level of the brain, they supply very complex and advanced programs of sensory intake, such as the tactile programming of complex walking movements, the auditory programming of human speech, and the visual programming of human reading. These procedures place great reliance upon the tactile, auditory, and visual pathways that are prerequisite to human walking, talking, and writing. All of these procedures address the brain at the appropriate level, in the sensory language that it understands, and concerning the function or functions for which it is responsible.

Procedures That Permit the Brain to Respond to Previous Programming

These procedures are sensory-motor in nature and provide an optimal opportunity for the brain to use the programs provided in the third principle. Since the programs were often repeated and included precisely coordinated large amounts of related information, the responses now elicited from the brain are holistic and will consist of precisely coordinated patterns of function. They include patterns of mobility function that range from crawling, through creeping, to the highest levels of human walking. They also include patterns of speech function ranging from meaningful sound to the highest levels of human speech, and patterns of human creativity emanating from a single, dominant cortical hemisphere, such as creative speech composition, creative writing, and creative manual accomplishments. These procedures provide an opportune environment in which to retrieve the specific patterns desired. For example, it is easiest for a human being to crawl on a smooth, flat surface. Therefore, a smooth, flat surface is provided if the goal is to retrieve a homolateral pattern of human crawling that has been programmed into the brain.

Procedures That Provide an Improved Physiological Environment in Which the Brain May Function

The best known of the procedures under this principle is called reflex masking. It is a response to the fact that in nearly every kind of brain injury, there is almost invariably an insufficient supply of oxygen to the brain. This is followed in minutes by the death of brain cells and brain injury. After many years of experience, the staff of the Institutes have been persuaded that all brain-injured children suffer from some degree of chronic hypoxia. This is demonstrated most clearly in the child who is diagnosed as having severe athetoid cerebral palsy, whose mouth is perpetually open as he or she gasps for air. These children are usually injured in the midbrain. They are frequently brilliant, as a result of their unhurt cortex, but have historically grown worse with each passing year as a result of their untreated midbrain injury. This process is reversed using the techniques described below.

The brain is entirely dependent upon a constant supply of nutrients, principally oxygen. The most important single step in child brain development is the provision of an adequate supply of oxygen to the brain to meet its needs under all circumstances, since without this nutrient, other methods of treatment, however ingenious, will fail.

In reflex masking, the child, under the closest parental observation, wears a small plastic mask over the nose and mouth. The mask is the type used to administer oxygen in hospitals. The child rebreathes his own expired air for periods ranging from 10 seconds to one minute. In each succeeding breath, the amount of carbon dioxide rebreathed increases. As a result, the chemoreceptors in the brain, which monitor every breath taken throughout life, detect the decreasing amounts of oxygen, and react by causing the child to breathe deeper and faster to increase the amount of inspired air and, thus, the amount of oxygen inspired. Simultaneously, the increasing amounts of carbon dioxide cause much greater amounts of blood to reach the brain, due to the fact that carbon dioxide is an extremely powerful vasodilator. Since the maximum time is one minute or less, the child reaps two rewards: great amounts of oxyhemoglobin reaching the brain and huge chest expansions and chest growth. This is vital since brain-injured children have markedly smaller chests than do well children. Reflex masking must *never* be attempted without prior consultation with the patient's medical doctor.

WHAT THE RESEARCH SHOWS

Following are results of the Institutes' program between 1972 and 1992. Results are published annually in the Institutes' publication, *The In Report*. These results were achieved entirely by parents treating their children at home, using the program of child brain development taught to them by the staff of the Institutes. The children were seen at the Institutes twice a year. Many of the children achieved victories in many or all of the categories listed.

Chest Growth

In a population of 987 brain-injured children consecutively admitted to the program, 888 had chests with circumferences below that of their well peers. Following the use of reflex masking, the average chest growth among the 888 children with below-average chest size was 167 percent greater than average chest growth among normal children, according to published charts used by pediatricians.

Mobility

1. Of the 2,164 individuals (ages seven months to 29 years, six months) who had never been able to move, 584 (26.98%) crawled across a room without help for the first time in their lives.

2. Of the 1,094 individuals (ages seven months to 19 years, four months) who were unable to creep, 471 (43%) began to do so.

3. Of the 1,222 individuals (ages 16 months to 26 years) who were unable to walk, 462 (37.8%) began to walk without help.

4. Of the 1,055 individuals (ages 20 months to 18 years, eight months) able to walk but not run, 364 (34.5%) learned to run at least 100 yards nonstop.

Speech

Of the 3,249 individuals (ages 17 months to 28 years, three months) who couldn't speak, 777 (23.9%) learned to speak consistently and meaningfully.

Vision

Of 624 individuals (ages 15 months to 24 years, nine months) who were blind, 212 (34%) attained useful vision.

Reading

Of 2,905 individuals who were unable to read, 2,334 (80.3%) learned to read. (They ranged in age from one-year-olds reading single words to three-year-olds reading books to five-year-olds reading newspapers to 24-year-olds reading age-appropriate materials.)

Writing

Of 1,160 individuals (ages 45 months to 30 years) unable to write, 388 (33.4%) learned to write.

Graduated to life

(The child is less than perfect on "The Profile," but such a graduation takes place when both staff and family are confident that continuing the program at home will result in the child completely recovering.)

80 individuals (ages 55 months to 23 years) graduated to life.

Graduated from the home program

(The child is totally successful neurologically, which is to say physically, intellectually, and socially. Such a child would be below average in no way and such a child is very often above average compared to a well child.)

52 individuals (ages 42 months to 19 years, five months) graduated from the home program.

Well Children

The approach taken with well children is based on the following observations:

- Our wildly variable intellectual differences are a result of the wide differences in the environments in which we were raised.

- Tiny kids would rather learn than eat or play, and they want to learn about everything right now.

- Given a choice, children will always choose the subject of greatest complexity. They are intensely curious.

- Tiny children use their five senses as laboratory tests to learn about every object with which they are not familiar. They use the same method of solving problems as do scientists.

- Children are superb learners. They are limited only by how much material they have to learn about and how it is presented.

- The ability to take in facts is an inverse function of age, so it is easier to teach any set of facts to a two-year-old than to a seven-year-old.

- If you teach a tiny kid the facts, he or she will discover the laws that govern them. But if you teach him the laws, the child cannot, as a result, discover the facts.

- Parents give their babies the degree of genius that each individual baby will possess by the amount and variety of visual, auditory, and tactile stimulation they give the child and the judicious use of the frequency, intensity, and duration with which they give it.

- The first six years of life are precious beyond measure. It is easy to make a baby a genius before six years of age, but extremely difficult to make a child a genius after that age. True geniuses are the kindest, most capable, most effective people around. The world has too few geniuses.

- Parents are the best teachers, but are in danger of having their natural instinct bullied out of them by professionals who believe that mothers are the problem.

Today there are hundreds of thousands of children who do one, many, or all of the following by age six or even younger: Read superbly; play the violin; read and speak several languages; do advanced math; are very familiar with classical art, music, zoology, history, linnaean classification, geography, and a host of other wonderful things; are splendid gymnasts; and are most especially warm, humane, sensitive, delightful human beings due to their parents' love and the Institutes' programs. We call this the "gentle revolution," and we assert that no child must be denied his or her birthright of being physically, intellectually, and socially excellent because his or her parents didn't know that their child could be.

REAL PEOPLE AND CHILD BRAIN DEVELOPMENT

Dawn was born in 1973 following 18 hours of labor, during which her mother received medication to hasten the birth. The doctors noted fetal distress and told the parents that the baby's survival was questionable. The baby survived the birth but at three months had poor use of her right hand and leg.

At age 45 months she began the Institutes' program, at which time she showed spasticity in her right arm and leg, could not walk in cross pattern, and had poor balance with poor manual dexterity in her right hand. Her intelligence, comprehension, and social behavior were at peer level. The diagnosis was a moderate, diffuse midbrain injury. An intense neurological program was created for Dawn, focusing on physical, physiological, and intellectual growth, with particular emphasis on the right side.

Dawn entered high school at peer level, where she succeeded academically, managed the field hockey team, swam for the varsity swim team, and served as an aid in special education classes. In 1995, Dawn graduated from college with a B.S. degree. In college, she was active in student government, was vice president of the biology club, taught swimming for the Special Olympics, and served as a peer counselor and tutor. Currently, Dawn works for a medical supply company and is contemplating returning to graduate school for a master's degree.

Jason's parents attended the "How to Multiply Your Baby's Intelligence" course and began a program of stimulation as soon as their son was born, with plenty of opportunity for him to be on the floor. As a result, Jason crawled many feet nonstop by the time he was six weeks old and enjoyed learning so much that one of his first words was "more!"

At six-and-a-half years old, Jason is home-schooled, reads at the high school level, and takes university classes for gifted children. He plays violin and piano, has an orange belt in karate, and enjoys gymnastics. He is a very sociable boy and easily establishes a relationship with everyone he meets.

HOW TO FIND A PRACTITIONER

The techniques described in this chapter are carried out exclusively by the families of the brain-injured and well children. The programs of the Institutes are entirely geared toward teaching people to administer the techniques at home. In addition to the courses (at varying levels of intensity) available at the Institutes, there are a number of books that contain detailed instruction in the techniques of child brain development. For more information, contact the Institutes directly at 8801 Stenton Ave., Wyndmoor, PA 19038, (215) 233-2050.

HOW TO LEARN MORE

Bennet, E. L., M. C. Diamond, D. Krech, and M. R. Rosenzweig. "Chemical and Anatomical Plasticity of the Brain." *Science* 146 (1964): 610–619.

Diamond, M. C. *Enriching Heredity: The Impact of the Environment on the Anatomy of the Brain.* New York: Macmillan, 1988.

Doman, G. "The Gentle Revolution." Paper presented to the International Congress for Early Education, Victoria, Spain, December, 1991.

Doman, G. *How to Give Your Baby Encyclopedic Knowledge.* Garden City Park, NY: Avery Publishing Group, 1984.

Doman, G. *How to Multiply Your Baby's Intelligence.* Garden City Park, NY: Avery Publishing Group, 1984.

Doman, G. *How to Teach Your Baby to Read.* Garden City Park, NY: Avery Publishing Group, 1986.

Doman, G. *Teach Your Baby Math.* Garden City Park, NY: Avery Publishing Group, 1979.

Doman, G. *What to Do About Your Brain-Injured Child.* Garden City Park, NY: Avery Publishing Group, 1974.

Doman, G. and J. M. Armentrout. *The Universal Multiplication of Intelligence.* Philadelphia, PA: The Better Baby Press, 1980.

Doman, G., M. Dimancescu, R. Wilkinson, and R. Pelligra. "The Effect of Intense Multisensory Stimulation on Coma Arousal and Recovery." *Neuropsychological Rehabilitation* 3, no. 2 (1993): 203–12.

Doman, G., D. M. Doman, and B. Hagy. *How to Teach Your Baby to Be Physically Superb.* Garden City Park, NY: Avery Publishing Group, 1988.

Doman, G., et al. "Children with Severe Brain-injuries: Neurological Organization in Terms of Mobility." *Journal of the American Medical Association* 174 (1960): 257–262.

Doman, G., et al. "Neurological Organization, the Basis for Learning." In *Learning Disorders*, edited by J. Helmuth. Seattle, WA: Special Child Publications, 1966.

Doman, R. and E. W. Thomas. "Brain-injury as a Diagnosis and the Results of Treatment in 335 Brain-injured Children," *Human Potential* 1, no. 5 (1968): 339–44.

Fay, T. "Neurophysical Aspects of Therapy in Cerebral Palsy: The Outcome of 177 Patients, 74 Totally Untreated." *Pediatrics* 29 (1962): 605.

Green, L. J. "An Ill Wind: A Discussion on Air Ionization and Its Effect on Our Environment." Proceedings, 12th annual meeting, World Organization for Human Potential, Philadelphia, PA, May 10, 1979.

Harvey, N. "The Relationship Between Stanford-Binet Test Scores and Doman-Delacato Developmental Profile Scores Achieved by Brain-injured Children." A research study conducted under the aegis of the Research Institute, Edward B. LeWinn, M.D., director. A master's thesis on file at the University of Pennsylvania, Philadelphia, PA, 1965.

Klosovskii, B. N. *The Development of the Brain and Its Disturbances by Harmful Factors.* Oxford: Pergamon, 1963.

Lee, E., G. Doman, and G. Kerr. "The Practical Results of a Program of Neurological Organization of the Institutes for the Achievement of Human Potential." Proceedings, 4th annual meeting, World Organization for Human Potential, Wyndmore, PA, April 28, 1971.

LeWinn, E. B. *Coma Arousal.* New York NY: Doubleday, 1982.

LeWinn, E. B. "Effect of Environment Influence on Human Behavioral Development." *New York State Journal of Medicine*, December 15, 1967.

LeWinn, E. B. *Human Neurological Organization.* Springfield, IL: Charles C. Thomas, 1969.

LeWinn, E. B. and M. D. Dimancescu. "Environmental Deprivation and Enrichment in Coma." *The Lancet*, July 15, 1978.

LeWinn, E. B. and W. Thomas. "Some Physical Characteristics of Brain-injured Children: Chest Circumference." *Human Potential* 3 (1970).

Morrow, J. *Mind Meets Brain: The Developmental Theories of Piaget and Doman.* Cambridge, MA: Harvard University, 1970.

Taylor, R., Jr. "Statistical Research at the Institutes for the Achievement of Human Potential: Measurement of Neurological Development." *Human Potential* 1, no. 2 (1968): 75–84.

Thomas, E. W. *Brain-injured Children.* Springfield, IL: Charles C. Thomas, 1969.

Wolf, J. M. *The Results of Treatment in Cerebral Palsy.* Springfield, IL: Charles C. Thomas, 1970.

ABOUT THE AUTHOR

Glenn Doman graduated from the University of Pennsylvania in 1940 and began pioneering the field of child brain development. This process was interrupted by distinguished service as a combat infantry officer in World War II. He founded the Institutes for the Achievement of Human Potential in 1955. More than 15,000 families from 135 nations have found their way to the Institutes. He has lived with, studied, and worked with children in more than 100 nations. He continues to spend all day, every day with "the finest parents on earth," deeply involved with the joyous process of getting hurt kids well. Among honors from many nations, he was knighted by the Brazilian government for his outstanding work on behalf of the children of the world. He is the author of *What to Do About Your Brain Injured Child* and numerous other publications.

Kevin V. Ergil, M.A., M.S., L.Ac., F.N.A.A.O.M., F.A.A.P.M.
William Prensky, O.M.D., L.Ac.

12 Chinese Medicine and Acupuncture

WHAT IS CHINESE MEDICINE?

Chinese medicine is an ancient system of healing that has been practiced, written about, thought about, and modified for at least 2,000 years. Acupuncture, herbs, diet, massage, exercise, and meditation are used to help the whole human being achieve a state of healthy balance. A basic assumption of Chinese medicine is that a human being is subject to the laws of nature and that he or she will be happiest and healthiest when living in accord with them.

Mental health in Chinese medicine is intertwined with physical health. There is no sense of the body and mind being split or separate from each other. Physical imbalance can be seen as a factor in mental problems, and proper mental equilibrium and healthy habits of thought are seen as important to good health. This perspective pervades all the approaches of Chinese medicine to mental health issues. Depression, substance abuse, anxiety, insomnia, irritability, and confusion are among the issues that yield to clinical approaches based on Chinese medicine. The optimization of health and the process of self-actualization can be enhanced and supported through the application of the principals of Chinese medicine.

It is not uncommon for patients to make use of Chinese medicine in combination with other approaches to health care. Mental health issues are no exception. A patient suffering from panic attacks might use psychoactive pharmaceuticals to bring the condition under control and then gradually reduce his or her dependence on pharmaceuticals. This approach makes a great deal of sense from the perspective of Chinese medicine, since the intent is to bring the patient back into balance and eliminate his or her need for drugs.

HOW IT BEGAN

As is the case with many systems of medicine in Asia, Chinese medicine has legendary teachers almost godlike in stature, who showed people how to practice medicine. The mythological originators of Chinese medicine are three ancient emperors. Fu Xi taught people how to domesticate animals and how to understand yin and yang. Shen Nong, or the Divine Husbandman, is said to have been born around 3494 B.C.E., and is considered to be the founder of herbal medicine. Huang Di, also known as the Yellow Emperor (born around 2674 B.C.E.), is known as the originator of the traditional medicine of China. He is the legendary author of the *Yellow Emperor's Inner Classic* (Huang Di Nei Jing), first compiled around 200 B.C.E., in which the traditional medicine of China is first described in a form that is still familiar to us today.

The earliest text sources available to us are the materials recovered from three tombs excavated at Ma Wang Dui in Hunan province, which date to 168 B.C.E. (Unschuld, 1985). These texts are considered to be older than the *Inner Classic*. They discuss magical and demonological concepts as well as some ideas about yin and yang in relation to the body. The texts present an early concept of channels in the body, but in a less developed fashion than the *Yellow Emperor's Inner Classic*.

The development of Chinese medicine as we know it began in the Han Dynasty. The Han created a stable aristocratic social order, expanded geographically and economically, and spread Chinese political influence in Vietnam and Korea. The Chinese today refer to themselves as the Han people after this dynasty. During the Han dynasty (206 B.C.E. to 219 C.E.) textual evidence appears that reveals the emergence of a medicine that is similar to the Chinese medicine we know today.

Chinese medicine continued to develop through the centuries. It is not a static tradition and it has not adhered rigidly to early ideas. Doctors used ideas from the ancient classics and combined them with their insights to compose new books. Ideas came into China from other countries and influenced the practice of medicine. Certain styles and approaches were emphasized and others were put aside. Rarely in Chinese medicine is anything discarded. Even today, ideas about therapy from 200 C.E. are used next to ideas that have emerged in only the last twenty to thirty years. All of this makes Chinese medicine very dynamic and rich. The skillful practitioner has a great deal to draw upon.

HOW CHINESE MEDICINE WORKS

Yin and Yang

Chinese medical thought begins with the theory of yin and yang. Yin and yang express the idea of opposing, but complementary, phenomena which exist in a state of dynamic equilibrium. The most ancient expression of this idea seems to be that of the shady and sunny sides of a hill. The sunny southern side is the yang side and the shaded northern side is the yin side. If you imagine the different environments that exist on either side of the hill you can begin to get an idea of yin and yang. The sunny side is bright, plants and animals that enjoy light are more prevalent, the air is drier and the rocks are warm. The shaded side is dim, the air seems moist and cool.

Chinese medicine believes that human beings have a nature which is inseparable from yin and yang. This means that they have a nature which is completely linked with the world around them. Just as life on the shaded side of a hill has characteristics which are different from those of the sunny side, our own life and body adjust to changes in the seasons, time of day, diet, and emotional states. Since yin and yang govern the world and the body, health is thought to be a result of living in harmony with yin and yang. An idea that is useful for thinking about yin and yang in relation to medicine is a burning candle. If one considers the yin aspect of the candle to be the wax and the yang aspect to be the flame we can see how the yin nourishes and supports the yang, how the yang consumes the yin, and in doing so, burns brightly. When the wax is gone, so is the flame. Yin and yang exist in dependence on each other.

Yin and yang are used to characterize all phenomena and to think about the kinds of symptoms a patient displays. A yin mental state is withdrawn, somnolent, depressed, or catatonic while a yang mental state is

Yang	Yin
light	dark
heaven	earth
sun	moon
day	night
spring	autumn
summer	winter
hot	cold
male	female
fast	slow
up	down
outside	inside
fire	water
wood	metal

Table 1. Yin and Yang Correspondences.

manic, hyperalert, or overexcited. The appearance of yang can be produced by too much yang or too little yin. The appearance of yin is produced either by too much yin or too little yang. In many cases states that are manifestly yang are actually produced by an insufficiency of yin aspects that normally balance the yang aspects.

Five Phases

Another idea that has played a significant part in the development of Chinese medicine is that of the five phases (*wu xing*), also sometimes referred to as the five elements. The five phases are earth, metal, water, wood, and fire. In general, the five phases speak to a set of dynamic relations that are found in many things. Five-phase thinking can cover almost everything from seasons to mental states.

Category	Wood	Fire	Earth	Metal	Water
Solid organ	liver	heart	spleen	lungs	kidney
Hollow organ	gallbladder	small intestine	stomach	large intestine	urinary bladder
Season	spring	summer	late summer	autumn	winter
Time of day	before sunrise	forenoon	afternoon	late afternoon	midnight
Climate	wind	heat	damp	dryness	cold
Direction	east	south	center	west	north
Development	birth	growth	maturity	withdrawal	dormancy
Color	cyan	red	yellow	white	black
Taste	sour	bitter	sweet	pungent	salty
Sense organ	eyes	tongue	mouth	nose	ears
Odor	goatish	scorched	fragrant	raw fish	putrid
Vocalization	shouting	laughing	singing	weeping	sighing
Tissue	sinews	vessels	flesh	body hair	bones
Mind	anger	joy	thought	sorrow	fear

Table 2. Five Phase Correspondences.

Anger, for instance, is a manifestation of the wood phase. If this idea seems strange, we should remember that wood is an emblem of plant life and that anger can arise quickly like a sprout bursting forth from the ground. Fire is associated with joy, which might be understood by thinking about expressions such as "it warms my heart" or "he gives me a warm feeling."

Qi and Blood

There is no concept more crucial to Chinese medicine than *qi* (pronounced: chee). This is the substance that makes the body move and the blood circulate. In this system of medicine, the body is pervaded by subtle material and mobile influences that cause most physiological functions and maintain the health and vitality of the individual. It is not unusual to see the idea of qi translated with the term "energy," but this translation hides the real idea of qi: It is a fine and mobile substance which acts differently in different places and can be nourished and stored. The character for qi is traditionally composed of two symbols. One is the image of breath or rising vapor, which is placed above the symbol for rice. Qi is linked with the concept of "vapors arising from food" (Unschuld, 1985). Over time the concepts associated with this character broadened, but never lost their distinctively material aspect.

The idea of qi is extremely broad, encompassing almost every variety of natural phenomena. There are many different types of qi in the body. Each type is related to the normal psychological and physiological activity of the body and mind. Qi helps us to breathe, to speak, to walk, to digest food, to think, and to feel.

Sometimes the analogy of wind captured in a sail is used to express the idea of qi. We cannot directly observe the wind, but we can infer its presence as it fills the sail. In a similar fashion, the movements of the body and the movement of substances within the body are all signs of the action of qi.

All illness in Chinese medicine is understood in relation to qi. Pain occurs when qi is blocked in its cycle through the body. When qi is insufficient, fatigue can occur or the functions of organs can be disrupted. When qi is congested or stuck, there can be pain and dysfunction.

Essence and Spirit

Together with qi, essence and spirit make up what are known in Chinese medicine as the three treasures. In brief, essence is the gift of one's parents, while spirit is the gift of heaven. Essence is the most fundamental source of human physiological processes: the bodily reserves that support human life and which must be replenished by food and rest, and the actual reproductive substances of the body. Spirit is the alert and radiant aspect of human life. We see it in the luster of the eyes and face of a healthy person and in their ability to think and respond appropriately to the world around them. The idea expressed by *shen*, or spirit, in Chinese medicine encompasses consciousness and healthy mental and physical function.

The health of the shen is considered fundamental to overall good health. In Chinese medical theory, mental disturbances, especially personality disorders and confusion, are considered disturbances of the shen. The health of the shen is produced by the healthy activity of the vital organs and the correct use of the mind.

The Organs and Channels

In Chinese Medicine, the word *channels* (meridians) refers to the pathways along which the qi flows, like water in underground rivers. At certain locations along the channels, the qi flows close to the surface and is easily touched and manipulated. These locations are called holes (*xie),* or acupuncture points. The channels travel up and down the body and along the arms and legs. They also go inside the body and connect with the internal organs.

The idea of an internal organ in Chinese medicine is a little different than in Western medicine. The physician of Chinese medicine encounters a body in which twelve organs function. These twelve are divided into six *zang* or solid organs — the viscera — and six *fu* or hollow organs — the bowels. The names and locations of the anatomical structures is familiar, but what is of utmost importance is the relationship between each organ and many physiological functions that are related to it. For instance, the spleen in Chinese medicine is related to digestion and to the process of thought and reflection. It is easy to think that, because this has nothing to do with the way in which we understand the spleen, the Chinese were wrong or confused. Instead we need to realize that the "spleen" in this case refers not to the organ specifically, but to the physiological and psychological processes that it is associated with. This is a system in which organs are important as markers of associated physiological functions rather than actual physical structures. Each organ is paired with another in a set of yin and yang pairs.

The organs are related to both physical and psychological functions. Ancient Chinese thought personalized the organs, giving them a title and set of actions that reflected their general characteristics and role in the body-mind.

The heart was the supreme controller that reflected its dominant role in physiological function and its role as the seat or home of the shen. The heart protector or pericardium was known as the "minister of leisure" because it created feelings of pleasure and joy. The liver was known as the "general in charge of making plans" and the home of the ethereal soul.

Chinese Medicine and the Mind

It is important to note that there is no distinct separation of body and mind in Chinese medicine. It is understood that the psyche and soma interact with each other and that aspects of mental and emotional experience can impact the body, and vice versa. In this sense, spirit is linked both to the health of the body and to the health of the mind. Similarly, aspects of human experience that are understood as predominantly mental in a biomedical frame of reference are linked to specific organs in Chinese medicine. Anger is related to the liver, while obsessive thought is related to the spleen, and joy to the heart.

As mentioned earlier, the fundamental idea in Chinese medicine is to establish the body in a balanced state of health. This does not mean that there is an ideal state of health that everyone must aspire to. It means that Chinese medicine seeks to create a situation where the person being treated becomes less prone to physical and mental disturbance because he or she is increasingly putting their lifestyle, physiology, and environment into an optimum relationship.

The key to this approach is the understanding and manipulation of qi. Diet, rest, exercise, and thought are all tools to manipulate qi. Beyond that, acupuncture, herbs, and massage can adjust the movement and density of qi in the body.

WHAT THE RESEARCH SHOWS

Research in the field of acupuncture and Asian medicine is a complex issue. It can be said that the 2,000-year history of acupuncture and Chinese herbal medicine represents a form of empirical research conducted by countless clinicians throughout China. In addition, its continued use in China and East Asia as a parallel medical system suggests a level of efficacy. However, the world in which we live often asks for a higher standard in the verification of the safety and efficacy of a medical technique or substance.

Systematic research on acupuncture has been conducted in China and

Japan for fifty years. Most of these studies are not randomized clinical trials (RCT) or even controlled studies, but what are called case series. A case series follows the treatment of a single condition for many patients and generalizes about the effectiveness on the basis of the total results. Although this method gives some information, it does not give us absolute scientific certainty about the usefulness of the intervention.

While most of the research in herbal medicine still falls into the above category, recently more research has been done on acupuncture in the West. As the result of this work, a large number of studies were gathered up and presented to the FDA to support changing the legal status of acupuncture needles from an experimental device to a standard medical device. In 1996, the FDA agreed that the acupuncture needle could be considered a class II medical device, no longer experimental.

Research has shown acupuncture to be clinically effective for conditions including respiratory tract disorders, stroke, acute and chronic pain, nausea, female infertility, menopause, and peripheral nerve injury. In terms of mental health, acupuncture has been scientifically shown to be useful in depression and substance abuse.

REAL PEOPLE AND CHINESE MEDICINE AND ACUPUNCTURE

Joan was a 36-year-old professional woman in the public relations field, who suffered from severe depressions that could last for months. Each round of these depressions began with a feeling of congestion in her chest and sudden awakenings at night, although no one could find any problem with Joan's chest or, for that matter, anything else medically wrong. The interruptions in her sleep continued, and the depression deepened during these bouts. Twice she had to be placed on a regimen of antidepressant drugs.

When Joan came to see me, upon referral from her psychiatrist, she was in the midst of a depression that had begun approximately two weeks before. She was not yet taking any drugs, and her sleep interruption patterns were worsening.

Joan had one child, a three-year-old girl, and also wanted to have another baby. She was afraid that her depression would deepen, and that she would have to be placed on a long course of antidepressant medication.

Examination showed Joan to be suffering from deficient kidney qi leading to deficient heart blood and a condition referred to as "cold in the upper burner." This caused the sleep problem, and the inability of her heart to maintain a proper residence for her spirit (mind) — leading to depression which tended to worsen over time. She was treated with a course of acupuncture to strengthen her kidney qi and to balance her kidney and heart, combined with herbs to strengthen her lungs and her spleen to aid in the balance of digestion, and to dispel the congestion from the cold afflicting her chest. She recovered completely within six weeks, did not require any antidepressant medication, and became pregnant two months later. She went through an uneventful pregnancy supported by regular (bimonthly) acupuncture, and gave birth to a healthy boy. She continues to be symptom-free after three years.

Malcolm was a 42-year-old construction worker with bipolar disorder who had been maintained for the past ten years on daily doses of lithium. His mania was the predominant pathological condition, causing him to go on wild buying sprees in which he emptied out his family bank account, and periods of elation, which led inevitably to exhaustion, some physical injury, and a subsequent period of severe depression.

Malcolm's examination revealed clear signs of deficient kidney, along with "heart's fire blazing upwards." His tongue showed clear signs of fire. The deficient kidney signs were confounded by the effect of ten years of lithium therapy, which can alter kidney signs, but the pattern of disturbance between the heart and the kidney was clear.

Acupuncture was initiated to restore the balance between kidney and heart and to strengthen the kidney yin. He received acupuncture twice a week for five weeks, then weekly acupuncture for five weeks, and then ongoing monthly acupuncture. Lithium therapy was not discontinued, but his daily dose was cut in half. Malcolm reported feeling "much more balanced" and "less frightened" about both his daily life and his dependence upon lithium. He has remained stable for five years under this treatment regimen.

∞

Tom was a very athletic 17-year-old boy, a football player in high school and a swimmer. He rather suddenly became extremely depressed and, subsequently, very anxious. He began to have trouble sleeping, and would awaken during the night with panic attacks, sweating profusely. He did not report remembering any nightmares or specific dreams.

Tom first came to see me upon the advice of his high school coach. After speaking for more than two hours, we began psychotherapy immediately, with counseling sessions three times weekly (and more often by telephone as needed) with a family and crisis intervention counseling psychologist specializing in adolescent psychotherapy. In addition, a psychiatric consultation was conducted and anti-anxiety medication was given twice daily.

In addition, we began acupuncture sessions three times a week, with traditional oriental medical herbal formulas directed to calming the spirit and to regulating emotional excesses. Tom responded very quickly to acupuncture, herbs, and the other therapies. His anxiety would be completely relieved during and following acupuncture sessions and the relief would last for up to twenty-four hours. Over the course of six weeks of continued therapy, he was able to stop all pharmaceutical drugs. He continued with counseling, acupuncture, and herbs for six months, during which time he regained his previous balance and stability.

∞

Louise was a 60-year-old woman who had recently lost her husband of thirty-two years. She was a legal secretary who had been working in the same rather large firm for twenty-four years, and had risen to the position of supervisor. She was known as a remarkably efficient and competent secretary who never forgot anything. She could recall the details of a meeting at which she had taken notes twenty years before.

About one year after she became a widow, she began to show signs of memory loss, confusion, and anxiety. The anxiety may have been a result of the other changes. She sought psychiatric evaluation from her company's Employee Assistance Program, but no conclusive diagnosis was made. It was unclear whether her condition was related to her recent loss, to advancing age, or to other causes. No specific physical findings led to any conclusion regarding electrolyte imbalances or other possible physical causes of her condition.

After exhaustive examinations and testing, she was referred to me by her psychiatrist. After speaking with Louise and examining her, it became apparent that she suffered from what is known in oriental medicine as "sudden shock" syndrome. The loss of her husband had been followed by a very minor accident during which she had been very frightened, although she suffered no physical injury. (She had been a passenger in a bus that had struck a young man riding a bicycle. There were no injuries to passengers on the bus, but the young man was permanently injured, suffering severe brain damage.)

The oriental medical strategy was to calm her heart and spirit and allow the spirit to find a safe abode in the heart once again. Herbal formulas were taken daily for seven days, then nothing for three days, then again for seven days for four cycles. In addition, Louise was given acupuncture twice weekly for three weeks, then once a week for six more weeks.

Following this regimen she recovered completely. She returned to her previous job (she had been on sick leave for nine weeks) and was able to resume her professional duties without any qualification or exception. Four years after treatment she remains completely without trace of her presenting condition.

WHAT TO EXPECT

When you first visit a practitioner of Chinese medicine you can usually expect several things to happen. You will be greeted and asked to explain the problem that you are trying to address. Generally, most practitioners will use what are called the four diagnoses to assess your situation. These are detailed below.

Asking Questions

The practitioner will ask you many questions. Some of these questions will address the specific problem and the conditions that make it worse or better. Many of the questions may seem unrelated. If you are there to discuss insomnia, you may be asked about your bowel movements, your diet, whether you prefer cold or hot climates, whether you perspire easily, if your back hurts, or if your knees are weak. You may be asked about your favorite foods, colors, or time of day. Questions that may seem unrelated to you are often very important to the practitioner, since your answers help him or her to understand your problem in relation to the overall functioning of your body and your specific situation.

Smelling and Listening

The sound of your voice and, in some cases, the odor of your body can give your practitioner important clues to your condition. A voice with a shouting strident quality can suggest a problem with the liver or the wood phase. A voice that is low and soft may suggest weakness of the qi while one that has a singing melodious quality suggests an involvement of the spleen or earth phase.

Looking

By observing the way you walk, your body's size and shape, and your general appearance, your practitioner can make many observations about your situation. Observation is also important in terms of learning about your shen and the health of your spirit.

Your tongue is also inspected to help with the diagnosis. The tongue can tell us a great deal about the state of the body and mind. Is heat present, and if so, where? Is the qi strong or weak? Is the blood circulating properly or stuck? Will the patient be easily angered or depressed? The tongue can help us to answer these questions.

Touching

This is perhaps the most famous diagnostic practice in Chinese medicine, but while it is important, it is only one of four. Even the most famous pulse diagnosticians state that pulse diagnosis is almost useless without the other three diagnoses. The practitioner will usually take your pulses, although this may not always be done. The process of pulse taking may last for several minutes. Besides counting the beats, the practitioner will feel subtle differences in size and quality at different positions and use this information to understand the way in which the organs (in the Chinese sense) are working and what needs help.

Depending on your condition and the style of practice used by the practitioner, he or she may want to palpate various areas of your body, especially the abdomen. Sometimes individual points or channel pathways will be touched as well. If this is the case, the practitioner will need you to partially undress and lie down during the diagnostic part of the visit.

Many practitioners of Chinese medicine will also use biomedical physical examination and laboratory diagnosis. Don't be surprised to see a blood pressure cuff and stethoscope or other diagnostic tools. These tools help the practitioner to follow up on his or her treatment and screen for serious health problems.

Once the diagnostic process is complete, the practitioner will try to gather all the information about you into a coherent diagnostic pattern in order to plan treatment. For example, a clinical approach to schizophrenia includes a pattern of "flaring of fire" with excess phlegm. A patient in this situation might have a sudden onset of mental disturbance, irritability, headache, insomnia, a flushed face, bloodshot eyes, and restlessness. The patient might become easily angered or violent. There might be instances of irrational behavior, shouting, and physical attacks on people and things. In this case, the pulse would be fast and stringlike and the tongue would have a purple color and be covered with slimy yellow fur (Cheung et al., 1981).

Treatment would include herbs that act to cool the body and to settle the disturbed qi. In addition, herbs that address phlegm and settle the mind would be added. Acupuncture would include points that would have similar actions, as well as points that are traditionally used to calm and treat a disturbed spirit.

In a normal office visit, treatment will begin after the diagnosis is complete. It is usually necessary to undress partially or completely for acupuncture treatment. The practitioner will provide a gown or sheet if necessary. Acupuncture is performed with very fine needles that are of different lengths and thicknesses. The average needle is about a quarter of a millimeter thick, about as thick as a hair. Unlike the hypodermic needle used for injections, the acupuncture needle has no hole in it and no cutting edge. Where the hypodermic needle cuts the skin as it is inserted, the acupuncture needle pushes tissue aside. This is why there is normally little or no bleeding after an acupuncture treatment.

The length of the needle depends entirely on where it is to be placed and on the method being used. Longer needles are used in areas where the muscles are thick or the point lies quite deep. Short needles, as short as half an inch, are used where the point lies close to the surface; the needle may be inserted only an eighth to a quarter of an inch. These areas include points on the face, wrists, and ears.

Generally there is little discomfort when an acupuncture needle is inserted, although some patients who are more sensitive may feel a sharp momentary prick. When there is not excessive sensitivity and the needle is properly inserted, there is usually very little discomfort on insertion. The needle is gently moved into place and when it reaches the proper location a sore or achy feeling is felt. This is known as "getting the qi." There can be some variation here according to the techniques used by the practitioner and the condition of the patient.

As few as one, or as many as thirty needles may be used by the practitioner depending on the patient's condition. Generally acupuncture needles are left in for a maximum of forty-five minutes, but twenty minutes is much more typical. Sometimes a needle is inserted only briefly and then removed.

A number of adjuncts to acupuncture treatment may be used. These include moxibustion, cupping, bleeding, skin stimulation, and massage. The most important of these is moxibustion, which involves burning the herb artemisia on or near the acupuncture point to influence the qi. Precautions are always taken to avoid burning the skin. Although this technique sounds a bit exotic, it is a very useful clinical tool that produces a sense of profound well-being and relaxation, and has measurable and beneficial effects on the immune system and other aspects of the body's function. Cupping is a technique of producing a vacuum in a bamboo, glass, or plastic cup that is then applied to the skin surface to increase local circulation. This method is used for many musculoskeletal conditions and for problems such as bronchitis. Skin stimulation is an important method in pediatrics, nervous system disorders, and skin conditions. There are a wide range of methods that involve lightly scraping the skin or tapping it with tools that stimulate and move the qi without piercing the skin.

A typical office visit will last from forty-five minutes to an hour and a half, depending on how the practitioner works, what you need, and other factors. The initial consultation may be longer and later consultations shorter. If you are going to receive an herbal prescription for your condition, it will usually be prepared while you are being treated. Herbs are provided in many different ways. The most effective and personal form is the formula of raw herbs that you take home and cook into a soup or tea. This method of formulation allows the skilled herbalist to adjust the dosage of each ingredient to your precise needs and to make the most of his or her herbal skills. Powders, granulated extracts, and pills are often used as well. Many of these offer substantial convenience to both patient and practitioner. In many cases they are combined to enhance effects.

How long you will need to see a practitioner of Chinese medicine and acupuncture depends entirely on your condition. If you are addressing a minor problem that is easily resolved, you may not need more than three or four visits. A chronic or long-standing problem may require a significantly longer time frame. In general, both you and your practitioner should expect to see some signs of progress after the first few treatments, even if these signs are very small. Ask your practitioner what you should expect and how he or she will evaluate progress.

HOW TO FIND A PRACTITIONER

Finding a good acupuncturist and herbalist may be as easy as opening the yellow pages of your telephone book, if you are lucky enough to live in a state that licenses acupuncturists and requires and tests for training in acupuncture and herbal medicine. At this time, about thirty-four states license or otherwise regulate acupuncture, but only California requires training in herbal medicine.

If you are beginning your search for a practitioner, you might start with friends or family members who have had a good experience with a local acupuncturist. If this information isn't available you may want to seek guidance from a state or national professional organization. State organizations will often have a referral number. Two national organizations provide referrals and information about the profession:

AMERICAN ASSOCIATION OF
ORIENTAL MEDICINE (AAOM)
433 Front Street
Catasauqua, PA 18032-2506
Tel: (610) 433-2448

NATIONAL ACUPUNCTURE AND
ORIENTAL MEDICINE ALLIANCE
(NAOMA)
14637 Starr Road S.E.
Olalla, WA 98359
Fax: (253) 851-6896

Deciding if a practitioner is well qualified is a matter of careful inquiry and good judgment. Is the practitioner licensed to practice? If he or she is not, and the state licenses acupuncture, do not use their services. If the state does not license acupuncture, the situation is more complicated since you will have to assess the practitioner without any help from the state. In this case the following concerns become even more important.

Is the practitioner well trained? Did he or she attend an accredited program in the United States or an official training program in China? Did they receive training in herbal medicine? Some practitioners will hold the NCCAOM Diplomate in Acupuncture and the NCCAOM Diplomate in Herbal Medicine. These are the only independent credentials available in the United States to assure you that a practitioner has met a minimum standard of competency. Today, most qualified practitioners hold these credentials, although some may not have bothered to get these credentials, especially in states such as California, where licensing standards are quite high.

If this sounds too complex ask the following questions:

- Is the practitioner licensed in your state?
- Does the practitioner have at least three years of formal training or have they been in practice for more than ten years?
- Can they tell you where and how they were trained?
- Do they use disposable needles or sterilize their needles after every use?

Don't accept a practitioner if you can't answer yes to every one of the questions above.

- Did they graduate from an accredited school?
- Is the practitioner NCCAOM certified in Acupuncture?
- Is the practitioner NCCAOM certified in Chinese Herbal Medicine?

- Does the practitioner carry professional liability insurance (malpractice insurance)?

"No" answers to these four questions should make you think or ask more questions.

- Do you know people who have been treated by the practitioner and are happy with him or her?
- Is the practitioner able to discuss your situation with you and understand what you need?

If you can answer yes to all of the above questions you should be in good hands.

HOW TO LEARN MORE

Cheung, C. S., U. Yat Ki Lai, U. Aik Kaw, and H. Harrision. *Mental Dysfunction as Treated by Traditional Chinese Medicine.* San Francisco: Traditional Chinese Medical Publisher, 1981.

Ergil, K. "China's Traditional Medicine." In *Fundamentals of Complementary and Alternative Medicine*, edited by M. Micozzi. New York: Churchill Livingstone, 1996.

Kaptchuk, T. *The Web That Has No Weaver.* New York: Congdon & Weed, 1983.

Hammer, L. *Dragon Rises and Red Bird Flies: Psychology and Chinese Medicine.* Barrytown, NY: Station Hill Press, 1990.

Unschuld, P. *Medicine in China: A History of Ideas.* Berkeley: University of California Press, 1985.

For information about research and scholarly initiatives in the field of acupuncture and Oriental medicine:

NATIONAL ACADEMY OF ACUPUNCTURE
AND ORIENTAL MEDICINE (NAAOM)
Box 62
Tarrytown, NY 10591
Tel: (914) 332-4576
E-mail: 75776.1734@compuserve.com

For information about educational programs and training in the field:

COUNCIL OF COLLEGES OF ACUPUNCTURE
AND ORIENTAL MEDICINE (CCAOM)
1010 Wayne Ave., Suite 1270
Silver Spring, MD 20910
Tel: (301) 608-9175

ABOUT THE AUTHORS

Kevin V. Ergil, M.A., M.S., L.Ac., F.N.A.A.O.M., F.A.A.P.M., is the Dean of the Pacific Institute of Oriental Medicine, where he directs the clinical program, teaches, and oversees the academic program. He maintains a private practice in New York City. As an acupuncturist (licensed in New York and California) and an herbalist, his research and clinical interests extend into the areas of chronic immunodeficiency disorders, women's health, substance abuse, and harm reduction acupuncture and general medicine. He has worked in the area of East Asian medicine since 1980.

He was previously President of the American College of Traditional Chinese Medicine in San Francisco. He is a medical anthropologist (University of Washington) whose research interests and activities have focused primarily on Chinese and Tibetan medicine. He is also a director of the Society for Acupuncture Research. Mr. Ergil is a fellow and founding governor of the National Academy for Acupuncture and Oriental Medicine. He chairs the committees for Research Information and Core Curriculum for the Council of Colleges of Acupuncture and Oriental Medicine.

William Prensky, O.M.D., L.Ac., is a licensed acupuncturist who lives and practices in New York City. Dr. Prensky has been practicing acupuncture professionally since 1972. He is one of the founders of the profession of acupuncture in this country; he was the first American licensed to practice acupuncture in the United States, and was one of the founders of the first university program to examine the efficacy of acupuncture.

Dr. Prensky is currently Associate Professor of Oriental Medicine and the Director of the Graduate Program in Acupuncture and Oriental Medicine at Mercy College, in Dobbs Ferry, New York. He is President of the National Academy of Acupuncture and Oriental Medicine, and Chairman of the Acupuncture Society of New York.

Carol Greiff Lagstein, C.S.W., A.T.R.-B.C.
Sandy Muniz Lieberman, M.M.T., A.D.T.R.
Jo Salas, M.A., C.M.T.
Patricia Sternberg, M.A., R.D.T./B.C.T.

13 The Creative Arts Therapies

INTRODUCTION TO THE CREATIVE ARTS THERAPIES

Creative arts have been part of human culture throughout time. Evidence of this can be seen in the music, dances, and rhythms of tribal rituals, the timeless history of storytelling, and the discovery of early cave paintings. The drive of people to communicate through the arts reflects the irrepressible urge of the mind, body, and spirit to create.

With the increased use of technology in all aspects of contemporary society, the need of the individual to create and communicate is sometimes seen as less important than efficiency and greater productivity (Warren, 1993). When the urge to create is denied, a valuable outlet for self-expression is lost. Creative arts therapists recognize the need for this outlet. They use their skills as artists and clinicians to guide the individual in creative exploration and expression. Through the process of creating, there can be a sense of release, freedom, healing, self-understanding, and personal growth.

A universal goal of creative arts therapists is an acceptance and respect for all aspects of the human condition. A safe environment is provided, where the individual can feel free to express him- or herself. It is a place where all confidences and disclosures are honored. The client is encouraged to explore every possibility of creative self-expression. An ideal goal is to reach the epiphany of the creative moment where time and thought surrender to the act of creating, and often the unconscious prevails. A more simple, but just as valued, goal is to make the mark, sound, act, or gesture that is authentic to oneself. All that is presented is received with appreciation, support, and at times, celebration.

Creative arts therapists work with adults, adolescents, children, and the elderly. They work with individuals, groups, and families. They treat people of diverse backgrounds and levels of need. Creative arts therapists may serve as guides for individuals who wish to enhance their creative abilities and achieve greater self-awareness. They also offer treatment for people who are physically, cognitively, and/or emotionally challenged. The creative arts therapist helps the individual to rediscover the freedom of self-expression found in children. In addition, the arts can create a pathway to repressed memories and feelings that might otherwise be censored. One finds expressive therapists in rehabilitation centers, counseling centers, psychiatric hospitals, schools, hospice programs, halfway houses, prisons, nursing homes, hospitals, private practice, and community centers, to name a few.

The choice of a traditional talk therapy approach to treatment versus an expressive arts therapy should be determined by the client or by others, such as the family or school, who may make decisions or recommendations for the client. Some people are more comfortable talking to a therapist than exploring creative modalities to promote growth and healing. Others may find it hard to use words to communicate thoughts and feelings, preferring more expressive methods. Sometimes an individual will respond to a combination of verbal and nonverbal therapies.

Creative arts therapists believe that the potential for healing is as boundless as one's imagination. This makes most creative arts therapists supportive of other alternative forms of treatment, such as homeopathy and meditation.

In this chapter, four creative arts therapists discuss the philosophy, background, and application of their particular approaches, in an effort to help the consumer gain a basic understanding of the method. The chapter focuses on art, dance/movement, music, and drama therapies. Keep in mind that there are several other forms of creative arts therapy not specifically described in this chapter, including poetry, sand play, puppetry, bibliotherapy, and story making, to name a few.

Art Therapy

Carol Greiff Lagstein, C.S.W., A.T.R.-B.C.

WHAT IS ART THERAPY?

The introduction of art to the therapeutic process adds a powerful dimension. Art therapy provides a vehicle for an inward journey through which thoughts, feelings, and images can be released in a concrete form. The act of creating this form is often as significant as the final product. The therapist and client can observe the tangible translation of the internal process as it evolves.

Art therapy has many potential goals. The process can be cathartic, where one releases feelings through the act of creating and/or through the images created. When one experiences catharsis there is a sense of relief and peacefulness. Sometimes this act of creating can carry with it a spiritual connotation because you are making substance out of something that did not formerly exist materially. Art can serve as a door to repressed experiences and feelings. At times there are images, shapes, or colors that convey unconscious material. The art therapist functions as a guide who helps the individual look at his or her artwork in an effort to understand what is being communicated.

A final goal would be to encourage the individual to explore his or her creativity in a safe, non-judgmental environment. The joy of creating has a curative function because it builds confidence and self-esteem. In addition, it allows you to experience a sense of freedom beyond all physical and emotional barriers.

A significant difference between art therapy and traditional verbal therapy is the creation of a final visual or tactile product, which serves as a permanent record of the experience. Its existence guarantees that the thoughts and feelings one portrays cannot be denied or forgotten. As you progress through treatment, you can review and reflect upon past stages of the therapeutic process. For many people, the art serves as a less threatening bridge for discussing inner feelings. Imagery can serve as a metaphor for personal concepts. Everyday symbols may be used to communicate profound ideas.

HOW IT BEGAN

Art has been used throughout history as an indicator of emotional, cognitive, and cultural life. The exploration of the meaning behind the symbols conveyed in dreams was introduced by Freud. Jung used art as evidence of his theory of a collective unconscious, with symbols that repeat throughout time and in various cultures (Wadeson, 1980). At the turn of the century, as part of a growing interest in psychoanalysis, several psychiatrists studied patients' artwork and its relationship to their state of mind. In this original context, the artwork was considered to be an enhancement to psychoanalysis, but not an independent form of treatment.

In this country, there were two pioneers in the field of art therapy. They presented two different perspectives on the curative process of art therapy. Margaret Naumberg, a psychoanalyst and educator, was the first to define the field in the early 1940s. She believed that art served as a passage to repressed thoughts, impulses, and memories. She felt that encouraging patients to create art and to understand the meaning of their creations would actually speed up the process of psychoanalysis. She stated, "When the therapist convinces the patient that he (she) accepts whatever the patient may express, the patient may project in images what he (she) dares not put into words" (Naumberg, 1966).

Ten years later, Edith Kramer pioneered a different theory of the effectiveness of art therapy. She proposed that the creation of art served as the sublimation of unconscious wishes and drives into a socially acceptable form. The healing aspect of art therapy occurs through the act of creating. In contrast to Naumberg, she did not feel it was necessary to verbally explore the symbols of the art. Most art therapists understand the two philosophies and have found a way to combine both approaches in their work.

In the 1960s, the American Art Therapy Association was founded. In this same period the association began publishing the *American Journal of Art Therapy*, and instituted an annual conference for professionals to share their work.

HOW IT WORKS

Each art therapist conducts art therapy sessions in a manner reflecting his or her professional style, although most sessions have some things in common. Most art therapists will have a wide assortment of art materials available during a session, allowing the client to choose. This also allows the art therapist to encourage the use of a material that will enhance, rather than hinder, an individual's ability to succeed in the creative process. For example, a child who is reluctant to get dirty would not feel at ease using clay or paints in initial sessions. Collage or markers may make the process easier. A goal may be to eventually guide the child to feel more comfortable with a messy material.

The art medium can also be used to help the individual expand his or her ability to be more expressive. A person who tends to be rigid and controlling may be guided by the art therapist gradually to explore materials that are more difficult to control. For example, it might be helpful to guide this individual from magazine collage to drawing, to pastels, and finally to paint. The impact of each material on therapy is often part of the process and can be discussed.

In a typical session, a client can expect to have the opportunity to create art. The art therapist will sometimes produce art with the client in an effort to respond to his or her nonverbal language. It is rare that an art therapist will add to or alter a client's art.

Often time is allotted for discussion of the client's experience. Art created during the session can be kept by the client or therapist, or continued in another session. Art therapists may recommend that clients continue to create art at home. This art is usually welcomed into sessions for further processing. Many individuals find art to be a gratifying form of expression and continue to be creative long after art therapy treatment ends.

When art therapy is conducted with a family or other group, the art therapist may introduce group projects that require social skills such as communication, sharing, and cooperation. In a family or group setting, the images can often help individuals communicate to others something that may have been too difficult to say in words.

WHAT THE RESEARCH SHOWS

Some art therapists have used traditional scientific research methods to measure the effectiveness of art therapy (for example, see Rosal, 1993; Neale and Rosal, 1993). More research has used subjective observation and qualitative assessment of the art therapy process in group, family, and individual case studies and through feedback from the clients, following a social science research paradigm. For example, Bowen and Rosal (1989) tested the effectiveness of three months of biweekly art therapy sessions to reduce the maladaptive behaviors of Karen, a cognitively challenged adult. The results reflected an increase in appropriate behavior, increased productivity, greater resources for satisfaction-seeking, greater body awareness, and a more integrated sense of self.

It is difficult to use traditional scientific scales to quantify the effectiveness of art therapy since the creation and the perception of art is greatly influenced by aesthetic and subjective experience. Art therapists have addressed this problem by using their creative ingenuity to develop new research paradigms that more accurately convey the art therapy process (Junge and Linesch, 1993; Edwards, 1993). Present and future research reflects these new research models (Schavarien, 1993; Quail and Peavy, 1994).

REAL PEOPLE AND ART THERAPY

One young woman covered the bulb of a lamp with papier-maché. She purposefully allowed a few strips of the papier-maché to peel off. She described it as a representation of herself, a recovering alcoholic. She added that, as she was healing, her light was beginning to shine through.

A young girl in an art therapy group displayed her abstract tissue paper collage for discussion. The art therapist and group observed that the collage looked like a burnt-down tenement building. The girl tearfully acknowledged that she had unknowingly portrayed the events leading to the death of her family.

An adolescent who was struggling with a conduct disorder was referred to an art therapist to work symbolically with limits and boundaries. This was done through the choice of media or themes. The client was encouraged to move from controlled to noncontrolled art materials, such as from colored pencils to paints. She was also asked to create a comic strip with a superhero who must confront situations analogous to those she experienced.

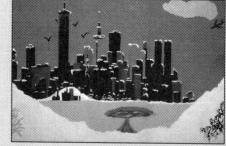

Figure 1 represents a group mural where eight individuals worked cooperatively to create a city scape. When one group member painted a significant part of the city, leaving others out, another

Figure 1

group member painted a bomber plane attacking the city. This nonverbal communication opened the door for more authentic verbal discussions.

Figures 2, 3, and 4 demonstrate projects done independently, but incorporating drama to unite the group. A mask-making project was introduced to a group of seven-to-ten-year old children diagnosed with learning disabilities. The children created characters to represent themselves. They wore their masks and assumed the identity of the created character. They also tried on and acted out one another's characters, and in the process, developed their sense of empathy and self-expression.

Art therapy was introduced to an in-patient in a psychiatric hospital, who was

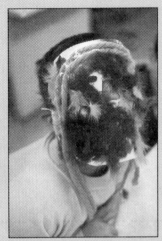

Figure 2

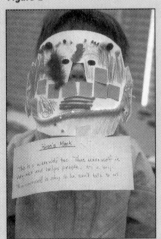

Figure 3

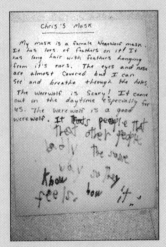

Figure 4

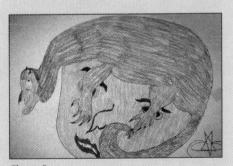

Figure 5

diagnosed as paranoid schizophrenic, and who suffered from hallucinations and delusions. His treatment plan included individual art therapy sessions several times a week to help him improve his reality testing. Materials such as clay and pencil drawing were suggested in order to help him gain a sense of control and to feel more grounded. It was a slow and painful process. At times he used the art simply to portray his internal experience where words failed. Figure 5 represents, through imagery, his experience of schizophrenia.

HOW TO FIND AN ART THERAPIST

The American Art Therapy Association established a credential of registration signifying an art therapist who had met specific professional criteria, including a minimum of 1,000 hours of supervised clinical experience. Art therapists of this level have the letters A.T.R. after their name. In 1994, the first certification exam in art therapy was administered to A.T.R.'s in an effort to help the public assess the level of competency of an art therapist. A credential of A.T.R.-B.C. (art therapist-board certified) is awarded to those who pass the exam.

An individual who is interested in learning more about art therapy could contact their local chapter of the American Art Therapy Association, or the national association for assistance. The address is:

AATA
1202 Allanson Rd.
Mundelein, Il. 60060
Tel: (708) 949-6064; Fax: (708) 566-4580.
The organization publishes a directory of art therapists.

HOW TO LEARN MORE

Anderson, F. E. *Art for All the Children: Approaches to Art for Children with Disabilities.* Springfield, IL: Charles C. Thomas, 1992.

Betensky, M. *Self-Discovery Through Self-Expression.* Springfield, IL: Charles C. Thomas, 1973.

Bowen, C. A. and M. L. Rosal. "The Use of Art Therapy to Reduce the Maladaptive Behaviors of a Mentally Retarded Adult." *The Arts in Psychotherapy* 16, no. 3 (1989): 211–218.

Edwards, D. "Why Don't Art Therapists Do Research?" In *A Handbook of Inquiry in the Arts Therapies*, edited by H. Payne. London: Kingsley Publishers, Inc., 1993.

Junge, M. B. and D. Linesch. "Our Own Voices: New Paradigms for Art Therapy Research," *The Arts in Psychotherapy* 20, no. 1 (1993): 61–67.

Kramer, E. *Art Therapy in a Children's Community*. New York: Schoken Books, 1978.

Kwiatkowska, H. *Family Therapy and Evaluation Through Art*. Springfield, IL: Charles C. Thomas, 1978.

Landgarten, H. B. *Clinical Art Therapy: A Clinical Guide and Casebook*. New York: Bruner/Mazel, 1981.

Levick, M. *They Could Not Talk So They Drew: Children's Styles of Thinking and Coping*. Springfield, IL: Charles C. Thomas, 1983.

Naumberg, M. *Dynamically Oriented Art Therapy: Its Principles and Practice*. New York: Grune & Stratton, Inc., 1966.

Neale, E. L. and M. L. Rosal. "What Can Art Therapists Learn from the Research on Projective Drawing Techniques for Children? A Review of the Literature." *The Arts in Psychotherapy* 20, no. 1 (1993): 37–49.

Quail, J. M. and R. V. Peavy. "A Phenomenologic Research Study of a Client's Experience in Art Therapy." *The Arts in Psychotherapy* 21, no. 1 (1994): 45–57.

Robbins, A. and L. B. Sibley. *Creative Art Therapy*. New York: Bruner/Mazel, 1976.

Rosal, M. L. "Comparative Group Art Therapy Research to Evaluate Changes in Locus of Control in Behavior Disordered Children." *The Arts in Psychotherapy* 20, no. 3 (1993): 231–241.

Rubin, J. *Child Art Therapy*. New York: Van Nostrand Reinhold, 1984.

Schaverien, J. "The Retrospective Review of Pictures: Data for Research in Art Therapy." In *Handbook of Inquiry in the Arts Therapies*, edited by H. Payne. London: Jessica Kingsley Publishers, Ltd., 1993.

Wadeson, H. *Art Psychotherapy*. New York: John Wiley & Sons, Inc., 1980.

Wadeson, H. *Dynamics of Art Therapy Psychotherapy*. New York: John Wiley and Sons, 1987.

Warren, B. "Introduction." In *Using the Creative Arts in Therapy*. Second Edition, edited by B. Warren. New York: Routledge, 1993.

RESOURCES

Journals

Art Therapy, the Journal of the American Art Therapy Association
1202 Allanson Rd.
Mundelein, IL 60060
Tel: (708) 949-6064; Fax: (708) 566-4580

American Journal of Art Therapy
Vermont College of Norwich University
Montpelier, VT 05602
Tel: (802) 828-8540; Fax: (802) 828-8855

Arts in Psychotherapy, an International Journal
Elsevier Science Inc.,
660 White Plains Rd.
Tarrytown, N.Y. 10591-515

Dance Therapy

Sandy Muniz Lieberman, M.M.T., A.D.T.R.

WHAT IS DANCE THERAPY?

Dance therapy is a form of psychotherapy that uses movement to further the development of the individual. Since our life stories reside in our bodies, the reality of who we are and who we have been is reflected in our movement. Dance therapists include this expression as part of the dynamic and creative process of therapy and inner growth. This can be transformative, for it may reach parts of ourselves that cannot be reached through talk alone.

It is well known that people do not always understand why they behave or feel in a certain way. In fact, unconscious unresolved issues may often motivate and control our behavior. But when we move, paint, sing, or dance, we are enlivening those aspects of ourselves that may be constrained by our everyday habits, speech patterns, or personality limitations. The dance can be particularly powerful due to the immediacy of feelings and sensations when felt in the body. This kind of exploration bypasses cognitive control, and taps into the unconscious material that needs to surface for healing to begin. This can be particularly powerful when "witnessed" by the therapist, as it provides confirmation to the emerging self that it has in fact been "seen."

HOW IT BEGAN

The use of dance in expressive release and healing has its roots in many ancient cultures. These societies used dance and community movement ritual as important aspects of daily life, providing a forum to express emotions, communicate cultural mores, and build community. This shared experience of movement expression no doubt eased feelings of isolation and supported the inclusion of the individual in society. It also supported the wholeness of the individual internally, as the creative, physical, and spiritual dimensions were expressed together. In contrast, Western society has traditionally seen people as more compartmentalized. Western medicine developed the medical model that focuses on symptom relief in physical health, while psychotherapy developed verbal approaches for mental health. Artistic expression was channeled into highly disciplined classical forms that required extensive training, such as ballet. The focus was on audience reception of the finished aesthetic product, rather than on the total healing experience of self/performer in relation to community.

In the early part of the twentieth century, this more compartmentalized experience of the individual began to shift. More holistic views were gradually explored in the fields of dance and psychotherapy. Modern dancers sought to communicate from their inner selves, emphasizing creativity, improvisation, and the spiritual dimension of the dance. Isadora Duncan and Ruth St. Denis were two such pioneers who experimented with new forms of dance as communication and communion with self and others. In the field of psychotherapy, there was a similar breaking away from convention, as psychologists explored the more nonverbal and expressive aspects of personality. Wilhelm Reich, an Austrian psychiatrist, worked extensively with the deep connections between the somatic and the psychic realms. His work on character armor, or body defenses, laid the groundwork for many theorists and clinicians who followed. Carl Jung, a Swiss psychiatrist, paid much attention to the creative process with emphasis on its therapeutic value. One of his major contributions was the development of the concept of "active imagination," a process whereby unconscious material becomes conscious through symbols in artistic experience. Each of these pioneering individuals contributed to the growing trend in society to seek a deeper, more holistic understanding of the individual in society. Dance therapy emerged in the 1940s out of this environment.

Marion Chace (1896–1970) is generally considered the "Grand Dame" of dance therapy. She was a gifted individual, a pioneering dancer who worked with hospitalized psychiatric patients, facilitating communication development and promoting social interactions with patients unreachable through verbal rapport alone. Her work with symbolism, group rhythm, and therapeutic movement relationships has greatly influenced the development of dance therapy theory and practice. Mary Whitehouse (1911–1979) was another major dance therapy pioneer who worked primarily in her private studio and placed a greater emphasis on helping her clients' unconscious material surface through movement. Integrating expressive movement and Jung's theory of active imagination, she developed a form of work called "authentic movement." In its essence, this is concerned with the embodiment of inner truth and the healthy integration of the individual. Many dance therapy initiatives were begun at this same time by others. Today, dance therapy has evolved as a form of psychotherapy that is widely recognized as working toward the wholeness of the individual. Its roots are still celebrated as coming from the spirituality of primitive dance ritual and modern dance's expression of the inner self.

HOW IT WORKS

The unity of body and psyche is a strong principle that underlies all dance therapy. Dance therapists understand that we are our bodies. Our biological predispositions combine with our life circumstances to develop the movement vocabulary and body image that shapes our personality, life habits, and coping styles. We carry themes from our childhood that become deeply embedded in our character structure and body image, affecting us throughout our lifetime. Dance therapists recognize and work with this information. For example, a child continually criticized and attacked by a parent may develop perpetually raised shoulders, as if in anticipation of the next assault. This holding pattern may be carried into adulthood, long after the threat is gone. In this example, the anxiety and apprehension of the child live on in the body of the adult, affecting that individual's ability to operate in the world. This nonverbal communication (raised shoulders) can signal to others on an unconscious level that here is a potential victim, thus continuing to define a person based on a past body holding pattern. Even when the psyche may forget or repress a part of our life story, our bodies do not forget. Some dance therapists call it "bone memory," the astonishing way our bodies remember an early trauma embedded in a physical movement habit. Body awareness and exploration can lead to the remembering of repressed memories and feelings, making previous unconscious material conscious and ready to be integrated into the personality. Through the therapy process, changes made by the client are reflected in both body and psyche.

Dance therapists enrich their understanding of clients' psyches through careful observation of their clients' body movements. Therapists train extensively in systems of "movement profiling" that can provide a tremendous wealth of diagnostic information about a client based on his or her movement. This information assists the therapist in working with a client for a deeper understanding of his or her experience and needs.

Another basic principle in dance therapy is that, when we change a body pattern, we directly impact the corresponding emotional and cognitive factors. For example, when a timid woman, who has only been able to whisper and tread softly through life, finds in movement therapy the impulse to stamp with strength around the room and assert her physical presence in space, this will have an impact on her psychological functioning. When a distractible scattered child with learning deficits experiences herself moving with prolonged directed attention across a balance beam, her newly discovered ability to focus in space will directly affect her general attention span. As people expand their movement range, and changes occur on a body level, growth and change occur in the psyche as well.

The movement therapist must create an environment that is safe enough for the client, so that a trusting relationship can develop. Only then can the mover feel secure enough to risk truly being "seen" by another, so that the growth process can begin. This is in contrast to some other body-oriented therapies that are more educational in nature, where a therapist might teach a movement prescription to solve particular ailments. In dance therapy, the developing relationship between the therapist and the client is a very integral part of the process.

WHAT THE RESEARCH SHOWS

Research studies have documented the efficacy of dance movement therapy as a treatment modality in specific situations. Brooks and Stark (1989) conducted a study which supported the premise that dance therapy can change how people feel. A single dance therapy session significantly changed the participants' affect, with depression and anxiety affected more than hostility. Movement therapy has been found to have a positive effect on body image by Franklin (1979) working with the mentally retarded, and by Christup (1962) with chronic schizophrenics. Another study (Kuettel, 1982) found that subjects receiving dance therapy will express less anxiety and greater affection than members of control groups. Westbrook and McKibben (1989) found that dance movement therapy improved movement initiation in patients with Parkinson's disease. They suggested that dance therapy may be equally useful for other groups of patients with neurological disabilities. Other studies have demonstrated the effectiveness of dance therapy with troubled youth (Payne, 1988), and with mothers and young children at risk of abuse (Meekums, 1991).

In 1993, the U.S. Senate appropriated money for research on the efficacy of dance therapy with older persons. The findings of this research project, submitted in 1996, strongly suggest that dance/movement therapy improved the functional abilities on a number of key variables for older adults who had sustained neurological insult (AOA Grant Number: 90 AM 0669).

Although there is pressure to prove the effectiveness of dance movement therapy both from within the field and from outside sources, serious issues have been raised by researchers that question whether the profession can be evaluated through the old paradigm model of traditional research (Meekums and Payne, 1993). Traditional research with its emphasis on objectivity, isolation of data, and strictly controlled parameters may not be relevant to the study of the effectiveness of a process which by definition is holistic, interactive, and difficult to isolate. Meekums and Payne (1993) present a strong case for the development and use of new paradigm methodologies in future dance therapy research, such as illuminative evaluation (Parlett, 1974, 1981).

REAL PEOPLE AND DANCE THERAPY

Specific client goals and what actually happens during a session vary considerably depending on the setting, population, and individual clients' needs. A few examples follow. For the autistic-like client who has severe social and communication deficits, the movement therapy usually is done one-on-one. As part of the process of relationship building, there are nonverbal techniques that dance therapists use to communicate empathy and establish trust. Dance therapists gain a deeper understanding of clients' experiences through such techniques as attunement in tension flow, adjustment in shape flow, and mirroring of basic body shape patterns. These often very subtle kinesthetic identifications are particularly powerful when used in relationship building with the nonverbal client, or the client who has difficulty relating to others. After a number of sessions, an autistic child who completely ignores the therapist might begin short and sporadic sequences of synchronistic movement with the therapist. Over time, fleeting eye contact and seemingly random touch would increase as the child actively begins to seek contact, increasing his or her level of tolerance for communication attempts. Using these active nonverbal techniques, the therapist encourages the specific goals of increased relatedness and increased ability to communicate needs.

For the average adult with intact ego boundaries, dance therapy can be done either individually or in a group. The structure can be minimal. Clients may improvise movements with freedom to explore their unconscious impulses. For example, an individual may discover a deep need to twirl around the space endlessly until all ability to maintain focus and balance is gone. She collapses in a heap and cannot move. Again and again she begins her sessions in this way. Eventually she may discover that her busy and successful lifestyle is quite similar, metaphorically. Her circular motions become frenzied and she loses her sense of stability. Then she lives in terror of that familiar place of collapse, fearing she may never rise again. Often the therapist will offer guidance to the client only as needed or requested. In this case, she might suggest the place of collapse as the starting point from which to begin exploring feelings, sensations, or impulses to move. Talking together after the movement, to process the experience, is often a very meaningful part of the therapy. This is when conscious verbal integration of the movement, feelings, and images can enhance the therapeutic experience. Goals specific to this way of working include self-awareness, empowerment, and integration of body and psyche.

Work with children may require much more structure and more therapist involvement. More formal activities, or movement games and exercises, are specifically designed to address the unique developmental needs of each child or group of children, stimulating social interaction, and self-expression. One example of this is a small group of preschool children, most of whom had been neglected or abused and were struggling to find ways to express their feelings without becoming overwhelmed by them. After moving with colorful silk scarves, which often facilitates movement due to their texture and flowing quality, the movement therapist suggested that the children pretend to be outdoors. One child drooped with passive weight and collapsed to the ground. Rocking slightly yet slumped over, the child said, "I am a dying flower." The other children were asked if there was anything that could be done for a dying flower. Their response was to move in parade-like fashion, delivering "flower food," water for the roots, and a great big yellow scarf "sun" to the child. Slowly, the dying flower child began to respond to the touch and stood up tall, twirling her scarf around. Goals here have included facilitating coping skills, stimulating social interactions, and expression of self.

Some dance therapists incorporate other creative modalities with their work in movement. Examples of this are using music to facilitate certain kinds of movement exploration, using art to visually express the symbols and imagery that may surface during movement, or using poetry to capture, in language, the spirit of the movement discovery. Whether or not other modalities are incorporated, dance therapy's unique distinction continues to be that it utilizes our very bodies as the instrument of self-expression, with every gesture and impulse choreographing our literal journey toward health. This immediacy and embodiment accounts for the powerful, often transformational nature of this work.

HOW TO CHOOSE A DANCE THERAPIST

The training for dance therapists is varied. At one end of the spectrum, there are therapists who see body and movement expression as first and paramount, with meaning in and of itself. They use terminology relating to movement, not to psychology, and they may or may not discuss the dance process. At the other end of the spectrum are therapists who have incorporated various psychological perspectives (ie: Jungian, psychoanalytic, developmental) into their movement therapy work with clients. Regardless of where a therapist is on this continuum, there are fundamental principles upon which all dance therapists agree.

Since its founding in 1966, the American Dance Therapy Association (ADTA) has worked to establish and maintain high standards of professional education and competence in the field. Dance Therapists hold masters degrees in Dance/Movement Therapy, and are eligible for a D.T.R. (Dance Therapist Registered). Alternate routes are available. There is an advanced level of registry, A.D.T.R. (Academy of Dance Therapists Registered) signifying that an individual may teach, provide training and supervision, and engage in private practice. For more information, contact the national office:

ADTA
2000 Century Plaza, Suite 108
Columbia, MD 21044
Tel: (410) 997-4040

HOW TO LEARN MORE

Adler, J. "Who is the Witness: A Description of Authentic Movement." *Contact Quarterly* 12, no. 1 (1987): 20–29.

Bernstein, P. *Eight Theoretical Approaches to Dance Therapy.* Dubuque, IA: Kendall Hunt, 1979.

Brooks, D. and A. Stark "The Effect of Dance Therapy on Affect: A Pilot Study." *American Journal of Dance Therapy* 11, no. 2 (1989).

Chaiklin, H. *Marian Chace: Her Papers.* Columbia, MD: A.D.T.A., 1975.

Chodorow, J. "To Move and Be Moved." *Quadrant Journal of the C. G. Jung Foundation for Analytical Psychology* 17, no. 2 (1984): 39–48.

_____ *Dance Therapy and Depth Psychology: The Moving Imagination.* New York: Routledge, 1991.

Christup, H. J. "The Effect of Dance Therapy on the Concept of Body Image." *Psychiatric Quarterly Supplement* 2, no. 36 (1962).

Franklin, S. "Movement Therapy and Selected Measures of Body Image in the Trainable Mentally Retarded." *American Journal of Dance Therapy* 3, no. 1 (1979): 43–50.

Kestenberg, J. and M. Sossin. *The Role of Movement Patterns in Development,* Vol. 2. New York: Dance Notation Press, 1979.

Kuettel, T. "Affective Change in Dance Therapy." *American Journal of Dance Therapy* 5 (1982): 56–64.

Levy, F. *Dance Movement Therapy: A Healing Art.* Reston, VA: The American Alliance for Health, Physical Education, Recreation and Dance, 1988.

Lewis B. P. and D. Singer, eds. *The Choreography of Object Relations.* Keene, NH: Antioch University, 1982.

Lewis, P. and S. Loman, eds. *The Kestenberg Movement Profile: Its Past, Present Applications and Future Directions.* Keene, NH: Antioch University, 1990.

Lewis, P. *Creative Transformation: The Healing Power of the Arts.* Wilmette IL: Chiron Publications, 1993.

Loman, S., ed. *The Body-Mind Connection in Human Movement Analysis.* Keene, NH: Antioch University, 1992.

Meekums, B. "Dance Movement Therapy with Mothers and Young Children at Risk of Abuse." *The Arts in Psychotherapy* 18, no. 3 (1991).

Meekums, B. and H. Payne. "Emerging Methodology in Dance Movement Therapy Research — A Way Forward." In *Handbook of Inquiry in the Arts Therapies*, edited by H. Payne. Philadelphia: Jessica Kingsley Publishers, 1993.

Muniz, S. "The Choreography of a Facilitating Environment: Movement Therapy with a Residually Autistic Latency Aged Child." In *The Choreography of Object Relations*, edited by P. Bernstein and D. Singer. Keene, NH: Antioch University, 1982.

Parlett, M. "The New Evaluation." *Trends in Education, Innovative* 34. London: HMSO/DES, 1974.

_____ "Illuminative Evaluation." In *Human Inquiry*, edited by P. Reason and J. Rowan. Chichester: John Wiley and Sons, 1981.

Payne, H. "The Use of Dance Movement Therapy with Troubled Youth." In *Innovative Interventions in Child and Adolescent Therapy*, edited by C. Schaefer. New York: John Wiley Interscience, 1988.

_____ ed. *Handbook of Inquiry in the Arts Therapies: One River, Many Currents.* Philadelphia: Jessica Kingsley Publishers, 1993.

Schwartz-Salant, N. and M. Stein, eds. *The Body in Analysis.* Wilmette, IL: Chiron Publications, 1986.

Siegel, E. *Dance Movement Therapy: Mirror of Ourselves.* New York: Human Sciences Press, 1984.

Westbrook, B. and H. McKibben. "Dance Movement Therapy with Groups of Outpatients with Parkinson's Disease." *American Journal of Dance Therapy* 11, no. 1 (1989): 27–38.

Whitehouse, M. "Physical Movement and Personality." Paper presented at the meeting of the Analytic Psychology Club, Los Angeles, 1963.

Drama Therapy

Patricia Sternberg, M.A., R.D.T./B.C.T

WHAT IS DRAMA THERAPY?

Drama therapy is defined by the National Association for Drama Therapy as "the systematic and intentional use of drama/theater processes, products, and associations to achieve the therapeutic goals of symptom relief, emotional and physical integration, and personal growth." Drama therapy uses structured and creative role-play to increase life skills. Its techniques deal with the here and now, enhancing problem-solving skills for the present and future, and illustrating alternative solutions to all problems.

Drama therapy can enrich the client's sense of self-worth through the discovery of his or her own inner resources as well as learning how to function in a group. Drama therapy can offer a vision of something outside the individual and beyond one's narrow view of the world. It is focused on the process rather than on a product, unlike theater education or theater performance, where artistic achievement rather than the actors' participation is the desired goal. However, some drama therapists are also theater directors who create productions for an audience, which then becomes involved in the process after viewing the product. Three such companies are Stop Gap Theater, Playback Theater, and Enact.

This active approach to behavioral, emotional, and cognitive change has been found to be effective with severely disturbed and disabled populations as well as others. It is a way to explore the creative potential in all people. It is a nonthreatening technique which promotes awareness of one's environment and one's inner resources, encourages self-worth, and expands problem-solving skills. It can be geared to varying levels of functioning.

HOW IT BEGAN

Drama therapy is the newest of the Creative Arts therapies. Although drama therapy has been practiced in Europe for many years, the National Association for Drama Therapy (NADT) was established in the U.S. in 1979, at Yale University with Gertrude Shatner as the first president. As of November 1997, the National Association for Drama Therapy had close to 400 members. Most registered drama therapists (R.D.T.'s) come to Drama Therapy from a drama/

theater background, and many theoretical frameworks are represented, reflecting varied backgrounds of training. These include Jungian, psychoanalytic, and Gestalt perspectives, as well as humanistic and cognitive psychology.

HOW IT WORKS

Drama therapy is practiced in a variety of settings and serves many different populations. It is used in mental health facilities, hospitals, schools, prisons, community centers, correctional facilities, rehabilitation programs, and businesses, as well as in private practice. Currently, drama therapists are working with special education classes, psychiatric patients, persons recovering from substance abuse, trauma victims, dysfunctional families, developmentally and physically disabled persons (including AIDS patients), prison and correctional facility inmates, anorexic and bulimic patients, the homeless, the elderly, children, adolescents, and others. Drama therapists provide services to individuals, groups, and families in addition to conducting clinical research.

Drama therapy uses many different techniques, from a full-fledged theater performance to stimulate the audience, as mentioned earlier, to simple sensory awareness exercises, depending on the population and its functional level. Drama therapists use techniques such as improvisation, role play, theater games, concentration exercises, mime, masks, and puppetry, as well as scripted dramatizations and opened-ended scripts. These techniques further emotional growth and psychological integration.

Drama therapists provide evaluation and treatment. They coordinate their efforts with psychiatrists, psychologists, nurses, social workers, and other personnel as part of a team treatment approach. One of the important assets of the drama therapist is that he or she is trained as a team player (as in the theater) and regularly works in conjunction with other therapists. In consultation with nursing staff and medical recommendations, the therapist conducts drama therapy groups to deal with problems, issues, and concerns of the patients. At times, specific recommendations are given to the therapist by a doctor, social worker, psychologist, or nursing staff for specific patient problems.

Emphasis is placed on problem-solving skills and role training, as well as ways and means to help achieve and maintain mental health. Through simulated life situations, patients get opportunities to try out new behaviors and methods of solving problems without the fear of any consequences. Sometimes, the drama therapist assists the group to identify common concerns or issues with which they would like to work. In addition, role-training situations are enacted, such as interviewing for a job or placement, asserting personal needs on the job or in a relationship, or handling anger, frustration, and stress in a constructive way. Patients can practice their verbal and problem-solving skills in a variety of spontaneous situations.

Drama therapists offer a variety of techniques that go beyond "talk therapy." They use many different kinds of objects in their work, such as dolls (life-size and otherwise), puppets, masks, hats, scarves, costumes, punching bags, Play-Doh, photographs, paintings, cubes, pillows, paper, crayons, and a myriad of other objects. Sound and music can also be a part of a private drama therapy session. But unlike the art therapist or music therapist, who follow through with these techniques, the drama therapist uses these articles as a stepping-stone to the drama. Through drawing or mask work, the client may actually become the image, and the role play could start there.

WHAT THE RESEARCH SHOWS

In David Read Johnson's work with schizophrenic patients (1980) the main issue has been the relationship between improvisational role playing and clear intrapsychic and interpersonal boundaries. His research focused on the problem of loss of the self and the potential of drama therapy in recovering it. Further studies on self-image have been conducted by Renee Emunah and Johnson (1983). Johnson's current research is focused on post-traumatic stress disorder.

Eleanor Irwin, who works mainly with children, has conducted research to determine how dramatic play can help the learning-disabled child and the emotionally disturbed child (Irwin, 1980).

Michiko Moriyama is currently using drama therapy to treat demented elderly patients in a nursing home in Japan (1994). Her results show that this therapy has produced rehabilitation effects on higher cortical functions, such as improved language and action abilities, and psychological effects, such as activating and stabilizing the patients emotionally, and reducing abnormal behavior.

REAL PEOPLE AND DRAMA THERAPY

A typical private drama therapy session would include some kind of a warm-up such as talking about what went on since the last meeting.

The client may want to replay any particularly difficult or emotional scenes. The therapist and the client may play out the situation as it happened, and/or play it again as the client wanted it to go. The therapist guides the client to understand his feelings and tries to help him understand those of the other people involved. The therapist may guide the client to realize that what the client said, and what he meant, were two different things. Communication skills are discussed, analyzed, and built upon. Possible alternative ways to handle feelings are explored.

A role play is enacted to give the client the experience of dealing with a difficult situation. The therapist creates resistance for the client, so that he is prepared for possible problems which may arise. Role reversal is used to give the client a chance to put himself in the other person's shoes, and to try to understand the feelings of that person. Future projection can be used, as well as inner monologue, or the empty chair technique. The client is given every opportunity to vent his emotions. Does he need to throw a couple of punches at the punching bag before he leaves? He laughs and realizes that most of what he came in with is gone or redirected. The therapist helps the client process what has happened during the session. They review what needs to happen next. Specific behavioral goals for the client are discussed and agreed upon for the next meeting.

∞

Let's take a look at a group session within a psychiatric facility, which is one of the most common work places for drama therapists. Most groups of psychiatric patients exclude anyone who is actively hallucinating, agitated patients who are non-directable, or patients who are actively suicidal.

Most therapists structure their session in a similar way with a warm-up of some kind, followed by the main action where role play is used, and a conclusion of sharing or processing. Sometimes a group meets over a long period of time and becomes cohesive. This is a goal in a long-term facility. However, in working in a short-term facility or crisis intervention groups, frequently there are newcomers to each session, so thata warm-up may consist of name games and "getting to know you" activities such as "My name is _____ and one thing I do well is _____."

The action segment is where role play is used. For example, a drama therapist may be contracted to work with a group of managers to help them become more aware of what constitutes sexual harassment today. One therapist was brought in to teach problem-solving skills to adolescents with behavior disorders. Drama therapy techniques, and specifically role play, have been used in sales training, hotel management, counseling, and crisis intervention even before it was recognized as drama therapy.

In some settings the group comes up with their own issues or problems to explore with the therapist. Sometimes the drama therapist is hired to work on skill building with a particular group, such as the adolescent group mentioned above, or with an incarcerated group. Here the therapist might focus on achieving social skills that would enable clients to be more effective in communicating when applying for a job, a place to live, or returning to a particular environment. An issue that comes up frequently with many behavior disorder groups is learning how to deal with anger using methods other than violence.

Once the problem is selected, volunteers act out the specific situation suggested by the therapist such as, "I want to be able to stand up for myself with my husband and not always have to do everything his way," or "Every time my kids have an argument I start screaming at them and make it worse. I want to handle the problem differently." Another common concern from patients about to be discharged from a psychiatric hospital is, "What do I tell people when they ask where I've been?" First, the problem to be worked on is selected, then the scene is set: location, time, place, etc. When everyone knows where they are and what they're doing, the players begin to improvise the scene. Sometimes prepared scripts are used to get the scene started or to get a discussion going, and then the players move to improvisation: "What would you say in that situation? Let's try the scene your way and see what happens."

When we move into the processing or sharing part of the session, the players talk about the feelings they had during the scene. Members of the audience are encouraged to express their feelings and responses.

Other possibilities are discussed, for instance, how else might the scene have gone or what else could the person have said? Everyone is encouraged to make some contribution. The processing discussion is as important as the action. One significant element stressed is that there is always more than one solution to every problem.

Often when a patient is warmed up to an issue, he or she becomes fully involved in the role play and has the same feelings and reactions that occur in the real situation. Comments frequently heard after a good role play are, "Now, I know how my husband feels!" Or, "I never thought of it that way before." Sometimes there's even more insight with comments such as, "I always thought he was a cold fish, now I see he could be just shy." The experience of being in someone else's shoes can be very insight-provoking. It is important to allow enough time for this processing at the end of the session.

Other types of group drama therapy include theater performances dealing with specific problem issues. These are most popular in school settings and usually offer the kinds of life choices facing students today in regard to drugs and alcohol, sexual conduct, violence, problems with parents, teachers, and their peers. Other groups present productions which offer information and/or education on a specific subject such as AIDS, drug abuse, illiteracy, dealing with violence, etc. Some groups offer workshops after the performance. These workshops can be anywhere from a month's residency to a one-session discussion to explore the issues dramatized in the performance. Others have a question-and-answer period at the end, and sometimes the players stay in role to answer such questions as, "Why didn't you want to go to bed with your boyfriend?"

HOW TO FIND A DRAMA THERAPIST

When choosing a drama therapist, verify that the person is an R.D.T. This is the only valid credential for drama therapists. These R.D.T.s are registered through the National Association for Drama Therapy and have met rigorous standards. R.D.T./BC denotes the added credential of board certification as a trainer. Standards of registration for R.D.T. include the following: expertise in dramatic, theatrical, and performance media; an understanding of psychotherapeutic process with different populations in a variety of settings; integration of the artistic and psychological aspects of drama therapy; and professional expertise in the field of mental health and/or special education. Many drama therapists in private practice hold other degrees in addition to their R.D.T. status (which denotes an M.A. as the minimum requirement), such as Ph.D., M.S.W., Ed.D., M.F.C.C., C.A.C., as well as credentials in the other creative arts therapies.

Unfortunately, there are people who call themselves drama therapists with no credentials other than their interest and/or experience in drama or theater, but without knowledge of the clinical background or study necessary to become registered. Some may have a degree in drama or in theater but that does not translate into being a drama therapist or holding the credential R.D.T. It's like a musician calling him or herself a music therapist just because he can play the piano.

The National Association for Drama Therapy is located at 5505 Connecticut Ave. NW #280, Washington, D.C. 20015. Their telephone number is (202) 966-7409. They keep an updated list of all R.D.T.s and R.D.T. /BCs, as well as all other members of the organization.

HOW TO LEARN MORE

Courtney, R. *Play, Drama and Thought.* New York: Drama Book Specialists, 1974.

_____ *Re-Play: Studies of Drama in Education.* Toronto: Ontario Institute for Studies in Education, 1982.

_____ *Drama and Intelligence.* Montreal: McGill-Queen's University Press, 1990.

Emunah, R. "Drama Therapy with Adult Psychiatric Patients." In *The Arts in Psychotherapy* Vol. 10. New York: Pergamon Press, 1985.

Emunah, R. and D. Johnson. "The Impact of Theatrical Performance on the Self-Images of Psychiatric Patients." *The Arts in Psychotherapy* 10 (1983): 233–239.

Irwin, E. "Introduction." Proceedings - First Annual Conference NADT, New Haven, CT: National Association for Drama Therapy, 1, 1980.

Irwin, E. C. and E. S. Portner. Proceedings-First Annual Conference NADT. New Haven, CT: National Association for Drama Therapy, 1, 1980.

_____ "The Diagnostic and Therapeutic Use of Pretend-play." In *Handbook of Play Therapy,* edited by C. Schaefer and K. O'Connor. New York: John Wiley & Sons, Inc., 1983.

Jennings, S. *Drama Therapy: Theory and Practice for Teachers and Clinicians.* Cambridge, MA: Brookline Books, 1987.

_____ *Creative Drama in Groupwork*. London: Winslow Press, 1986.

_____ "Drama Therapy with Families, Groups, and Individuals." in *Waiting in the Wings*. London: Jessica Kingsley, 1990.

_____ and S. L. Sandel. *Waiting at the Gate: Creativity and Hope in the Nursing Home*. New York: Haworth Press, 1987.

_____ "Drama Therapy and the Schizophrenic Condition." In *Drama in Therapy*, Vol. 2, edited by G. Schattner and R. Courtney. New York: Drama Book Specialists, 1981.

Moriyama, M. "Drama Therapy with Alzheimer Patients." National Association for Drama Therapy Conference, New Orleans, LA: Unpublished paper, 1994.

Landy, R. *Drama Therapy: Concepts and Practice*. Springfield, IL: Charles C. Thomas Publishers, 1985.

_____ *Persona and Performance: The Meaning of Role in Drama, Therapy, and Everyday Life*. New York: Guilford Press, 1993.

_____ "Training the Drama Therapist: A Four-Part Model." *The Arts in Psychotherapy* 10 (1983): 175-185.

Read Johnson, D. "The Other Room." *Dramascope* 11, no. 2 (1991): 7.

Read Johnson, D. "Effects of a Theater Experience on Hospitalized Psychiatric Patients." *The Arts in Psychotherapy* 7 (1980): 265–272.

Salas, J. *Improvising Real Life: Personal Story in Playback Theater*. Dubuque, IA: Kendall/Hunt Pub. Co., 1993.

Shatner, G. and R. Courtney. *Drama Therapy* Vol. I and Vol. II. New York: Drama Book Specialists, 1981.

Sternberg, P. and A. Garcia. *Sociodrama: Who's in Your Shoes?* New York: Praeger Press, 1989.

Music Therapy

Jo Salas, M.A., C.M.T.

WHAT IS MUSIC THERAPY?

Music therapy is the use of music, in the context of a therapeutic relationship, to meet treatment goals. It usually involves making music, and uses the qualities of music itself — rhythm, melody, timbre, harmony, pattern, and so on. Music therapy is built on the presence of order and form in music. Self-expression, communication, and integration, the central goals of most forms of therapy, take place within the framework of this artistic medium that is in itself integrated, expressive, and communicative.

Music therapy is used with a wide range of clients, including physically and mentally handicapped adults and children, psychiatric patients, emotionally disturbed children and adolescents, the elderly, and normally functioning people seeking self-awareness and growth. The method and techniques that a music therapist chooses will depend on the needs, capabilities, and musical interests of the clients, as well as on the therapist's own musical and therapeutic background. A music therapist working with a group of elderly women in a nursing home may sit at the piano and play songs carefully chosen from the era of their young womanhood. As they are drawn into the familiar melodies, they also experience connection to one another and to their past; their respiration deepens; memories and emotions are stimulated and shared verbally. Another therapist working individually with a patient in a psychiatric hospital may offer a selection of simple percussion instruments — drums, shakers, a xylophone. With very little talking, the patient and the therapist improvise together, saying things with the music that cannot be said in words. Other possible activities might include group instrumental improvisation; choosing popular songs and relating them to one's life, perhaps by rewriting the lyrics; learning how to play the piano, guitar or trumpet (with the emphasis on the therapeutic process); or songwriting, either full-fledged original songs or "fill-in" songs, where the clients supply words or phrases that require their expressiveness and creativity.

HOW IT BEGAN

Music therapy was developed in the U.S. after World War II (although, of course, music's healing effects have been noted for centuries and in all cultures).

Staff working in VA hospitals observed that their patients improved physically and emotionally after the visits of musicians who came to entertain them. Exploring the use of music in a more deliberate way, musicians and theorists evolved the first methodologies of music therapy. In 1950, the National Association for Music Therapy was formed. Music therapy grew as people realized that it was effective with many different kinds of clinical populations. In 1971, a second association, the American Association for Music Therapy, was created to support broader training and research. As of early 1998, the two associations have merged, becoming the American Music Therapy Association, which will encompass their combined spectrum of philosophies and practices.

HOW IT WORKS

The experience of creativity and mastery is a powerful step in building self-esteem, an important goal for many music therapy clients. Creating a musical piece, learning to sing a song, or simply producing a drumbeat at the right moment may lead to a lasting sense of affirmation. An unsuspected musical talent may be discovered — not as rare as you might think, and particularly valuable for someone who has believed herself to be without talents. Whether a client is especially gifted or not, it is the therapist's task to frame musical activities so that they will be successful and satisfying. This satisfaction can occur on every level, from the chromosomally damaged three-year-old breaking into a crooked smile as he hits the tambourine, to the opera singer recovering from a stroke who finds the courage to use her voice once again.

As in other modalities, music therapy begins with a process of assessing the client's needs and strengths. The therapy will be more effective and enjoyable — and enjoyment is healing in itself — if the therapist is aware of the client's abilities, experience, and interests, especially those directly related to music. Based on that assessment, treatment goals are identified, with the client's participation and agreement, if possible. A goal for a withdrawn adult client in a music therapy group might be to relate to others through vocal and instrumental music. For a troubled adolescent who has been referred for individual music therapy, a goal might be to develop self-esteem and creative self-expression through improvisation and song composition. The therapist establishes an understanding about measuring progress during treatment, either with the client, the client's family or clinic staff, or with the primary therapist, if music therapy is being used adjunctively.

WHAT THE RESEARCH SHOWS

Music therapists have researched the processes and effectiveness of music therapy with many different client groups. In this field, as with the other arts therapies, researchers are still learning the most effective ways to record and investigate their work. Many reports on traditional quantitative research are statistically inconclusive, even though the work they describe is interesting and apparently of value to the clients. The problem lies in accurately describing the phenomena of music therapy, usually too diverse and subtle for quantification. Qualitative case study research methods, increasingly adopted by researchers, tend to yield a clearer picture. One article presents a study of music therapy with a dying cancer patient. The author finds that music therapy can accomplish not only clinical goals, such as reduction of anxiety, but can also engender profound and healing interactions between the patient and family members (Martin, in Bruscia, 1991). Another article presents a four-phase model of early-childhood musical development and discusses the parallels with major models of developmental psychology (Briggs, 1991). In an exploration of music therapy with alcoholics, the researcher reports that participation in group music sessions allows clients to express feelings without their usual recourse to alcohol. Their enjoyment of the sessions leads them to attend consistently, an important factor in the success of the treatment (Dougherty, 1984).

REAL PEOPLE AND MUSIC THERAPY

When Sam was three, he was diagnosed with a malignant brain tumor. He was treated successfully, and he's now a healthy, active, bright six-year-old. But the experience of his horrifying illness has left a mark. He was much too young to understand the pain, the surgeries, the experience of being physically restrained, the strictures of convalescence. He is deeply angry, and most of his anger is aimed at his mother. He refuses to talk at home, although he has an unusually good vocabulary. He has tantrums when it is time to go to school. In spite of being angry at his mother, she's the only person he wants to be with. She understands the causes of his rage, but she's at a loss to know how best to help him. She brings him to me for music therapy, in the hope that Sam might find new ways to express himself.

In his first sessions, Sam flits from one instrument to another. He's especially entranced by the child-size guitar, small enough for little fingers but with a mellow, beautiful sound. He doesn't talk or make eye contact. I listen to him, play with him, accept his choice of verbal silence, invite him — with music — to consider new ideas. He shows himself to be a creative child and, like any artist, he is gratified by his own creations. He begins to look at me directly. He volunteers a question or a comment here and there.

Sam's way of being in the world has been shaped to a large extent by his experience of illness and treatment. Guessing that it must have been an outrage to his spirit to be so helpless and uncomprehending during that time, I design activities that give him a chance to assert the control that he had lost as a three-year-old. He readily accepts the invitation to be the conductor who tells me when and what to play, and when to stop. He learns to exercise a conscious choice over how we spend our time in the sessions. He learns that I will listen when he says what he wants. He talks more and more. His playing becomes increasingly organized and sustained. Together we develop a repertoire of activities that he chooses to return to in each session, often involving vigorous improvisation with drums, cymbal, and other percussion. His music is very expressive, very creative and adventurous, and well-controlled. Sometimes we'll improvise for ten or twelve minutes without stopping.

After about three months, Sam's mother reports that he's less angry at home and more amenable to going to school. He continues to come to therapy, playing his favorite instruments, singing his favorite songs, and playing the games we have devised together.

HOW TO FIND A MUSIC THERAPIST

Music therapists are trained in three areas: clinical theory and practice, music therapy theory and practice, and music itself. Music therapists are required to have enough practical musicianship, including repertoire, to be able to guide and support their clients' musical expression. There are currently four accepted credentials for music therapists: Certified Music Therapist (CMT) or Advanced Certified Music Therapist (ACMT) for graduates of AAMT-affiliated schools; Registered Music Therapist (RMT) for graduates of NAMT-affiliated schools; and Music Therapist, Board Certified (MT-BC), the credential issued by the new association AMTA. To find a music therapist in your area, contact:

AMTA
8455 Colesville Road, Suite 930
Silver Spring, MD 20910

HOW TO LEARN MORE

Boxill, E. H. *Music Therapy for the Developmentally Disabled.* Austin, TX: Pro-Ed., 1985.

Briggs, C. A. "A Model for Understanding Musical Development." *Music Therapy* 10 (1991): 1–21.

Bruscia, K. E. *Case Studies in Music Therapy.* Phoenixville, PA: Barcelona Publishers, 1991.

Dougherty, K. M. "Music Therapy in the Treatment of the Alcoholic Client." *Music Therapy* 4 (1984): 47–54.

Martin, J. A. "Music Therapy at the End of a Life." In *Case Studies in Music Therapy*, edited by K. Bruscia. Phoenixville, PA: Barcelona Publishers, 1991.

Nordoff, P. and C. Robbins. *Music Therapy in Special Education.* New York: John Day, 1971.

Nordoff, P. and C. Robbins. *Creative Music Therapy.* New York: John Day, 1977.

Payne, H., ed. *Handbook of Inquiry in the Arts Therapies: One River, Many Currents.* London: Jessica Kingsley, 1993.

RESOURCES

Journals

Journal of Music Therapy
Publication of the National
Association for Music Therapy
8455 Colesville Road, Suite 930
Silver Spring, MD 20910

Music Therapy
Publication of the American
Association for Music Therapy
P.O. Box 80012
Valley Forge, PA 19484

The Arts in Psychotherapy
Elsevier Science Inc.
660 White Plains Road
Tarrytown, NY 10591-5153

ABOUT THE AUTHORS

Introduction and Art Therapy: Carol Greiff Lagstein, ATR-BC, CSW, has a master's degree in Art Therapy from Pratt Institute and a Masters of Social Work from Columbia University. She is a registered, board certified art therapist and a certified social worker. She has extensive post-graduate training in psychodynamic psychotherapy and family therapy. Currently she is an adjunct professor and coordinator of the undergraduate art therapy program at St. Thomas Aquinas College. She is also in private practice and is the co-director of Teen Power, an organization providing discussion groups and services for adolescent girls and their families, and she works as a social worker in a middle school.

Ms. Greiff Lagstein gratefully acknowledges the generous contributions and support of her friend and mentor, Nana Koch, Ed.D., D.T.R.

Dance Therapy: Sandy Muniz Lieberman, M.M.T., A.D.T.R., is a registered dance therapist with a master's degree in Dance Movement Therapy from Antioch/New England Graduate School. She has had extensive post-graduate training with Janet Adler (authentic movement training) and with Dr. Judith Kestenberg (The Kestenberg Movement Profile). She has worked extensively as a therapist, staff development trainer, and consultant to agencies serving autistic, developmentally disabled people, and preschoolers at risk. She also maintains a private practice in Rockland County, NY. Her current specialization is working with groups of women using the creative arts for personal empowerment and the development of community ritual forms.

Music Therapy: Jo Salas, MA, CMT, holds a master's degree in Music Therapy from New York University. She has worked with emotionally disturbed and learning disabled children and adolescents, and with developmentally disabled adults, in residential treatment, day treatment, and private practice. Her published work on music therapy includes her article "Aesthetic Experience in Music Therapy" (*Music Therapy* Vol. 9, 1) and "Like Singing with a Bird: Improvisational Music Therapy with a Blind Four-Year-Old," co-authored by David Gonzalez (*Case Studies in Music Therapy*, Kenneth Bruscia, ed., Barcelona Publishers, 1991). She is a former member of the editorial board of *Music Therapy*, the professional journal of the AAMT. She is also the author of *Improvising Real Life: Personal Story in Playback Theater* (Kendall/Hunt, 1993).

Drama Therapy: Patricia Sternberg, RDT/BC (Registered Drama Therapist Board Certified), chairs the National Association for Drama Therapy Board of Examiners and serves as a drama therapy consultant to hospitals and schools. She received her master's degree from Villanova University and is a full professor of Theater and Film at Hunter College in New York City. She is currently at work on her eighth book, *Theatre for Conflict Resolution.* Her other books include *Arts for the Handicapped* and *Sociodrama: Who's in Your Shoes?* (with Antonia Garcia). She is a well-known workshop leader, both nationally and internationally.

Fran Segal, Ph.D.

14 Ecopsychology and Holistic Health

WHAT IS ECOPSYCHOLOGY?

Ecopsychology is a holistic clinical practice that acknowledges the importance of meaningful personal relationship with the natural world, both for the healthy functioning of the human psyche and for physical life support. Recognizing that this psychological relationship between nature and people has been severely damaged for much of modern humanity, ecopsychologists have developed theories and practices to help restore this bond, and the resulting sense of belonging to and being a part of the world. In this way, ecopsychology brings the concept of holistic healing into a larger arena than that of just the individual. The ecopsychological view calls for cultural therapy as well as individual therapy. As such, it frees and encourages people to work in both areas.

While ecopsychologists do not encourage reverting to ways of life from the ancient past, there is a growing recognition that valuable ancient wisdom has been lost. By gradually removing ourselves from physical contact with nature, we have lost touch, quite literally, with where we've come from, what sustains us during our lives, and where we return to after death. From a holistic health point of view, this is clearly a psychological and spiritual loss, as well as a physical one. When a baby is permanently separated from a nurturing mother, it loses not only physical sustenance but also a deep psychological and spiritual bond with the life it came from. In this same sense, the urban dweller's separation from nature, our "earth mother," has led to a break of psychological and spiritual bonds to the land, leading to a chronic sense of rootlessness and a feeling of not truly belonging anywhere.

Humanity has gradually separated itself from the rhythms, images, and sensations of nature, so that many people complain of a deep emptiness inside but no longer know what is missing. The break with nature is a devastating form of alienation which, added to other social pressures, has left many, in American society in particular, with no ground to stand on. It has caused instead a profound instability leading to increasing incidences of homicide, suicide, family violence, substance abuse, depression, schizophrenia, and other "mental diseases."

The field of ecopsychology is developing in response to a growing recognition that we are in the middle of an ecological and a psychological crisis, and that these two crises are deeply interrelated. Many ecopsychologists believe that the only way to solve these crises is by bringing individuals and their cultures back into a meaningful relationship with the ecological systems within which they exist. This is most often accomplished through wilderness trips, the use of ritual in natural settings, and the integration of principles of ecopsychology into psychotherapy.

The ideas of ecopsychology represent not just another subfield within psychology, but a set of realizations that must be incorporated into all aspects of theory and practice, if we are to move toward greater holistic health (in the most inclusive sense of mind, body, and planet) in the coming century. The point is well made by Vietnamese Buddhist monk and Nobel peace prize-winner Thich Nhat Hanh, who writes:

> Restoring mental health cannot be simply efforts to adjust man to the modern world with its galloping pace of economic growth. The world is ill. Adaptation to an ill environment cannot be the way to real mental health. Many people who need psychotherapy, as you all know, have been victims of the contemporary life with its lack of meaning . . . Psychiatric treatment requires environmental change and psychiatrists must participate in efforts to change the environment, but that is only half the task. The other half is to help man to be himself, not by helping him adapt to an ill environment, but by providing him with the strength to refuse it and change it. (1985)

HOW IT BEGAN

At one time in human history, nature and culture were intimately related. All human activity was carried out in nature, and the natural rhythms and images that were perceived through the senses filled the human mind, inspired the emotions, and were reflected in the culture through art, ritual, mythology, or other means. This allowed people to feel connected to and a part of the world around them, as indeed they were.

In the European tradition, the forces enlivening these aspects of nature, such as thunder, sun, or sea, were conceived of as "gods" and "goddesses," as in the Greek and Roman pantheons. In other traditions, such as Taoist or Native American, which are still alive today, these life forces were sometimes called "nature spirits." In these traditions and others, qualities in nature were realized to be so related to aspects of the human condition that their culture developed in ways that honored this relationship and the cohabitation of humans and nature on the earth. This aspect of culture was viewed as important for physical, psychological, and spiritual well-being.

The theoretical roots of ecopsychology can be traced to these origins and to the responses that developed when Western culture began turning away from nature. In Europe, nature-oriented literary and philosophical traditions arose in the nineteenth century in reaction to the alienation felt as a result of the Industrial Revolution. The so-called Romantic poets of the British Isles strove to keep alive an emotional sensitivity to nature, writing odes and ballads that expressed the importance of the natural world around them in relation to their inner life. In the realm of philosophy, phenomenologists such as Heidegger described a belief that consciousness is rooted in a particular place in the physical world. Finally at the turn of the century, as the new discipline of psychology was forming, Freud's student Carl Jung began developing concepts such as "anima mundi" or "soul of the earth" reflecting a deep respect for the natural world and the human relationship to it.

The literary tradition continued in the U.S. with Henry David Thoreau's book *Walden Pond*. In 1851 he wrote: ". . . life consists of wildness. When I would recreate myself I seek the darkest wood, the thickest and most interminable and to the citizen, most dismal swamp. I enter as a sacred place, a Sanctum sanctorum. There is the strength, the marrow of nature. In short, all good things are wild and free." Thoreau knew the value of wilderness for healing and rejuvenation, and even in his time he was concerned about the encroachment of civilization into wild areas and the uncaring attitude of the "citizen" toward wilderness.

After Thoreau came other "nature writers" who based their work on their personal inner experiences in wilderness. The insights described in this rich literary tradition, which continues even today, were beginning to ring true with large numbers of readers by the early twentieth century. Perhaps the most well-known and influential of these writers was John Muir, the mountaineer, writer, and activist who founded the Sierra Club and was involved in the creation of the national park system in the 1940s. He wrote in his time that "thousands of tired, nerve-shaken, overcivilized people are beginning to find out that going to the mountains is going home; that wilderness is a necessity; and that mountain parks and reservations are useful not only as fountains of timber and irrigating rivers, but as fountains of life" (Nash, 1967). At the Sierra Club's ninth biennial it was stated that "the parklands of America are the greatest mental health guardian we have" (Nash, 1967).

As this sentiment continued to grow, the disciplines of philosophy, ecology, and psychology came together under various contemporary names such as ecosophy and deep ecology, the latter being a movement founded by Norwegian philosopher Arne Naess. The concept of deep ecology, which quickly spread to the U.S., is perhaps the closest forerunner to the emergence of ecopsychology, because it recognizes that contact with healthy ecosystems is a requirement for human quality of life. Deep ecology also stresses that humanity itself is only one part of an ecosystem in which all parts have value in their own right (i.e., not simply for humanity's use).

Expanding upon these ideas, Bill Devall and other American deep ecology philosophers looked ahead to a possible future for humanity in a sustainable and respectful relationship with nature. Devall states that this relationship, once achieved, will lead humanity toward enhanced creativity, greater time spent in contemplation, and ultimately, to human spiritual development.

Feminist theory, and what is often called feminist earth-based spirituality, which looks to early European paganism, has also played a part in the development of ecopsychology. Feminist historians have brought to light relational, earth-honoring ways of looking at and being in the world, which existed in the European past. These ways were destroyed with the rise of a more patriarchal, Christian culture that denied that nonhuman life was imbued with a soul, and which limited spiritual worship to a "God" who resided only in the sky.

Important historical research has been done in this area by Merlin Stone, Marja Gimbutus, and Riane Eisler. "Ecofeminist" writers, including Carolyn Merchant and Susan Griffin, have pointed to ways in which the oppression of the natural world has been analogous to the oppression of women in the history of male-dominated Western societies.

The contemporary field of transpersonal psychology, based on the premise that all life is inherently related, has also created a fertile ground for the ideas of ecopsychology to grow and develop. Some of the theoretical work in this area draws from Jung's writings, but much is also based directly on Eastern philosophies and on spiritual traditions worldwide.

The deep ecologists' philosophical principles, ecofeminist research and theory, and transpersonal psychology together have set the foundation for the ecopsychological work of nurturing the reemergence of a healthy human/nature relationship.

HOW IT WORKS

Ecopsychology practice has most often taken the form of wilderness trips and nature outings for the purpose of psychological and physical well-being. This began in the 1940s with the formation of Outward Bound. While originally conceived as a survival skills course for young sailors, the Outward Bound programs now aim for "personal development, interpersonal effectiveness, and [the development of] philosophy and values" (Bacon, 1983). These programs and many others that have been developed in recent years are based on physical challenge in the wilderness setting as a means for expanding the boundaries of experience and, ultimately, expanding participants' self-esteem. These programs are now available not only for the general population, but also for various clinical populations such as abused women, delinquent youths, business management teams, and other groups.

There is a second orientation toward use of wilderness experience that is outwardly more spiritual and involves the use of ritual. Probably the most popular of this type of format is the "vision quest," though other ritual forms involving meditation, art, and group process exist as well. The term "vision quest" originally referred to a Native American tradition, although this type of activity has been a part of many earth-based cultures around the world. The use of the term "vision quest" by non-Native Americans has evoked a great deal of controversy, so this phrase is being used less and less by wilderness trip leaders. Vision quest involves preparing to go to the wilderness in search of meaning with the help and support of a group of peers, spending time alone and fasting in the wilderness to seek wisdom or a "vision," and returning to share it with the group and one's society.

The two orientations to wilderness experience, physical challenge and psycho-spiritual ritual, can be seen as two poles on the body/mind continuum in relationship to nature. What becomes clear in their practice is that both are necessary in order to relate to nature as a whole person. Physical challenge helps us go beyond our usual limitations so that we can have a broader range of experiences, and ritual gives meaning to the experience. When physical challenge is used alone, it can easily become a task of "conquering" nature rather than achieving a balanced relationship with it. When ritual is not grounded in exploring physical boundaries, it can become empty theatrics.

Many ecopsychologists have found that there must be continued activity after the conclusion of the wilderness trip that honors and keeps one in touch with the experience, for the sake of the emotional well-being of the participant. Robert Greenway, who led and researched wilderness trips as Professor of Psychology at Sonoma State University throughout the 1970s and 1980s, found that unless there is follow-up of some sort, trip participants could fall into depressions or other emotional/mental states that were less healthy than their states prior to the experiences. He attributes this to the experience of a new level of aliveness in the wilderness being followed by a return to a culture which does not honor these insights. Greenway encourages participants to learn meditation before such a trip, and then to use it as a means of staying in touch with all aspects of one's self after the trip. Creative arts therapies and environmental activism also seem to be effective for this purpose. Devall and Sessions (1985) point out an "obligation to act directly or indirectly to create change in the world toward a greater appreciation of life"; this may mean politics, art, ritual, or another field of endeavor.

The wilderness journey or pilgrimage has been the primary way that the principles of ecopsychology have come into practice. Many other orientations are possible and are developing as the field grows and expands. For example, Joanna Macy and John Seed have developed an ecopsychological form which they call a "Council of All Beings." The council helps participants identify with the natural world by asking each person present to represent one nonhuman life form at the "council," and to advocate for it. As a part of the process, which usually lasts one or two days and includes some outdoor activities, participants are also aided in finding their individual power to act for change.

An ecopsychological perspective also can be brought into the psychotherapy session. While this may not always be the method of choice for the use of ecopsychological concepts, it can often be an important means of introducing clients to an aspect of their lives that may be undervalued or overlooked. How this happens will vary depending on the theoretical orientation of the therapist. For example, a psychodynamically oriented therapist may explore the client's childhood experiences with nature as they relate to current life issues. A behaviorally oriented therapist might begin to incorporate exercises in nature that a client could do on her or his own, as part of a therapeutic treatment plan. The humanistic or expressive arts therapist has the opportunity to bring an ecopsychological orientation to the healing that takes place through creative expression; and the transpersonal therapist can bring a new dimension of meaning to dreams and myths, which so powerfully incorporate universal images of nature. All of these methods are currently being explored.

When we begin to see wilderness as a life partner who mirrors our own depth and richness, supports our growth, and is a part of us at the transpersonal level, then we begin to see how the earth is involved in an ongoing organic process of its own, having inherent value in and of itself. Working with this stage of awareness is now an area of much focus as the theory and practice of ecopsychology continue to develop.

WHAT THE RESEARCH SHOWS

In a review of challenge-based therapeutic use of wilderness experience with emotionally disturbed children and adolescents, delinquent adolescents, and adult psychiatric patients, Peter Gibson (1979) stated that "while many of the empirical studies are of questionable validity due to methodological shortcomings, it is clear that wilderness programs can and do result in positive changes in the self-concepts, personalities, individual behaviors and social functioning of the program participants." In 1987, Willis and Drebing completed a comprehensive research project called "Wilderness Stress Camping as an Adjunctive Therapeutic Modality." In this study they looked at the "virtual explosion" in the number of mental health programs making use of what they call "wilderness stress camping" as a treatment modality. They found that working through the anxiety and fears brought about by these programs served to build self-esteem, enhance self-concept, develop trust, and provide other psychological and sociological benefits. In addition, they felt that the programs were beneficial in providing development of leadership skills, awareness of self in community, and spiritual or mystical experience. Under the category of wilderness stress camping they included a wide range of activities such as rock climbing, group problem-solving, and solitary outings lasting several days. While the authors found that wilderness programs can benefit "just about anyone," they state that they are not advised for "any person who is acutely psychotic, on heavy medications such that balance and other basic functions are severely impaired, highly disorganized, a medical risk as with the possibility of severe seizures, organically impaired as with Alzheimer's disease, undergoing a course of ECT, patients with very poor impulse control who are risks for suicide or homicide, and patients who would otherwise be disqualified due to age or disability" (Drebing and Willis, 1987).

In my own transpersonally-oriented study of people who felt they had meaningful experiences of "communing with nature in wilderness," four major stages of the process could be identified. The stages are 1) an enhanced sensory/perceptual awareness; 2) an enhanced emotional awareness accompanied by an emotional catharsis; 3) a direct experience of union or oneness with the environment (what may be called an enhanced "spiritual" awareness); and 4) an enhanced sense of individuality and creativity accompanied by a desire to somehow "give back" to the world.

In the first stage, heightened sensory awareness is brought about by a rich environment offering unlimited stimulation from an endless variety of sources, e.g., the smell of pine cones, a view of a lake, the feel of a rock, etc. This leads to a fuller integration of the life of the body into consciousness, but can also lead to inner conflict if feeling in the body is blocked by certain mental self-images or ego. As in other holistic bodywork therapies it can be said that certain "blocks" or denials are held in the body and when that part of the body is touched in a certain way, it comes back to life by releasing these blocks. In the wilderness experience, one might say that the body is experiencing the therapeutic touch of nature in an intensive and ongoing way. The process of release is the emotional catharsis, the second stage in the transformational process. The catharsis may focus on life events, past behaviors, or acceptance of one's mortality, for with a true acceptance of the body must also come an acceptance of death. Once consciousness becomes stable in its integration of body awareness, one can move into a realization of the even broader identity of the transpersonal self, beyond the time/space boundaries of ego and body.

This experience has parallels in various spiritual traditions whereby one comes to experience that "I have a mind and body and emotions, but I am not a mind and body and emotions." If one is open and ready for the experience, this type of consciousness seems to occur almost naturally in wilderness settings. In the research, subjects spoke of a "mirroring" quality of the wilderness that allowed them to see themselves with new awareness. They also described having a new awareness of synchronicity between events in the environment and their internal worlds of thoughts and feelings. One subject who had experience with a sense of connectedness that came from meditative practice stated, "When you're meditating . . . what's in you is doing the meditation, but out there the whole thing is a meditation and it's coming into me instead."

The specific mirroring occurrences serve as teachers fostering greater self-awareness, and at the same time fostering the expansion of self-identity into the transpersonal realm. There is a sense of being an integral part of the environment, of being a part of something greater than one's physically separate self, because of the undeniable sensation of everything working together. As human beings, each one of us has a vast internal depth and richness. Wilderness can match this depth and richness and, in this sense, be a partner in our personal growth.

REAL PEOPLE AND ECOPSYCHOLOGY

The following are excerpts from an interview with a woman about her "vision quest" experience.

> I was on this real rocky knife-like ridge and it dropped off very sheerly in both directions. I was getting more scattered, looking at this as a dangerous place, it would be easy to fall off — all that was running through my head. To look down and see these crystals was a way of getting back, literally, in contact with the earth again. . . . I could relax and look at these rocks, and the more I looked at them, the more fascinated I got with them. They were

like clear bubbles of quartz that came out of this real dark, denser kind of lava. So the rock itself was going through this major change . . . and was frozen in that moment of transformation from very dark and dense to much lighter and clearer. . . . My fears had been alienating me from my environment. [I was] in this tense, constricted kind of state like 'oh my God, what am I doing up here?' and the rocks were just so beautiful and striking that they pulled me out of [this condition]. There was a tremendous shift in my attention and my fears were dispelled I know, by the beauty of the rocks. . . . A little bit later I got shaky and looked down and there were the crystals again, so a similar thing happened to me twice on that ridge. [The rocks] became real symbolic for me in terms of expressing for me what I had learned on that trip, going into the dark places within and bringing them to light. So I attached lots of meaning to the whole trip . . . there was a real kind of heart connection for me . . . a sense of loving and being loved, that kind of a flow . . . it's like it's trustworthy, I'm trustworthy. The two really go together. That kind of trusting experience allows for a lot of creativity . . . being able to step out and look at things and not be real afraid. . . .To me being creative is also being able to take risks.

In this scene, the primary sensory input was visual and, as in many wilderness experiences, the enhanced perception involves a sense of beauty. This quality cannot be overestimated in its power to heal by drawing consciousness into the body. Some ecopsychologists believe that the negative sensory stimulation that surrounds modern urban dwellers, such as traffic sirens, dirty air, and even certain "ugly" consumer products, are responsible for the dulling or closing down of the senses. Conversely, in a healthy natural environment, the beauty and harmony of what is perceived encourages the senses to more fully open.

The second stage, or emotional catharsis, in the above example takes place around fear, risk-taking, and being able to trust. In this case, as the experience progressed, the subject began to see her fear as an "internal judge or critical parent that was running rampant . . . my protective little constricted ego." This is not to say that her situation may not have been truly dangerous, but that, in her particular case, she was getting in touch with a more expanded view of herself that helped her feel capable of the attempt she was making, and inspired her to complete it. The beauty of the rocks allowed her to keep her senses open and thus stay in touch with this part of herself.

The third stage, or the transpersonal aspect, is described in this account as a "heart connection." Other people have used words such as "oneness," "belonging," etc., when they had similar experiences. It is also generally described as a point of relaxation and sometimes a sense of being "home."

The fourth stage, wanting to creatively reciprocate or give back to nature, is one which may occur immediately, or not until much later when one has left the wilderness. This woman described this as a very subtle process for her, first manifesting in a greater ability for risk-taking "in order to look at the world" around her, and then as an enhanced feeling of respect and honor for the other life around her. This latter was particularly inspired by an episode which occurred after seeing the rocks. She states:

> I remember being on this one ridge and seeing a juniper tree; and my mother just loves juniper trees. This tree was just beautiful the way it was sculpted by the wind; and it just reminded me very much of my mother and other women from that side of the family, women I would consider really exceptional. They've also endured some severe elements too and so just like the tree has a really unique shape, a unique beauty, not the picture perfect kind of postcard tree or something like a pine or fir with a geometric triangular shape. It was weird and contorted and weathered in some ways and not everybody would find it very beautiful, but I found it very beautiful. That was a real, real special moment to see that again. A strong feeling of reverence and respect, honoring this living thing came up for me.

Trees and animals that appear to mirror human life is a recurring theme in wilderness accounts. Another woman whose entire wilderness experience was centered around a particular tree said, "It looked real wise, and I thought of all the storms it must have weathered that had shaped it the way it was. I thought of some of the storms in my own life and how they had shaped me."

HOW TO FIND A PRACTITIONER

There are no uniform training standards for ecopsychologists, nor are there licensing or certification procedures. Practitioners of ecopsychology come from varying backgrounds and use a variety of clinical practices.

The following organizations can direct you to practitioners with specific kinds of training. Ask for details of the training of the recommended practitioners.

CENTER FOR PSYCHOLOGICAL
AND SOCIAL CHANGE,
HARVARD MEDICAL SCHOOL
Sarah and Lane Conn
51 Winthrop St.
W. Newton, MA 02165
Tel: (617) 965-4893 or -5097

COLORADO OUTWARD BOUND
SCHOOL
945 Pennsylvania St.
Denver, CO 80203-3198
Tel: (303) 837-0880
(Challenge-oriented)

THE INSTITUTES FOR
DEEP ECOLOGY EDUCATION
The Tides Foundation
Box 2290
Boulder, CO 80306
(Education and "Council of All
Beings")

INTERNATIONAL SOCIETY FOR ECOLOGY
AND CULTURE
P.O. Box 9475
Berkeley, CA 94709
Tel: (510) 527-3873
(Combines ecopsychology study and
social/political action groups.)

THE SCHOOL OF LOST BORDERS,
S. FOSTER AND M. LITTLE
Box 55
Big Pine, CA 93513
E-mail: lostbrdrs@telis.org
("Vision Fast" and ecopsychology
trainings)

WILDERNESS GUIDES COUNCIL
P.O. Box 482
Ross, CA 94957
Tel: (415) 456-4370
(A national organization of wilderness
guides who offer ecopsychologically-
oriented wilderness trips.)

Ropes Courses: Usually one day long challenge-oriented courses. Offered through hospitals, camps, and various non-profit organizations.

Private practitioners: Individual practitioners advertise locally. Check references and speak with past clients or participants.

Ecopsychology academic programs: Some psychology programs are beginning to recognize ecopsychology and may be helpful in referring people to practitioners. Current course work or programs exist at California Institute of Integral Studies, San Francisco, CA; JFK University, Orinda, CA; Naropa Institute, Boulder, CO; and Prescott College, Prescott, AZ.

ECOPSYCHOLOGY NEWSLETTER ONLINE:
http://isis.csuhayward.edu/ALSS/ECO/index.html

HOW TO LEARN MORE

Bacon, S. *The Conscious Use of Metaphor in Outward Bound.* Denver, CO: Colorado Outward Bound School, 1983.

Berman, M. *The Reenchantment of the World.* New York: Bantam Books, 1981.

Berry, T. *The Dream of the Earth.* San Francisco: Sierra Club Books, 1988.

Badiner, A. H., ed. *Dharma Gaia.* Berkeley: Parallax Press, 1990.

Brown, M. H. "Wilderness Vision Quest." Proceedings of the Third Annual Wilderness Psychology Group Conference, Morgantown, WV, 1982.

Buber, M. *I and Thou.* Translated by Walter Kayfmann. NY: Charles Scribner's Sons, 1970.

Capra, F. *The Turning Point.* NY: Bantam Books, 1982.

Cass, A., ed. *The Soul Unearthed: Celebrating Wilderness and Personal Renewal Through Nature.* NY: Jeremy P. Tarcher, 1996.

Devall, B. and G. Session. *Deep Ecology.* Layton, UT: Gibbs M. Smith, Inc., 1985.

Drebing, C. E. and S. C. Willis. "Wilderness Stress Camping as an Adjunctive Therapeutic Modality." Western Psych. Assoc., 67th Annual Convention, Long Beach, CA, 1987.

Eisler, R. *The Chalice and the Blade.* San Francisco: Harper and Row, 1988.

Foster, S. and M. Little. *The Book of the Vision Quest: Personal Transformation in the Wilderness.* New York: Prentice Hall, 1980.

Foster, S. and M. Little. *The Roaring of the Sacred River: The Wilderness Quest for Vision and Self-healing.* Big Pine, CA: Lost Borders Press, 1997.

Gablik, S. *The Reenchantment of Art.* NY: Thames and Hudson, 1991.

Gibson, P. M. "Therapeutic Aspects of Wilderness Programs: A Comprehensive Literature Review." *Therapeutic Recreation Journal.* Arlington, VA; National Therapeutic Recreation Society, 2nd quarter. (1979).

Glendinning, C. *My Name is Chellis and I'm in Recovery From Western Civilization.* Boston and London: Shambhala Publications, 1994.

Griffin, S. *Woman and Nature.* NY: Harper and Row, 1978.

Halifax, J. *Shamanism.* NY: The Crossroad Publishing Co., 1982.

Hanh, T. N. "Man and Nature." In *The Path of Compassion*, edited by F. Eppsteiner and D. Maloney. Berkeley, CA: Buddhist Peace Fellowship, 1985.

Heidegger, M. *Being and Time.* NY: Harper and Row, 1962.

Highwater, J. *The Primal Mind.* NY: Harper and Row, 1981.

Hillman, J. and M. Ventura. *We've Had a Hundred Years of Psychotherapy and the World's Getting Worse.* San Francisco: HarperCollins, 1993.

Jung, C. *Two Essays on Analytical Psychology.* Princeton: Princeton University Press, 1966.

Kimball, R. O. "The Wilderness as Therapy." *The Journal of Experiential Education* 5, no. 3 (1983): 6–9.

La Chapelle, D. *Earth Wisdom.* Silverton, CO: Finn Hill Press, 1978.

La Chapelle, D. *Sacred Land, Sacred Sex.* Silverton, CO: Finn Hill Press, 1988.

Macy, J. *World as Lover, World as Self.* Berkeley, CA: Parallax Press, 1991.

Metzner, R. *The Well of Remembrance: Rediscovering the Earth Wisdom Myths of Northern Europe.* Boston and London: Shambhala Publications, Inc., 1994.

Nash, R. *Wilderness and the American Mind.* New Haven and London: Yale University Press, 1967.

Roszak, T. *The Voice of the Earth.* NY: Simon and Schuster, 1992.

Roszak, T., M. E. Gomes, and A. D. Kanner, eds. *Ecopsychology: Restoring the Earth, Healing the Mind.* San Francisco: Sierra Club Books, 1995.

Segal, F. "Ecopsychology: Toward an Integration of Nature and Culture." *Creation Spirituality,* Vol. 9, No. 2. Oakland, CA: Friends of Creation Spirituality, Inc., 1993.

Segal, F. *Wilderness Experience: A Phenomenological Study.* Ann Arbor, MI: University Microfilms International, 1989.

Shepard, P. *Nature and Madness.* San Francisco: Sierra Club Books, 1982.

Spretnak, C. *The Spiritual Dimension of Green Politics.* Santa Fe, NM: Bear and Co.,
    Inc., 1986.

Stone, M. *When God Was a Woman.* NY: Harcourt, Brace, Jovanovich, 1976.

Wilber, K. *No Boundary.* Boston, MA: Shambhala Publications, Inc., 1979.

ABOUT THE AUTHOR

Fran Segal is a writer, artist, and clinical (eco)psychologist in private practice in
Berkeley, CA. Major influences on her work include Jungian/transpersonal psy-
chology, Taoist, Buddhist, and Native American philosophies and disciplines;
and hiking, climbing , skiing and being in the back country of the high Sierra.
She has been leading personal growth-oriented wilderness trips since 1985
when she trained with Outdoor Leadership Training Seminars in Colorado.
Her Ph.D. dissertation research was on "The Experience of Communing with
Nature in Wilderness"; and she has taught "Wilderness Experience and Deep
Ecology" at John F. Kennedy University. As an artist, she is currently designing
and building slate murals, using the natural colors and textures of stone to
enhance the spirit of natural place in urban garden settings.

David McMillin, M.A.

15 Edgar Cayce on Mental Health

WHAT IS THE EDGAR CAYCE APPROACH TO MENTAL HEALTH?

The Edgar Cayce approach offers a comprehensive resource on the prevention, causes, and treatment of mental illness. This body of information covers the full spectrum of mental health problems including depression, anxiety, schizophrenia, personality disorders, relationship difficulties, and childhood behavioral problems. This approach also covers developmental issues such as personal growth and the fulfillment of human potential.

Edgar Cayce provided this information from an altered state of consciousness similar to self-hypnosis. When an individual came to him for a "reading," he entered into this altered state of consciousness, after a brief period of preparation, and then he would verbally describe the cause of the condition and suggest a treatment plan to restore health. Over 14,000 of these psychic discourses were stenographically transcribed, and they have been preserved in the archives of the Edgar Cayce Foundation in Virginia Beach, VA, where they are available for public use. These readings are the foundation of the approach described in this chapter.

In the readings, Cayce recommended a wide variety of modalities and techniques for the treatment of mental and emotional disorders, including physical, mental, and spiritual modalities. Although Cayce recommended a vast array of therapeutic techniques, he consistently maintained that treatments of any kind do not heal. They can only assist the body to heal itself. The therapies, then, were also suggested as preventive measures and for health maintenance for persons recovering from mental illness.

HOW IT BEGAN

Although Cayce (1877–1945) had no formal training either as a medical professional or a psychic diagnostician, he is widely regarded as the father of holistic medicine. Edgar Cayce's career as a medical intuitive began at the age of fifteen, when he spontaneously entered an altered state of consciousness and diagnosed an illness acquired as a result of an accident he suffered while playing baseball. He prescribed a treatment for himself that consisted of a poultice made up of simple, natural ingredients from his mother's kitchen. His parents followed his instructions to create the poultice and he recovered quickly. As he matured and became aware of his potential for helping others, he dedicated his life to alleviating suffering, especially in children. Over a period spanning five decades, Edgar Cayce gave thousands of readings to persons suffering from almost every type of disease. Hundreds of these readings were for persons suffering from mental illness in its myriad forms.

James C. Windsor (1969) and Charles T. Cayce (1978), grandson of Edgar Cayce, later focused on the mental health applications of the Cayce material. Their important work laid the foundation for further development of Edgar Cayce's approach and are highly recommended reading in this area.

HOW IT WORKS

Cayce's approach is a holistic one, in that it addresses the body, the mind, and the spirit. To address the physical pathology associated with mental illness, Cayce commonly prescribed chiropractic treatment, osteopathy, massage therapy, nutrition, exercise, herbal teas, hot packs, electrotherapy (including use of the radial appliance and the wet cell battery, described below), and hydrotherapy. Castor oil packs were recommended to improve assimilation of foods and elimination of wastes from the intestinal tract. For the mental aspects of the illness, he used "suggestive therapeutics" (a form of naturalistic hypnosis), behavior modeling, thought monitoring (mindfulness), visualization, bibliotherapy, and a cognitive restructuring exercise called the "ideals exercise." The spiritual dimension of the approach emphasized awakening the inner self, and included therapeutic milieu, companion therapy, prayer, meditation, color therapy, and music therapy. Following are examples of how these treatments might be applied for two specific types of mental illness.

The Treatment of Depression

Edgar Cayce consistently acknowledged the strong biological aspects of depression in his readings. He defined depression as a "lapse in nerve impulse," a description strikingly similar to the modern medical view that links depression to a chemical imbalance in the nervous system.

Edgar Cayce noted numerous causes of depression. At a physical level, he stated that hereditary predisposition was sometimes a factor. Glandular imbalances (particularly involving the adrenal, thyroid, and pineal glands) were often cited as causes of depression. Injury to the spine was another common causal factor in cases of depression.

From a psychological perspective, depression can be caused by negative thought patterns such as self-condemnation. He often stated that "mind is the builder" and quoted the Biblical verse "as a man thinketh in his heart, so is he" (Proverbs 23:7). Destructive thought patterns are sometimes associated with stressful life events and environmental influences (such as traumatic childhood experiences). Edgar Cayce frequently described the processes by which negative thought patterns are translated into nervous system pathology (hence the "lapse in nerve impulse" in cases of depression).

The spiritual aspects of depression relate to the purpose and meaning of life. Why are we here? What is life about? Edgar Cayce observed that spiritual malaise was often the source of depressive feelings. A lack of spiritual awareness and commitment to growth and development can contribute to depression.

Cayce believed that regardless of the cause(s) of the depressive symptoms, the nervous system is usually involved, so physical therapies such as spinal adjustment, exercise (outdoors in the open), and hydrotherapy (the therapeutic use of water such as steam baths, colonics, etc.) were common recommendations given by Edgar Cayce. He recommended the use of a device called the radial appliance, which operates somewhat like a magnet, redistributing and equalizing the body's own energy, resulting in improved sleep and relaxation.

At the mental level, Cayce suggested various techniques including positive affirmations, bibliotherapy (inspirational reading material), and meditation. From a spiritual perspective, individuals were told to find a purpose in life. He described a technique called the "ideals exercise," in which an individual focuses on the purpose of life and the importance of integrating a spiritual ideal with the mental and physical aspects of living. Also, individuals were encouraged to be of service to others.

Naturally, this holistic approach has to be adapted to the individual. For high functioning persons with mild depression, the treatment is largely a matter of self-care. Other than bodywork (e.g., spinal adjustments and massage) and hydrotherapy, most of the work is done by the individual. For severe depression, more support by health care professionals is required. A residential program such as a clinic may be helpful.

The Treatment of Schizophrenia

As with depression, Edgar Cayce was decades ahead of modern medical science in recognizing the strong biological aspects of schizophrenia. He provided graphic descriptions of the nervous system pathology in this illness. He listed the various causal factors including genetic predisposition, physical insult to the nervous system, biochemical imbalances (often involving the glands), and the role of stress in precipitating psychotic episodes. As with depression, he recommended a holistic therapeutic approach including physical, mental, and spiritual modalities. However, due to the severity of the illness, the role of the health care provider shifted to a more team-oriented model. Edgar Cayce made frequent referrals to the Still-Hildreth Osteopathic Sanitarium in Macon, Missouri (no longer in existence). At this institution, individuals were treated with dignity and respect (in contrast to the state hospitals of that era). They received the full range of treatments including spinal adjustments, hydrotherapy, electrotherapy, diet, and psychosocial rehabilitation.

Edgar Cayce's recommendations for electrotherapy were particularly noteworthy. While recognizing the degeneration of brain nerve tissue in schizophrenia, he stated that the nervous system could be regenerated through the application of electrotherapy. Most often, he prescribed the use of a simple chemical battery (the "wet cell battery"); it produces a very minute direct current and, combined with various medicinal solutions, would he said, stimulate nerve tissue.

In some instances, if families were unable to send their relatives to Still-Hildreth, Edgar Cayce provided recommendations for home treatment. In a couple of exemplary instances, families were able to bring the individuals home from the mental institution, provide the treatments, and gain excellent results with the assistance of their local health care professionals (Smith, 1991).

WHAT THE RESEARCH SHOWS

The health concepts advocated by Edgar Cayce have been researched in a variety of ways, directly and indirectly. For example, the Still-Hildreth Osteopathic Sanitarium (to which Edgar Cayce made frequent referrals in cases of major mental illness) reported very impressive results on the treatment of schizophrenia in an extensive research project involving 860 subjects. Sixty-eight percent of patients admitted within the first six months of the illness were treated and assessed as recovered. The reported recovery rate for people with schizophrenia for over two years was twenty percent (Hildreth, 1938).

Contemporary research has focused on some of the specific therapeutic techniques recommended by Edgar Cayce. Grady (1988) reported an increase in the level of certain hormones and neurotransmitters (chemical messengers of the nervous system) in subjects using the radial appliance (also referred to as the "impedance device"). In a double-blind study of the radial appliance, McMillin and Richards (1995) reported a tendency for improvement of circulation in subjects using the appliance.

Cayce and Thurston (1974) studied Edgar Cayce's recommendations for treating children with behavioral problems. They found that a combination of massage, castor oil packs, and pre-sleep suggestions were helpful in decreasing problems such as fighting, poor sleep, anxiety, etc.

Pecci (1972) reported notable improvement in a study of sixteen children with hyperactive behaviors and seizure problems. Castor oil packs were the primary therapeutic intervention.

The Meridian Institute is a research group dedicated to the scientific study of Edgar Cayce's approach to healing. Research reports are provided free to anyone requesting them. Although the primary research focus is currently on medical disorders, mental and emotional symptoms are often present and are measured in the research protocol.

REAL PEOPLE AND THE EDGAR CAYCE APPROACH TO MENTAL HEALTH

Following is a description of two cases of major mental illness treated by Edgar Cayce himself (Smith, 1991).

The first individual had been a postal worker who became mentally ill and was a patient at the Rockland State Hospital in Orangeburg, New

York. Edgar Cayce's reading for this man stated that he had injured his spine when he slipped and fell on ice while doing his job. As was typical for such cases, Edgar Cayce recommended spinal adjustments and the wet cell battery. The treatments were given as recommended by Edgar Cayce and the man recovered without further hospitalizations or relapse.

The second case cited was a young artist who was physically assaulted and subsequently confined in a mental asylum on Ward's Island in New York. She was psychotic (out of touch with reality) and exhibited the mood swings typical of manic-depressive disorder. As with the previous case, Edgar Cayce described the incident that produced the injury and recommended spinal adjustments and the wet cell battery. Also, in this particular case, noting the psychological damage resulting from the attack which produced the illness, he recommended a change of environment (therapeutic milieu) and companion therapy until she was able to take care of herself. This woman received the treatments advised by Edgar Cayce and was cured of her mental illness.

Contemporary application of Edgar Cayce's approach has also produced positive outcomes. An example is the case of J. K., a middle-aged woman suffering from severe anxiety and suicidal depression. J. K. was recently divorced, struggling financially, and suffering significant gastrointestinal symptoms. She was referred to a medical doctor for an antidepressant medication to address the severe depression. Although she was hesitant to take the medication, she was reminded that it was a temporary measure to help her immediate crisis. This is an example of complementary medicine, as practiced by Edgar Cayce. When people were in crisis, he would utilize whatever therapies were helpful in getting the person stabilized and then pursue a more natural course of healing.

J. K. participated in weekly counseling sessions for about three months to address her attitudes about herself and life. She was able to accept herself and become more empowered by using her will to choose the attitude and behaviors that she wanted to express, rather than feeling victimized.

She was referred to a chiropractor experienced with Cayce's approach. He diagnosed and treated problems with her spine that were contributing to her anxiety and gastrointestinal symptoms. She began using herbal teas (yellow saffron and slippery elm bark) and castor oil packs, therapies recommended by Cayce to heal the gut.

The gastrointestinal connection is often significant in cases involving depression and/or anxiety. As Cayce noted, the abdomen contains its own nervous system and brain, called the enteric nervous system, that "sends and receives impulses, records experiences and responds to emotions. Its nerve cells are bathed and influenced by the same neurotransmitters. The gut can upset the brain just as the brain can upset the gut" (Blakeslee, 1996) This is one of the hottest areas of modern medical research and yet one more example of how the information provided by Edgar Cayce was (and still is in many respects) on the leading edge of medical research and application.

The pattern of healing for J. K. was typical in many ways. Within six to eight weeks she no longer was anxious and depressed. The gastrointestinal symptoms had been eliminated. She went back to school and became a professional massage therapist. She has followed the Edgar Cayce approach for maintaining health and has not had significant emotional symptoms since her recovery (over five years).

As a final example, the case of P. H. illustrates the application of the Edgar Cayce approach for a person suffering from severe and persistent mental illness. P. H. had been in the public mental health system for over fifteen years with multiple and lengthy hospitalizations in psychiatric institutions. At various times she had been diagnosed as having schizophrenia, bipolar disorder, and schizoaffective disorder. She had used the full range of medications and psychiatric rehabilitation procedures typically prescribed for such disorders.

When P. H. came to me for counseling and consulting, she had been involved in an Edgar Cayce study group for several months and was receiving significant support there. The members of the study group (aware of the importance of a healthy spine) recommended that she receive chiropractic treatment, and she did. I provided counseling and consulted with her on the use of the wet cell battery. Within a year of the onset of this treatment regimen, she had obtained a full-time job and gotten married. After four years, she is still married and working. She has not received further psychiatric treatment. Under the supervision of her psychiatrist, she was able gradually to decrease and eventually eliminate psychiatric medications. P. H. reported to me that she believes the wet cell battery and spinal adjustments made a significant contribution to her recovery.

WHAT TO EXPECT

As is evident from the above discussion, there is considerable variability in the application of the Edgar Cayce approach. Depending on the severity of the condition, this approach can vary from being highly self-care–oriented to the involvement of a team of health care professionals.

Whatever the application, it is important to recognize that all healing comes from within. The best that a healer can do is to stimulate and encourage the healing process. In other words, the client/patient must accept responsibility for the healing process. Even in cases of severe disability (such as schizophrenia), the individual is encouraged to be as responsible as possible. If the person is so incoherent as to be irresponsible (e.g., acute psychosis), the persons providing treatment must accept the responsibility for the healing. A spiritual orientation by all persons involved is essential.

The time frame for healing varies depending on the condition. Mild depression and anxiety will often respond within a few weeks. More severe conditions (such as schizophrenia, manic-depressive illness, Alzheimer's disease, etc.) by their nature require long-term application involving months and even years of treatment. Childhood problems such as bed wetting, simple phobias (such as riding a school bus), and thumb sucking are often corrected within a few days or a couple of weeks.

Edgar Cayce utilized the full range of therapeutic options available during his life. Although the treatment recommendations were usually for relatively natural remedies, he was flexible in dealing with each individual. In certain cases he suggested surgery or very strong medications. In modern terminology, the Edgar Cayce approach is an excellent example of complementary medicine. Complementary medicine can be thought of as treatment "in addition to" standard medical practice. Complementary medicine emphasizes cooperation between health care professionals of conventional and alternative therapies. (Budd et al., 1990; LaValley and Verhoef, 1995).

The health care professionals who use the Edgar Cayce approach in their clinical practice will spend time talking with their clients about what is happening in the clients' lives. They will listen closely to the choice of words and how they are spoken to get a sense of the mental and spiritual aspects of the presenting problem. Some practitioners follow Edgar Cayce's example and enlist a medical intuitive to provide input into the therapeutic process. Practitioners often develop their own intuitive abilities to complement their medical training.

HOW TO FIND A PRACTITIONER

The Association for Research and Enlightenment (ARE) maintains a list of health care professionals who utilize the therapeutic principles and techniques recommended by Edgar Cayce. The ARE operates a substantial library, which is open to the public. This library contains all of the Edgar Cayce readings plus numerous books, and audio and video tapes on health related topics. The ARE also operates a bookstore.

Most of the practitioners utilizing the Cayce approach are chiropractors and massage therapists. Massage therapists can receive training in this approach at the Reilly School of Massage Therapy in Virginia Beach (which is associated with the ARE). Atlantic University in Virginia Beach (also associated with the ARE) offers holistic health classes with a strong emphasis on the Edgar Cayce approach. Otherwise, health care professionals educate themselves by studying the Cayce readings and numerous health books and resources available from the ARE. There is no certification process for persons applying this approach.

Practitioners vary in their knowledge of, and experience in, working with the Edgar Cayce approach. Health care practitioners who apply Cayce's system of healing must study the Cayce readings and integrate that information into their clinical practice. They may have limited experience treating major mental illness. It is a good idea to do some background reading to familiarize yourself with Cayce's approach to treating mental illness (see How to Learn More). This can help you to choose a practitioner as well as provide useful information for the self-care aspects of the approach.

The ARE Clinic operates a limited residential program where individuals can receive the full range of therapies recommended in the Edgar Cayce readings.

RESOURCES

THE MERIDIAN INSTITUTE
1168 First Colonial Rd., Suite 12
Virgina Beach, VA 23458
Tel: (757) 496-6009

THE ASSOCIATION FOR RESEARCH
AND ENLIGHTMENT CLINIC
4018 N. 40TH ST.
Phoenix, AZ 85018
Tel: (602) 955-0551

THE ASSOCIATION FOR RESEARCH
AND ENLIGHTENMENT
67th Street and Atlantic Ave.
Virginia Beach, VA 23458
Tel: (757) 428-3588

HOW TO LEARN MORE

Blakeslee, S. "Complex and Hidden Brain in the Gut Makes Cramps, Butterflies, and Valium." *The New York Times,* January 23, 1996, C1-C3.

Budd, C.; B. Fisher; D. Parrinder; and L. Price. "A Model of Cooperation Between Complementary and Allopathic Medicine in a Primary Care Setting." *British Journal of General Practice* 40, no. 338 (1990): 376-378.

Callan, J. P. "Holistic Health or Holistic Hoax?" *Journal of the American Medical Association* 241, no. 11 (1979): 1156.

Cayce, C. T. "Concerning a Physical Basis for Mental Illness." Paper presented at the A.R.E. Medical Symposium in Phoenix, AZ. Available as *Child Development Series No. 9.* Virginia Beach, VA: A.R.E., 1978

Cayce, C. T. and M. Thurston. "Child Behavior Problems." *ARE Journal* May (1974): 108–116.

Grady, H. *Study of the Cayce Impedance Device.* Phoenix, AZ: Fetzer Energy Medicine Research Institute, 1988.

Hildreth, A. G. *The Lengthening Shadow of Dr. Andrew Taylor Still.* Third Edition. Kirksville, MO: Osteopathic Enterprises, Inc., 1938.

LaValley, J. W. and M. J. Verhoef. "Integrating Complementary Medicine and Health Care Services into Practice." *Canadian Medical Association Journal* 153, no. 1 (1995): 45–49.

McGarey, W. A. *Physicians Reference Notebook*. Virginia Beach, VA: ARE Press, 1983.

McMillin, D. *Alzheimer's Disease and the Dementias*. Virginia Beach, VA: LifeLine Press, 1994.

McMillin, D. *Broken Lives: Case Studies in Schizophrenia*. Virginia Beach, VA: LifeLine Press, 1995.

McMillin, D. *Living Nightmares: Case Studies in Anxiety*. Virginia Beach, VA: LifeLine Press, 1992.

McMillin, D. *Principles and Techniques of Nerve Regeneration: Alzheimer's Disease and the Dementias*. Virginia Beach, VA: LifeLine Press, 1995.

McMillin, D. *Shades of Sadness: Case Studies in Depression*. Virginia Beach, VA: LifeLine Press, 1995.

McMillin, D. *The Treatment of Depression*. Virginia Beach, VA: LifeLine Press, 1991.

McMillin, D. *The Treatment of Schizophrenia*. Virginia Beach, VA: LifeLine Press, 1991.

McMillin, D. and D. G. Richards. *The Radial Appliance and Wet Cell Battery: Two Electrotherapeutic Devices Recommended by Edgar Cayce*. Virginia Beach, VA: LifeLine Press, 1995.

Pecci, E. F. "The Relationship Between Emotion and Function in Children." A paper presented at the ARE Medical Symposium in Phoenix, AZ, Jan. 13–16, 1972.

Smith, A. R. "Rachel's Nightmare." *Venture Inward* 7, no. 6 (1991): 12–14.

Windsor, J. C. "A Holistic Theory of Mental Illness." In *Physician's Reference Notebook*, edited by W.A. McGarey. Virginia Beach, VA: ARE Press, 1983.

ABOUT THE AUTHOR

David McMillin, M.A., is a mental health professional living in Virginia Beach, VA. Mr. McMillin received a B.A. in Psychology from Greenville College and an M.A. in Clinical Psychology from Sangagmon State University in Springfield, IL. Mr. McMillin is a researcher with the Meridian Institute and a professor at Atlantic University where he created and taught a course entitled "Principles and Techniques of Energy Medicine." He is the author of six books addressing the treatment of mental illness from the perspective of the Edgar Cayce material. He co-authored a book with Douglas Richards entitled *The Radial Appliance and Wet Cell Battery* and wrote a treatment manual entitled *Principles and Techniques of Nerve Regeneration*. David McMillin lectures and provides workshops on his research and on the clinical application of the Edgar Cayce material.

Doris Rapp, M.D.

16 Environmental Medicine

WHAT IS ENVIRONMENTAL MEDICINE?

The emotional well-being and the learning ability and memory of some children and adults can be adversely affected by what they eat, touch, and smell. Environmental medical physicians estimate that approximately 25 to 50 percent of the population are affected by environmental illness, although many do not know it. This chapter will discuss how to find out which substances trigger these reactions and how to correct the condition.

People affected by allergies and sensitivities often note some of the following on a daily or intermittent basis, depending on the allergen, and the duration and type of exposure:

1. Sudden changes in affect and mood including hyperactivity, irritability, anger, aggression, depression, and vulgarity. Some become excessively tired and withdrawn, or retreat to dark tiny spaces or under furniture.

2. Many of the above complaints are associated with physical illness such as headaches, abdominal pain, muscle aches, asthma, congestion in the nose or eyes, itchy skin, and/or twitches. Excessive infections, especially of the ears, sinuses, and lungs are common. Many of those who are affected appear to have a strong personal or family history of common allergies such as hay fever, asthma, eczema, or hives.

3. Inexplicable changes in their writing or drawing. The letters or numbers

can be abnormally small, large, deformed, in mirror images, upside down, or very different from normal.

4. Periods of poor comprehension of written or spoken information. Some can only read print if it is upside down. Some cannot tell time. Some see letters that whirl about or roll off the page.

5. Changes in speech, such as speaking unusually fast or too loudly. Some repeat the same phrase over and over. Others babble, become hoarse, or cannot speak clearly or at all.

6. The senses of hearing, smell, and touch in environmentally ill persons can be abnormally acute. They may cringe, pull away, and scream if someone tries to touch them. They may be unable to tolerate the sound of normal speech.

7. Some walk with a strange gait, almost falling or tipping over.

8. A few have extreme irrational and unusual behavior. They scream, claim to be out of their bodies, see spiders on the walls, and feel that they have lost control of their bodies.

Multiple chemical sensitivities are a new illness in today's world. This can be debilitating and devastating for those who are affected, and parents, educators, psychologists, and health professionals are often skeptical or unaware of the scope and severity of environment-related illnesses. At the rate that this illness is becoming evident, this will surely change.

HOW IT BEGAN

In our modern society, we are increasingly exposed to large amounts of chemicals that interfere with our health and well-being. In the 1930s, Drs. Albert Rowe and Albert Rowe, Jr. began to study the effects this exposure has on our health. They described a condition called allergic toxemia. They clearly showed that many emotional and physical illnesses could be caused not only by foods, but also by molds, pollen, and dust. They recommended dietary changes and avoidance of known offenders. In the 1940s, Theron Randolph, M.D., wrote about how chemicals can similarly affect the body and mind causing many health complaints such as arthritis and depression. He discussed a condition called allergic fatigue which is increasingly prevalent today. In the 1950s, Fred

Speer, M.D., coined the term Allergic Tension Fatigue Syndrome in children, which was strikingly similar to the illness currently referred to as attention deficit disorder (ADD) or attention deficit hyperactivity disorder (ADHD) seen in both children and adults. He again emphasized diet as a means of relief.

In spite of the fact that fifty years have passed since these revelations, there is still little acceptance on the part of the medical establishment that allergies cause a wide range of physical and mental illnesses. Instead, many highly sophisticated drugs are used as the preferred therapeutic modality. Medicines certainly provide quick temporary relief and their costs are covered by insurance companies. But it is preferable to find and eliminate the cause of an illness.

Insurance carriers will typically pay large sums for drugs and procedures that are scientifically documented but not helpful for many people, while they arbitrarily refuse to pay for alternative methods that relieve symptoms more quickly, effectively, and inexpensively. They claim that the medical literature does not verify the efficacy of these treatments to the satisfaction of the medical establishment in spite of a plethora of scientific evidence (Rea, 1992, 1997).

In recent years, precise, efficient methods of allergy testing have been developed, such as provocation/neutralization testing. This method enables environmental medical specialists to pinpoint medically significant cause-and-effect relationships in minutes. Increasingly, scientific data validate and more fully explain the effectiveness of these methods, which are fast, safe, effective, and inexpensive.

HOW IT WORKS

The human body is now exposed to many chemicals on a daily basis. Our stressed bodies react by eliminating certain chemicals in the urine, feces, perspiration, and exhaled air, but the load of toxins is so heavy that many have to be stored, particularly in the fatty areas of the body. This is damaging, particularly to our immune, endocrine, and reproductive systems. The children and adults of today are not nearly as healthy as those of fifty years ago. They may live longer but the quality of life has suffered. New illnesses have arisen and others have become much more prevalent, such as asthma, cancer, birth anomalies, autism, Alzheimer's disease, Tourette's Syndrome, panic disorder, learning disabilities, and endometriosis, to name only a few.

Let us take a simple example of how the body can be affected. Suppose you breathe in some dust or a mold. This can swell the tissues of your nose and lungs, causing congestion. This decreases the blood supply so infection often develops in the ears, sinuses, or lungs. If you are given antibiotics for the infection, the delicate balance in the intestines is altered, allowing an overgrowth of undesirable yeast and a loss of the necessary lactobacillus organisms. This yeast overgrowth can change how you feel and act. Common manifestations are a white tongue, bloated abdomen, red anus, itchy genitals, and depression.

Chemicals are even more harmful because there is a direct line between the olfactory nerve in the upper part of the nose and the brain. The chemical goes directly into this critical body area and can alter how you think, feel, and act. We can strengthen the body with nutrients and provide basics such as filtered or pure water, proper bowel elimination, and exercise. We can use the newer form of neutralization allergy therapy, so that many allergenic substances, and even a few chemicals, can be tolerated with less or no illness. But the key challenge still remains: How can we avoid or eliminate the rapidly expanding number of allergenic and chemical offenders that surround us? We also need to alter the structure of the health care and insurance industries so that people will be able to afford the care that will help them to get well.

What can you do? Much of the work of detecting and eliminating food and chemical sensitivities can be done at home as self-care. In certain people, there is a need for the intervention of a medical specialist who is knowledgeable about the treatment of multiple sensitivities. You can begin to find and eliminate the cause of your sensitivity by asking yourself what was eaten, touched, or smelled prior to the onset of the symptoms. Ask if the change is due to something inside a home, school, or workplace, outdoors; or due to a food. For example, when exactly did the troublesome symptoms begin? Are they noted mainly after a snack or meal? Is your health a problem during weekdays at school or work, and not evident when you are home, or vice versa? Look around and find out what is special, new, or different in the area where symptoms occur. If it is a food, your symptoms will probably occur shortly after eating. If changes in how you feel, look, or act occur after smelling an odor, think "chemical sensitivity."

To pinpoint the cause, go through the five steps discussed below. Do this before and after entering each room in your home, workplace, or school, before and after meals and chemical exposures. Changes due to foods, beverages, or dust, mold, pollen, or something in the environment usually occur within fifteen minutes to an hour after exposure. Symptoms caused by chemical exposures often occur within seconds to a very few minutes. Once symptoms develop they can last for minutes to days. This varies from individual to individual and on different occasions in the same person. If major changes occur as a result of the following techniques, you are probably very close to finding specific answers to help yourself. One word of caution, however: Do not test for any food that you know causes an alarming or frightening reaction such as severe asthma or unconsciousness.

1. Write your name, the alphabet, or the numbers one to ten. If your ability to do any of these things alters, it indicates that your brain has been affected by exposure or food. For example, if you write well when you go to bed, but cannot write normally when you wake up in the morning, something in the bed or bedroom can be the cause of your learning problems.

2. If you have breathing problems, blow into a Peak Flow Meter. (Please see the Resources section for information about how to order this and other products referred to in this chapter.) This is a plastic tube with an indicator or gauge that moves as you blow into it. A drop of 15 percent is significant. For example, if you blow 400 before you eat and an hour later you can only blow 300, a 25 percent drop, you probably ingested something that diminished your lung function. If you find that a food is the cause of physical or emotional problems, it is often your favorite. Make a list of the five foods and beverages you "cannot live without." If a food item is a problem, you probably included it on your list.

3. Take your pulse for a full minute using a watch with a second hand. A change of 20 when you are quiet and relaxed is unquestionably significant. Also, note if the pulse is regular. It should not suddenly become very fast and then slow down or miss beats. A change in the pulse often indicates that the whole body has suddenly been put into an "alert" mode. It is similar to a smoke alarm that is set off when there is a fire in a room. For example, suppose your pulse rate is routinely 80. You can check an odor in the following manner. Smell the suspect tobacco, perfume, marking pencil, or gasoline for a few seconds. Does your pulse increase to 100 or higher? This degree of change strongly suggests a sensitivity to that exposure. Such individuals will often smell odors before others notice them and complain that odors, such as gasoline, make them ill.

4. Notice how you look. Are your ears or cheeks abnormally red and hot, do you have dark circles under your eyes, or are your legs restless or weak? Were these changes first evident only after the exposure? Such changes provide fast clues. For example, many children and some adults develop brilliant red earlobes and restless legs just before they become uncontrollable, or there is a change in how they act or feel. Some also develop a spaced out or somewhat frightening look in their eyes.

5. Spend a few moments to consider how you felt before exposure to a food or chemical. Compare it to how you felt after you were exposed. This refers to your physical as well as emotional well-being. You may have felt certain emotions (sadness, fear, desperation, etc.) for so long that they seem normal to you, but they may actually be caused by sensitivities more than you realize. Take note of whether these changes occur throughout the course of the day, week, or year, and on an intermittent or constant basis.

Once you have carried out the five steps listed above, before and after various exposures, you can often tell what is causing your illness. One of the benefits of this process is that it helps you realize that some troubling symptoms may be caused by sensitivities, rather than simply being aspects of your personality. On the other hand, some people are so constantly exposed to toxins that they might require a detoxification process before they can properly assess their situation. The next step is to try to eliminate the specific cause.

If the suspected toxin or offending agent is inside a building, look around and find out what is new, different, or unusual in that area. Is there too much dust, mold, or evidence of some chemical? Think of carpets, new construction materials (paint, wallboard, shellac, etc.), new furniture (plywood, vinyl, etc.), pesticides, or scented body or cleaning agents. Are the furnace filters clean? Are the air ducts clean? Try to eliminate the specific cause. An air purifier that can remove dust, molds, pollen, and chemicals might be the answer and it can sometimes help overnight. One can be obtained on a short trial basis and returned if it does not help (see Resources).

For symptoms that occur outdoors, think of pollen, mold, factory pollution, pesticides, fresh asphalt, or other chemicals. If the symptoms are mainly noted on damp rainy days or in wet places, molds may be the cause. If it is the damp or pollen season of the year, you may need an air purifier in your bedroom, in particular, but if this does not relieve the problem, seek allergy treatment for pollen and/or molds from a nearby specialist.

The ideal answer is always to try to eliminate the source. If the cause is pollution, such as outside pesticide spraying, switch to natural lawn care. If the neighbor's lawn pesticides are a problem, and they won't use safer, more natural methods to control their weeds, avoid being home at the time when these chemicals are applied, and keep the windows closed when you are at home. Again, an air purifier might be helpful.

There are a number of methods to help relieve health concerns due to foods and beverages. First you must find the cause. If you suspect a single item, eliminate it in *all* forms from your diet for five to twelve days, and then add it back. If you found that the symptoms stopped when it was avoided and recurred when you reintroduced it, you have found an answer. Avoid that food, or receive allergy extract treatment from a physician familiar with this technique.

If you suspect several foods, try the Multiple Food Elimination Diet discussed in my books *Is This Your Child?* and *Is This Your Child's World?* for one week (see the Resource section). This diet allows most fruits, meats, and vegetables, but it excludes common allergens such as milk, wheat, eggs, chocolate, corn, sugar, orange juice, food dyes, preservatives, and additives. Adults can use the same diet, but should be aware that they must also avoid coffee, tea, alcohol, and tobacco. During the second week, add the foods back one at a time and see which food causes symptoms to reappear. Many people will improve in three to seven days.

Once you become aware of which foods cause symptoms, you can use a rotation diet. This enables you to eat gradually increasing amounts of certain problem foods, but not more than once every four days. In time, certain foods will no longer cause symptoms. Books by Golas (1983) and Powell (1989) can be helpful with implementing this diet. If this diet is combined with neutralization allergy extract treatment, many problem foods can be ingested in normal quantities within a relatively short period of time.

Another way to help diminish food allergies is to aid digestion and detoxification so the body can better utilize various nutrients and foods. There are various dietary programs and supplements that enhance bowel function, the efficiency of the liver, and the normal pathways of the body to eliminate unwanted substances. These include, for example, Dr. Steven Levine's Permavite and Dr. Jeffery Bland's series of "Ultra" products (see Resources).

For a chemical sensitivity, try to remove or avoid the problem chemical whenever possible. If that is impractical or difficult, obtain a Dust-Free air purifier or a Personal Air Purifier on a trial basis for your home, school, or work area.

WHAT THE RESEARCH SHOWS

Space limitations prevent a detailed account of the current research on food and environmental sensitivities, but the interested reader can see Dr. Rea's books, *Chemical Sensitivity, Vol. 1–4* (1992–1997), for a detailed review. The P/N (provocation/neutralization) testing itself often provides convincing proof of the cause-and-effect relationships between foods and chemicals and symptoms. In many cases, when a suspected allergen is introduced into a person's system, a symptom immediately results. When the correct neutralization dose is found, the symptoms abate. For many patients, this is enough "proof."

REAL PEOPLE AND ENVIRONMENTAL AND FOOD SENSITIVITIES

Ryan was initially seen in our medical center when he was four years old. His mother noticed that after he attended school two afternoons a week, he became so fatigued he could barely stand up and he clung to her. His teachers complained that he had other periods when he was unbelievably hyperactive and uncontrollable. His face tended to twitch or tic frequently.

Because his symptoms seemed much worse when he was at school, his mother was advised to go to his classroom and look around. She observed that the table tops in his room and his nap area were sprayed with a popular phenol-containing aerosol disinfectant several times each afternoon. To evaluate this factor, we sprayed a four-inch spot of this aerosol onto a paper towel and then placed it near him. In thirty minutes, his behavior changed. He could not hold a pencil, clung excessively to his mother, whined, and appeared exhausted. These were exactly the types of complaints that were noted during and after school. Oxygen relieved his symptoms in minutes.

The disinfectant for the table tops was switched to Aqueous Zephiran and an air purifier was placed in his classroom. It is of interest to note that the teacher felt there was significantly less infection and absenteeism in that room after these measures were taken. Other teachers have made similar observations after air purifiers were placed in their classrooms.

At one year of age, Liza began to cry and whine constantly for no apparent reason. She also had repeated bronchitis, which perplexed her doctors. Liza's ability to learn was also impaired at certain times. This was first evident at age four when she could not concentrate and remember during swimming lessons. Even though she normally learned easily, she could not concentrate or follow the simplest swimming instructions when she was in the pool. Learning problems due to a chlorine sensitivity were not obvious again until she was twelve years old, and a teacher noted a marked deterioration in the content and the penmanship of a composition she had written. These changes were later traced to the bleach used in the family laundry. The air from the laundry room was vented into the room where she wrote the paper. Liza suffered from chronic recurrent infections and headaches, mainly during the cold months. Her major complaint, however, was severe leg aches. Usually this complaint suggests a dairy allergy, but this was not the case for this child. Since she was a toddler, Liza's parents had to rub her legs every evening or during the night. At times she cried for as long as sixteen hours at a stretch. By the time she reached six years of age, her mother recognized that many foods seemed to cause headaches, vomiting, and problems with learning. It was clearly evident that riding the school bus made her so sick that she would vomit, faint, and sometimes subsequently fall asleep for as long as forty-eight hours. There were periods when she was too weak to walk more than a block or two. No one knew why.

She also had recurrent nosebleeds, easy bruising, and rectal bleeding. When she was only six-and-a-half years old, she had vaginal bleeding. Her knees were black and blue, not from a fall while running or playing, but from unexplained bleeding inside her joints. Repeated medical evaluations did not provide relief or answers.

Liza's mother and father also complained of a number of physical symptoms, many of which were worse in the winter. Her brother had depression and problems with memory and concentration that were also worse during the cold months.

During the summer, four years after they moved into their new home, the family became aware that there was a gas leak in their stove. At that time, it was suggested that they acquire an electric stove. Three days later, Liza's brother stopped having temper outbursts, and his disposition improved remarkably. Liza's legs stopped aching for the first time in years; she no longer cried with leg pain each night. It was apparent that the stove's natural gas leak had caused these problems.

However, later that year, when the weather became colder, the gas furnace was turned on again. Once more the entire family had another flare-up of their previous complaints. They recognized clearly for the first time why their medical symptoms recurred each winter. The cause was a leaking furnace and improper venting of the exhaust fumes. Once they recognized the cause-and-effect relationship, they bought a new furnace, switched their heat to electricity, and corrected their ventilation problems. After this was completed, the winter medical complaints of each family member quickly subsided.

Liza, however, continued to have intermittent illness. The "spreading phenomenon" had become clearly evident. This refers to the reaction noted every so often after certain individuals develop chemical sensitivities because of an initial excessive or prolonged exposure to some chemical. Once sensitized, they find that very little exposure to any chemical odor will cause immediate and sometimes quite severe and prolonged symptoms.

∞

Anita was initially seen when she was thirteen years old. A few weeks before her examination she had been so despondent that she had tried to slash her wrist. She had been ill her entire life, possibly, in part, because her mother had been exposed to many strong chemical cleaning agents at work while she was pregnant. In the uterus, the baby kicked and hiccuped excessively. During that time her nursery was being remodeled, exposing the fetus and later the infant to the chemical odors associated with paint, particleboard, new carpeting, etc. As an infant, she had a feeding problem and vomited frequently. This situation improved when she was switched to a soy-based formula. She had allergies that caused nasal congestion and she did not sleep properly until she was taken from her newly decorated nursery and placed in the living room, which had a wooden floor and older furniture.

Throughout childhood, she suffered from a number of physical complaints. By the age of twelve she rarely felt well. She cried easily and often. When she entered a new school in the fall of that year, she developed a visual problem. She said that the letters seemed to roll off the page and to twirl around, turn upside down, and become double. In spite of her high IQ, she had tremendous difficulty reading and could not learn. She had periods of irritability and hostility and many other symptoms. She was often too tired to get out of bed, and became extremely depressed.

She tried a four-day rotation diet for a few weeks and determined that certain foods made her feel worse. In our office, we tested the suspect foods. After the first day of tests, she noticed improvement in her symptoms. The next day, when we tested her for a mold, suddenly she could not read at all. When we found the correct neutralizing dose of mold allergy extract, she was again able to read. The third day, after we treated her for soy allergy, her normal vision returned. For the first time in weeks, she could read print that was not upside down. By the fourth day, she was remarkably improved and had hope for her future. She was smiling and a totally different young lady than when she entered the office a few days earlier.

Nancy is a young, vibrant, well-trained special education teacher whose symptoms became progressively more evident over a period of about eight years. At first, no one recognized why she was ill, and she wondered why she felt so badly and "out of control" at certain times. Although her complaints were particularly evident when she was in her classroom, it was years before she realized that excessive chemical exposures at work were part of her problem. For example, she repeatedly inhaled the odor of disinfectants because her classroom happened to be located next to the children's lavatories. She did not recognize the obvious cause-and-effect relationship. The combination of chemicals used during school renovations, aerial pesticide spraying, fresh paint in her new apartment, and molds, both at her school and in her waterbed at home, created havoc in her immune system. These various exposures exceeded the level that her body could tolerate, and the result was severe debilitating illness.

She was seen by one physician after another. No one recognized the true cause of her sickness. After many tests, she was told that she was stressed, and her health problems would go away if she would just calm down. At one point, she was advised to see a psychiatrist who told her to "tough it out" when she felt dizzy. Her extreme exhaustion, muscle weakness, constant ear ringing, and severe depression finally forced her to take a leave of absence for ten weeks in the spring of 1991. At that time, she was too tired to get out of bed, take a shower, or prepare a snack. She cried most of the time and became so ill that it took twenty minutes for her to crawl the few steps from her bedroom to the bathroom. She lost her self-confidence and thought she must be a weak or bad person because she couldn't control her moods or regain her physical health. Little did she realize that her depression was biochemical and could be helped by dietary regulation and environmental changes.

When Nancy was seen by an environmental physician, she was complaining of the following symptoms: extreme fatigue, muscle aches/spasms, mood swings, excessive crying, leg cramps and pain, numbness of fingers and face, ringing in the ears, irritability, dizziness and blackouts, headaches, a heavy head, difficulty concentrating, nausea, abdominal pain, and difficulty focusing. Most physicians who hear a list of complaints of this type have been taught that such patients have a psychological problem, but this variety and number of symptoms are typical of many chemically-sensitized adults and children.

Challenge Testing with individual allergy extract solutions easily reproduced some of the above symptoms. Most notable was the trouble she had thinking clearly and the depression, anger, and crying that resulted from a test with the air from Nancy's school. A single drop of several standard allergy extracts (dust mites, molds, phenol) provoked symptoms. Within eight to ten minutes she experienced facial numbness; heaviness in her head; fatigue; swelling of the mouth and cheeks; itching and burning of her eyes; pressure in her ears; pain and tightness in her jaw; cramping of her hands and feet; facial pain; a hot feeling in her face; dizziness; vertigo; numbness in her hands, feet, and face; difficulty talking; a rapid heartbeat; extreme fatigue; and a metallic taste in her mouth. These reactions all subsided in about ten minutes after Nancy received one drop of the correct neutralizing dilution of the same allergy extract that caused the response. At one point she was given a placebo, a mock injection, which caused no change in how she felt or acted. At no time was she aware of which item was being tested.

At the end of the last test, she had a frightening response of the type that had previously occurred at school. She suddenly ran wildly, from the office into the parking lot, using vulgar language and screaming. Her car keys had to be taken from her because her companion was aware that in the past she had driven at a reckless speed when this happened.

After a thorough clinical evaluation, she was found to be sensitive to foods, dust, molds, pollen, and chemicals. She also lacked some essential nutrients. After she received allergy extract treatment for the various substances to which she was sensitive, her symptoms markedly improved. This comprehensive environmental medical therapy was combined with detoxification, which included exercise, massage, saunas, and frequent intravenous nutrient therapy. For a year she also drank a formulation called Ultraclear, an oral detoxification formula. After two years of this type of therapy she stated, "I feel so well that it is a foreign feeling for me. I honestly look forward to what is yet to come. It's all up from here!"

She was fortunate because her family provided positive support during her ordeal. In time, they realized that she had a genuine illness, and they learned how to detect the cause of her unusual responses to specific inadvertent exposures. For her and her family, it was a relief to understand what caused her reactions.

In September 1994, however, she found she was without funds or a job. She could not afford the allergy extract therapy that had helped her maintain her health. She did not want to fight for insurance coverage, social security, worker's compensation, or disability aid. She decided to investigate alternative methods of help, trying shiatsu, a form of acupressure, and energy balancing. Shiatsu was so helpful that, in time, she was able to discontinue her allergy extract therapy, her extremely strict rotation diet, and all her nutrients except for vitamin C. However, she found that she had to continue to avoid chemicals, drink purified water, and eat organic foods while limiting or avoiding certain major food offenders. At times, she finds that she can tolerate certain exposures that previously caused devastating and debilitating effects. If she is very cautious, she can now go to church. She can shop in a mall for about ten minutes, something she had dared not consider for many months. She can visit friends, have a real Christmas tree, and even cautiously attend a concert. She is rarely without her charcoal mask and is constantly on guard and fearful that she will be exposed to something that will cause a setback. If her symptoms flare because of an exposure, especially if she is stressed, she uses vitamin C, alkaline trisalts, shiatsu, and meditation. Although she continues to find certain exposures impossibly challenging and incapacitating, she is encouraged because she is gradually improving. She is presently back at school, in a different room, and, by using good judgment, extreme caution, and avoidance, she has adjusted to a different, but far more normal, and acceptable lifestyle.

WHAT TO EXPECT

If you visit a physician trained in environmental medicine, he or she will typically study your previous records, and do a very detailed history and physical examination. A number of blood tests are often indicated to check for common illnesses and allergies. In addition, provocation/neutralization or special titration allergy skin tests can be most helpful. These tests can document whether or not allergies are a problem. For the provocation/neutralization (P/N) test, one drop of a strong extract of a suspected allergen is injected into the arm. If you are allergic to this substance, symptoms often appear. Then, one drop of this same extract, which has been diluted five fold, is administered. This process of administering weaker dilutions of the extract will be repeated every eight minutes until the symptoms disappear. This dose is called the neutralization dose. P/N testing enables a physician to pinpoint specific cause-and-effect relationships. By injection of this dilution into the arm, you can prevent or treat the allergy. Titration skin tests are a more complex version of this test that allow for more precise testing and treatment for allergies to dust, pollen, and mold in particular.

A typical program of environmental evaluation and patient education will include recommendations for dietary changes, and ways to make a home more safe and allergy-free. Exercise, adequate hydration with pure water, and excellent bowel function are given detailed consideration. Special additional tests also might be indicated for certain patients who have particularly complex problems that have not responded adequately to the above program.

HOW TO FIND AN ENVIRONMENTAL MEDICAL SPECIALIST

There are physicians scattered over the United States who are trained in environmental medicine. You can call The American Academy of Environmental Medicine at (215) 862-4544, or write to them at P.O Box CN 1001-8001, 10 East Randolph Street, New Hope, PA 18938 to find the nearest trained specialist. These physicians are usually board-certified in one or more other specialties in medicine. In addition, they have taken special courses, and passed oral and written examinations.

RESOURCES

For more details about any aspect of this chapter, it is strongly suggested that you read, *Is This Your Child's World?* or *Is This Your Child?* These books are listed below and are as valuable for adults as they are for children. In addition, a video, "Environmentally Sick Schools," is available which vividly demonstrates how exposures to dust, molds, pollen, chemicals, and certain foods can alter how some people feel, act, learn, and behave.

Call Practical Allergy Research Foundation (PARF) at (716) 875-0398 for Dust Free or other air purifiers, for Peak Flow Meters to detect causes of breathing problems, and for many of the resource books listed below (marked with an asterisk). Or write to PARF at 1421 Colvin Blvd., Buffalo, NY, 14223.

Call National Ecological and Environmental Delivery System (NEEDS) at

(800) 634-1380 for the Personal Air Supply and many other products useful to chemically sensitive people. Their address is 527 Charles Ave., Suite 12 A, Syracuse, NY, 13209.

The detoxification preparations referred to above can be ordered from Allergy Research Group, 400 Preda St., PO Box 489, San Leandro, CA, 94577-0489, (800) 545-9960, and from HealthComm International, 5800 Southview Dr., Gig Harbor, WA 98335, (206) 851-3943.

HOW TO LEARN MORE

Ashford, N. and C. Miller. *Chemical Exposures: Low Levels and High Stakes.* New York: Van Nostrand Reinhold, 1991.*

Colborn, T., D. Dumanski, and J. P. Myers. *Our Stolen Future: Are We Threatening Our Fertility, Intelligence, and Survival? A Scientific Detective Story.* New York: Dutton, 1996.

Dunford, R. and K. May. *Your Health and the Indoor Environment.* Dallas: NuDawn Publishing, 1991.

Durnil, G. *The Making of a Conservative Environmentalist.* Bloomington, IN: Indiana University Press, 1995.

Golas, N. and F. G. Golbitz. *If This Is Tuesday, It Must Be Chicken.* New Canaan, CT: Keats Publishing Co., 1983.*

Green, N. S. *Poisoning Our Children: Surviving in a Toxic World.* Chicago: Noble Press, 1991.

Krohn, J. *The Whole Way to Allergy Relief & Prevention.* Second Edition. Point Roberts, WA: Hartley and Marks, Inc., 1996.*

Krohn, J. *The Whole Way to Natural Detoxification.* Point Roberts, WA: Hartley and Marks Publishers, 1996.*

Lawson, L. *Staying Well in a Toxic World.* Chicago: Noble Press, 1993.

Matthews, B. L. *Chemical Sensitivity.* Jefferson, NC: McFarland and Co., 1992.*

Moses, M. *Designer Poisons.* San Francisco: Pesticide Education Center, 1995.

Powell, D. *Why 5? A Complete Food Allergy Diet Book.* Waterdown, Ontario: Cobra Limited, 1989.*

Randolph, T. and R. Moss. *An Alternative Approach to Allergies.* New York: Harper & Row Publishers, 1989.*

Rapp, D. J. *Is This Your Child?* New York: William Morrow, 1991.*

Rapp, D. J. *Is This Your Child's World?* New York: Bantam Publishing, 1996.*

Rapp, D. J. *The Impossible Child at School and at Home.* Buffalo, NY: PARF, 1989.*

Rea, W. *Chemical Sensitivity,* Vols. 1, 2, 3 and 4. Boca Raton, FL: Lewis Publishers, 1992–1997. Available through the American Environmental Health Foundation, 8345 Walnut Hill Lane, Suite 225, Dallas, TX 75231. (800) 428-2343 or (214) 361-9515.

Regenstein, L. G. *Cleaning Up America the Poisoned.* Washington, DC: Acropolis Books, 1993.*

Rogers, S. *Tired or Toxic?* Syracuse, NY: Prestige Publishing, 1990.*

Rousseau, D., W. Rea, and J. Enwright. *Your Home, Health and Well-Being.* Vancouver: Hartley & Marks, 1989.*

Wilson, C. *Chemical Exposures and Human Health.* Jefferson, NC: McFarland and Co., 1993.

Tate, N. *The Sick Building Syndrome.* Far Hills, NH: New Horizon Press, 1994.

Thrasher, J. and A. Broughton. *The Poisoning of Our Homes and Workplaces.* Santa Ana, CA: Seadora, 1989.

* Can be ordered through PARF, see the "Resources" section.

ABOUT THE AUTHOR

Doris Rapp was born in Erie, PA, and knew from the age of four that she wanted to be a physician. She earned her B.A. degree, magna cum laude, and an M.A. degree from the University of Buffalo. She studied medicine at New York University, Bellevue Medical Center, followed by training in Pediatrics and a fellowship in Allergy and Immunology. She practiced conventional pediatric allergy medicine until 1975, when she attended a conference on newer approaches to allergy detection and treatment. This changed her life and her method of treating patients. Since that time, she has used these newer, more effective techniques to help patients. She also has written books about their effectiveness; she believes the public should not have to wait to hear about more effective treatment techniques due simply to the medical establishment's reluctance to acknowledge newer ways that have repeatedly proven beneficial. She presently lives, practices, researches, and writes in Arizona.

Wes Sime, Ph.D., M.P.H., Ph.D.

17 Exercise Therapy:
Working Out the Problem

WHAT IS EXERCISE THERAPY?

Exercise therapy (also called walk/talk therapy) is the practice of combining a program of exercise with traditional psychotherapy. The exercise is carried out within the session, under the guidance of the therapist. In addition to the weekly walk/talk therapy sessions, the client is encouraged to establish a regular program of daily exercise which, ideally, would continue long after the therapy has concluded.

Adding exercise to psychotherapy can be beneficial for people suffering from a wide variety of mental health issues and interpersonal problems. These include depression, anxiety, addictions, irritability, and confusion. It is also good for overall health and for self-actualization.

Exercise therapy can be combined successfully with a number of other traditional, mainstream therapies, as well as nontraditional health care procedures. This is particularly true of healing arts that might help with physical recovery from the traumatic aspects of exercise, help people get in touch with bodily reactions to outside influences or recognize subtle changes in body position and alignment. It is advisable to use caution when combining exercise therapy with methods that dramatically alter biochemistry of the body; it is possible that dietary or pharmaceutical interventions may influence the blood sugar levels in such a manner as to compromise or intensify exercise effects.

It should be emphasized that walking is not the only effective method of exercise during psychotherapy, but it is the most convenient and readily accessible safe method. Jogging is effective, as long as the pace is slow enough to allow comfortable conversation. Hiking up mountain trails is perhaps more aesthetically desirable and physically stimulating than walking on flat ground, and biking is certainly feasible, though somewhat dangerous if the conversation detracts from attention to the path or roadway.

HOW IT BEGAN

Since the time of Hypocrites (460–377 B.C.), exercise has been viewed as a primary component of the "healing power of nature." Throughout history, many other medical philosophers have declared the virtues of exercise without necessarily offering a rational scientific explanation about the mechanism by which it works.

In the last half century, technological advancements in labor-saving conveniences have reduced the need for physical exercise in daily living. Motorized transportation has virtually eliminated walking or bicycling to work. Most tasks in factories and industry have become at least semi-automated, so that what previously had been a physically demanding task, such as lifting or pushing, now is accomplished by some hoist, lift, or other powered device.

The first recorded sessions of exercise (walk/talk) therapy were conducted in the middle of this century by Thaddeus Kostrubula, a psychiatrist who practiced in San Diego, California. He took many of his patients walking on the beach and eventually wrote the book *The Joy of Running* (1976). Kostrubula firmly believed that the cathartic ("getting it off your chest") effects of physical exertion carry over into psychological catharsis. He felt it only logical that he, as a trained clinician, should be on the scene to effectively process the rich source of emotionally-charged material as it came forth. Many other health care professionals have taken to recommending exercise for their clients, but one in particular has written about the objective procedures needed to prescribe exercise for depression and anxiety (Johnsgaard, 1989).

The modern history of exercise therapy is defined by the professional careers of Kostrubula, Johnsgaard, and Sime. There are very few others who have clinical credentials to treat mental health issues and who opt to conduct the combined walk/talk therapy.

HOW IT WORKS

Johnsgaard (1989) reports that during exercise, his clients loosen up, become less inhibited, less self-conscious, and more in touch with their immediate feelings and experience. He says they tend to become more energized and seem more inclined to talk about their own needs and feelings. At a brisk pace of walking, clients are more likely to get in touch with their anger and their need to assert themselves, which is extremely helpful for those who tend to repress their anger and defer to the needs and concerns of others.

As a therapist, I find that brisk activity (such as walking side-by-side with the client) helps to break down barriers and encourages people to engage in difficult topics of conversation. In addition, it is highly therapeutic and cathartic (aids in "getting it all out") when the issues are complicated or entangled. Walking helps stimulate both the client and the therapist to be alert and creative in the problem-solving process. In addition, the constantly changing scenery seems to be refreshing for most clients. There is less face-to-face interaction when both client and therapist are walking. This allows the therapist to pose difficult questions or confrontive interpretations without inadvertently putting added pressure on the client due to direct eye contact, which might seem to call for an immediate reply. Similarly, if the client is having difficulty formulating a response, gazing at the scenery or focusing on walking seems to help create an informal atmosphere that allows more spontaneous responses.

WHAT THE RESEARCH SHOWS

Numerous scientific studies have documented the association between habitual exercise and positive mood and affect (Steptoe et al., 1993; Berger and Owen, 1992; Byrne and Byrne, 1993; Daniels et al., 1992). Groups of individuals accustomed to a regular routine of physical labor on the job, or to moderately intense leisure exercise or competitive games (basketball, racquet ball, jogging, etc.), report that they feel better when they exercise. In most cases, they experience mild withdrawal symptoms if they stop due to injury or if they fail to maintain a regular schedule of exercise (at least once every two or three days) (Rajala et al., 1994; Weyerer, 1992). Part of the benefit associated with exercise is an increase in self-esteem (McAuley et al., 1991). Feeling good about one's self comes through accomplishment as well as through a change in body tone or fitness (Fisher and Thompson, 1994).

There are many possible reasons why exercise benefits mental health. The first is the so-called thermogenic theory, which states that the increased metabolism associated with exercise generates body heat and perspiration, which, in turn, causes biochemical changes in the body that are associated with mood elevation (DeVries et al., 1968). Both heat and cold tolerance have been shown to improve with enhanced emotion stability as an outcome of exercise training (Dienstbier et al., 1987). Another theory is that the increase in respiration due to exercise has some potential benefit. Individuals who have a tendency to hyperventilate or who have other breathing problems (Fried, 1990) seem to benefit from an exercise program.

The physical fatigue associated with an extended program of exercise helps people relax, improves the quality of sleep (Bliwise et al., 1992), and minimizes the immediate impact of stress and the frustration of daily living. To a certain extent, it may be that the distraction of enjoyable movement or the mild discomfort of physical labor keeps one's mind off other problems (Roth et al., 1990). Note here that the enjoyment of music, movement, and dancing also is associated with mood elevation.

There are two specific biochemical changes associated with mood and exercise. Endorphins, the body's natural painkillers, are released during any form of mild, moderate, or severe trauma (such as injury, childbirth, or surgery.) This includes exercise, which necessarily elicits very small tears in the muscle and other soft tissues surrounding joints that are under physical load. It seems that the body releases endorphins to accommodate the muscle/joint discomfort, and this simultaneously causes mood elevation in most people (Lobstein and Rasmussen, 1991). Secondly, several other chemicals (serotonin, dopamine, and norepinephrine) that are essential in normal nerve communication and sensory awareness (touch, pressure, motion) also have a positive influence on sleep quality and duration (Dey, Singh, and Dey, 1992). It also should be noted that the interaction of the physical effects of exercise (thermogenic, tension reduction, and biochemical anesthesia), together with a feeling of accomplishment and a sense of well-being about weight loss and a fit, trim body, are a part of the positive effects. (Some people might experience the added satisfaction of saving money on commuting by walking to work, or on errands).

It appears that aerobic (running, swimming) and anaerobic exercise (weight lifting, strength training) are equally effective for achieving mental health benefits (Johnston et al., 1993; Folkins and Sime, 1981; Norvell and Belles, 1993).

Regarding the dosage required (frequency, intensity, duration), it does not appear that there is a direct relationship between the amount of exercise and the mental health benefits (Hobson and Rejeski, 1993). In fact, it appears from some studies that high-intensity aerobic activity is not absolutely required to achieve mental health benefits (Blumenthal et al., 1991). However, there is recent evidence showing that regular exercisers (six days/week for forty-five minutes of moderately intense activity) who are deprived of exercise arbitrarily suffer substantial withdrawal symptoms (muscle tremor, sleep disturbance, anxiety, depression, fatigue and confusion) after just twenty-four to forty-eight hours (Mondin et al., 1996). These symptoms subside quickly upon return to regular exercise.

REAL PEOPLE AND EXERCISE

Don was 30 years old and unemployed when he came for therapy due to depression. He had a history of marijuana usage that compounded his depressive symptoms. His financial problems were such that he had no form of transportation to use in looking for work. His only motivation for work was to satisfy his basic needs and that of his recreational drug habit. His psychiatrist insisted on counseling, in addition to the medications prescribed for depression and for a mild form of anxiety, which also is often present among depressed patients. Don verbalized his sincere intent to find work and to reduce or stop the marijuana use, but he was very discouraged about his prospects. Circumstance brought him a job in the parts department of a company owned by a distant family member. He still had a transportation problem and lived about five miles from work. He found a neighbor who would drop him off on the way to do other errands on most of his work days. There was no ride home, so Don was obliged to walk the distance. He agreed with the therapist that walking would be good for him, but he also resisted initially, thinking that it would be distasteful, boring, and would make him sweat, something he hated. After the first few days of work and walking home, the client sheepishly revealed in the counseling session that he rather enjoyed being outside by himself. He had discovered a quiet route by a railroad track and he found that he definitely enjoyed the walk and his shower upon arriving home. The unexpected benefit was that Don found that his urge to use marijuana diminished also, as he was more relaxed and content upon completing the walk home from work. Later he was able to buy a bicycle, so he was not dependent on the neighbor for his ride to work in the morning. Don's experience was not a complete success, since he did fluctuate in his discipline to maintain the exercise habit and his abstinence from the marijuana. His strongest motivation to continue or to renew the practice was the absence of his depression symptoms.

Amy is a 53-year-old female client who suffers from severe anxiety attacks and mild depression. She is married with no children, and had a fairly distasteful childhood as her father was an alcoholic and her mother contracted throat cancer when Amy was an adolescent. She had to care for her mother, who lost her voice and her physical attractiveness rapidly with the progression of the cancer. Both of her parents died very early, and her marriage was a mess. Her blood pressure was elevated, which I treated with relaxation, biofeedback, and counseling for several months with only modest success. The client preferred the counseling sessions and showed good progress in facing her marital situation.

Her job was the single most satisfying element in her life. Her boss, with whom she had had an affair in previous years, was something of a father figure to her. She was in awe of him, partly because she could gain his considerable recognition by performing her executive secretarial duties exceptionally well. Her life was not fulfilling and her ability to confront issues was extremely limited. She had a dependent personality style. Upon the discovery that this client loved the outdoors and loved to walk, I offered this mode of interaction as part of our therapy sessions. We agreed, however, that the walk/talk therapy would continue only as long as Amy was willing to remain open to confronting issues related to her lifestyle and her childhood issues of abuse, neglect, etc. She responded exceptionally well. It became quite common for her to lash out at me with a line of colorful swear words as she responded to my provocative questions and interpretations. This grew into a wonderful banter of teasing remarks, followed by her swearing at me. But in the midst of the swearing she began to acknowledge that those issues did, in fact, bother her a great deal and that it was permissible for her to vent her anger at the father figure through me. In essence, the walk/talk therapy opened new dimensions to therapy than those available in the stifling confines of a cramped clinical office with dead air and no change in scenery. This client moved away about four years ago, but returns once or twice each year to check in with me and she insists that our sessions be active.

WHAT TO EXPECT

Most clients under the age of 40 who have not had prior medical complications (neurological disorder, orthopedic limitations, back injury, endocrine disorder such as diabetes, or heart attack symptoms) can usually make the decision for themselves that a moderately intense, gradually increasing program of exercise is safe for them. In general, if you have a typical lifestyle that includes walking while shopping, climbing stairs as needed and conducting routine leisure activities without compromise, then you can probably assume that the walk/talk therapy, together with a well-designed personal exercise program, is safe. On the other hand, if you are over 50 years old and have experienced any symptoms of compromised cardiovascular functioning (shortness of breath, slight chest pain, fatigue, etc.), it is very important to see a physician and perhaps have an exercise tolerance test.

Your exercise plan need not be overly ambitious or vigorous in order to be effective in providing mental health benefits. Enjoyment of the activity is more important than intensity. While "no pain, no gain" may be the theme for weight lifters and marathon runners, it is not essential for the average, previously sedentary person and, in fact, it could be detrimental for some individuals who seek physical and emotional relief from their symptoms. The bottom line is that every person is unique and the response he or she has to a particular bout of exertion should be evaluated in order to adjust the next bout of exercise. To be specific, if you hope to jog as your friends and neighbors do, but you can't seem to continue running for more than a couple of minutes without stopping to rest — that's okay. The idea is to run as slowly as possible until something is uncomfortable (shortness of breath or your legs hurt), then walk until you are bored or eager to get going. Then run again and this time you may be able to tolerate a longer bout of exercise before needing to rest. This is the natural process of working up to a fast pace of running. If exercise makes your legs sore and stiff, or if you are persistently fatigued the day after your exercise session, then you have probably overdone it and you should ease back a little in the next session. By contrast, if you do not experience any emotional symptom relief, then perhaps the intensity and duration is insufficient or the type of activity you have chosen is simply not appropriate for you.

If you go to see an exercise therapist, he or she will likely ask about your previous experiences with exercise, and about the history of the emotional issues that you want to work on. I have developed the following questionnaire that can be used to help you think about your own history with exercise.

Lifestyle Survey of Past and Present Activity Patterns

- What memories do you have about playing games outdoors as a child? Did you play vigorous and prolonged games involving running that were enjoyable, satisfying, or fun? If so, do you ever seek to relive those experiences in some way that reproduces the sensation of the fun and some of the movement and activity?

- In your adolescent years, what kinds of competitive games or recreational activities did you participate in on a regular basis? Were these vigorous games or leisure activities that required some endurance on your part? If so, do you ever wish to relive those experiences for the competitive or recreational value that you enjoyed at the time?

- What kind of physical activity is a part of your regular habit pattern these days? Do you walk your dog, play games with children, work on the lawn and in the garden, play recreational games, go on walks or bike rides, or swim?

- Does your current employment require any type of vigorous physical activity?

- In your past work history, what kinds of jobs required fairly heavy amounts of physical work (lifting, carrying, sweeping, etc.)? Were these jobs reward-ing in ways other than monetary compensation (i.e., did you feel a sense of satisfaction upon completion of a job well done, or did you appreciate the sense of relief and well-being associated with the end of a hard day)? If so, do you ever long to again experience some aspect of the hard-work ethic and feeling of accomplishment?

- Are there alternative ways to commute to your job (i.e., can you take a bus or train part way and walk some distance; can you drive part way and save on parking by walking the additional distance; can you get a ride with someone and then walk or ride a bike home on some occasions)? If so, would you be willing to make some accommodations in order to build an exercise program into your regular "get to work" time?

- Do you recall any positive experiences (pleasure, joy, satisfaction, reward, energy) with walking, jogging, running, biking, swimming, stair climbing, etc. that would influence you to establish or renew a pattern of exercise that includes those activities?

- Do you recall any very negative experiences (fatigue, discomfort, irritabili-ty, aggravation, bad feelings about sweat/perspiration, etc.) that would make it hard for you to start some kind of regular exercise program?

- Does your spouse participate in exercise programs, or does he or she encourage you to exercise? Would your spouse be willing to help you find opportunities for exercise and resulting rewards?

- Do you have a friend with whom you would enjoy participating in an activity (besides fishing) that requires some vigorous, perhaps friendly competition? If so, would you be willing to get him or her to participate with you on a regular basis?

The course of exertional talk therapy might be as short as one or two visits (for a highly receptive and low-risk client), or it might take a regular program over six to eight weekly visits to work up to a sufficient duration and intensity of exercise to produce the desired effects.

Risks and Pitfalls

- There is a strong tendency for many people to overdo therapeutic exercise. This can cause strain, pain, or injury and will not be productive, as they will not feel that the benefits outweigh the costs in terms of effort, time expenditure, respiratory discomfort, sore feet and muscles, joint pain, etc.

- People who have been very sedentary for a long time, or who have medical complications (heart, lung, gastrointestinal problems), should be seen by a physician before beginning a graduated exercise program. It is also important to recognize individual differences in motivation, ability, and restrictions. Clients who have orthopedic limitations, back pain, arthritis, etc. will have to adjust the intensity of their activity. Failure to attend to this concern will eventually result in poor follow-through when they are on their own.

- It is important for most clients to alternate between two or more kinds of activity, some of which must be enjoyable. For example, even the most resistant client may find it acceptable to walk or jog if it means that they will be in better shape to ski, dance, or compete in some recreational activity such as basketball.

- Be aware of how external factors might interfere with a continuing exercise plan. If your spouse hates exercise or is unwilling to cooperate with child care, sustaining a long-term exercise plan will be difficult.

- Use daily behavioral reinforcements to solidify habits. For example, sign a pact with yourself agreeing that you will not eat dinner or watch TV until you have performed your daily dosage of exercise.

- Plan for the first bout of laziness, and report to a partner or use a log to prompt you during difficult periods of job pressure and family conditions that might get in the way of your regular enjoyable pattern of exercise.

- Using a log to document benefits versus costs of exercising can be helpful. Be sure to include your mood and changes in life circumstances along with other more obvious benefits (weight loss, more productive and efficient work patterns). This will help you maintain a rigorous pattern of exercise over the long term.

HOW TO FIND A PRACTITIONER

If you have an uncomplicated history (no serious anxieties, depression, or other mental health problems) and are simply looking to prevent problems and boost general well-being, you may find appropriate benefits at a local YMCA or health club or with a personal trainer. However, if you are trying to overcome a mental health problem you will need to work with a professional counselor or psychotherapist.

Although many psychotherapists believe that exercise is beneficial to their clients, systematically conducting exercise during therapy is rare among traditional counselors. Stuck in a high-rise office building in a downtown urban area, or accustomed to the face-to-face talk format, many therapists find it difficult to suggest an active vigorous therapy session. That is why you might want to take the initiative to suggest a brisk walk as part of a counseling session. You will need to find a competent counselor who will engage in a counseling session while walking, climbing stairs, or whatever the environment will permit (such as a stationary bicycle in the office.) It is essential that the therapist have some understanding of the physiological principles of exercise prescription (starting slow, using modest goals, establishing a progressively increasingly pattern of duration, frequency, and intensity) even if you are also using a personal trainer to help design home exercise sessions.

It is important to recognize your need for additional kinds of therapy in treating this condition. It might be desirable to include biofeedback, massage, acupuncture, creative arts therapies, dietary changes, and/or naturopathy, for example, in addition to the exertional talk therapy. A good therapist should encourage you to do so in order to amplify the results of the treatment.

Unfortunately, there is no state or national directory of individuals who are certified as competent in both exercise prescription and counseling. You may have to interview several psychotherapists in order to find one who appreciates exercise (ideally, they would exercise regularly themselves) and who is willing to engage in walk-talk therapy in the same session. To my knowledge, there are no specific training programs that prepare therapists for conducting exercise therapy. Rather there are numerous exercise physiology programs that prepare educators to become fitness leaders and personal trainers with excellent skills in exercise prescription (helping people to maintain safe yet challenging levels of exercise over time), and to motivate participants to continue in a regular program of exercise. Unfortunately, these individuals rarely have mental health or counseling skills and they do not routinely engage in the exercise along with the clients. The American Association for Applied Sport Psychology (AAASP) has a subsection devoted to "Health Psychology." Many of the individuals listed have some experience in exercise as a healthy behavior, and some have the requisite counseling skills to provide walk/talk therapy if requested by the patient. You can call me at (402) 472-4305 or (402) 472-1161 for referrals to practitioners in your area listed in the AAASP membership directory. You might also contact the American College of Sports Medicine, as they have a listing of personal trainers and fitness leaders who can provide safe and effective exercise planning. Their telephone number is (800) 638-6423.

HOW TO LEARN MORE

Bahrke, M. S. and W. P. Morgan. "Anxiety Reduction Following Exercise and Meditation." *Cognitive Therapy and Research* 2 (1978): 323–333.

Berger, B. and D. Owen. "Mood Alteration with Yoga and Swimming: Aerobic Exercise May Not Be Necessary." *Journal of Perception in Motor Skills* 75, no. 3 (1992): 1331–43.

Bliwise, D., A. King, R. Harris, and W. Haskell. "Prevalence of Self-reported Parsleep in a Healthy Population Aged 50 to 65." *Social Science Medicine* 34, no. 1 (1992): 49–55.

Blumenthal, J.; C. Emery; D. Madden; S. Schmiebolk; M. Walsh-Riddle; L. George; D. McKee; N. Higginbothan; F. Cobb; and R. Coleman. "Long-term Effects of Exercise on Psychological Functioning in Older Men and Women." *Journal of Gerontology* 46, no. 6 (1991): 352–361.

Bosscher, R. J. "Running and Mixed Physical Exercises with Depressed Psychiatric Patients: Exercise and Psychological Well Being." *International Journal of Sports Psychology* 24, no. 2 (1993): 170–184.

Byrne, A. and D. Byrne. "The Effect of Exercise on Depression, Anxiety and Other Mood States: A Review." *Journal of Psychosomatic Research* 37, no. 6 (1993): 565–574.

Choi, P. "The Psychological Benefits of Physical Exercise: Implications for Women and the Menstrual Cycle." *Journal of Reproductive and Infant Psychology* 10, no. 2 (1992): 111–115.

Daniels, M., A. Martin, and J. Carter. "Opiate Receptor Blockade by Naltrexone and Mood State After Acute Physical Activity." *British Journal of Sports Medicine* 26, no. 2 (1992): 111–115.

DeVries, H.; P. Beckman; H. Huber; and L. Dieckmeir. "Electromyographic Evaluation of the Effects of Sauna on the Neuromuscular System." *The Journal of Sports Medicine* 8 (1968): 61–69.

Dey, S., R. Singh, and P. Dey. "Exercise Training: Significance of Regional Alterations in Serotonin Metabolism of Rat Brain in Relation to Anti-depressant Effect of Exercise." *Psychological Behavior* 52, no. 6 (1992): 1095–1099.

Dienstbier, R. A., R. L. LaGuardia, and N. S. Wilcox. "The Tolerance of Cold and Heat: Beyond (Cold Hands-Warm Heart)." *Motivation and Emotion* 11 (1987): 269–295.

Doyne, E., D. Schambless, and L. Beutler. "Aerobic Exercise as a Treatment for Depression in Women." *Behavior Therapy* 41 (1983): 434–440.

Dua, J. and L. Hargreaves. "Effects of Aerobic Exercise on Negative Affect, Positive Affect, Stress, and Depression." *Journal of Perceptual and Motor Skills* 75, no. 2 (1992): 355–361.

Fisher, E. and J. Thompson. "A Comparative Evaluation of Cognitive-Behavioral Therapy (CBT) Versus Exercise Therapy (ET) for the Treatment of Body Image Disturbance: Preliminary Findings." *Behavioral Modification* 18, no. 2 (1994): 171–185.

Folkins, C. H. and W. E. Sime. "Physical Fitness Training and Mental Health." *American Psychologist* 36, no. 4 (1981): 373–389.

Fried, R. *The Breath Connection.* NY: Plenum Press, 1990.

Greist, J.; M. Klein; R. Eischens; J. Faris; A. Gurman; and W. Morgan. "Running as a Treatment for Depression." *Comprehensive Psychiatry* 20 (1979): 41–54.

Gronningsaeter, H.; K. Hyten; G. Skauli; and C. Christensen. "Improved Health and Coping by Physical Exercise or Cognitive Behavioral Stress Management Training in a Work Environment." *Psychology and Health* 7, no. 2 (1992): 147–163.

Hobson, M. L. and W. J. Rejeski "Does the Dose of Acute Exercise Mediate Psychophysiological Responses to Mental Stress?" *Journal of Sport and Exercise Psychology* 15 (1993): 77–87.

Johnsgaard, K. W. *The Exercise Prescription for Depression and Anxiety.* New York: Plenum Press, 1989.

Johnston, J. L., L. M. Petlichkoff, and W. K. Hoegger. "Effects of Aerobic and Strength Training Exercise Participation on Depression." *Medicine & Science in Exercise & Sports* 25, no. 5 (1993): 135.

Klein, M.; J. Greist; A. Gurman; R. Neimeyer; D. Lesser; N. Bushnell; and R. Smith. "Comparative Outcome Study of Group Psychotherapy Versus Exercise Treatments for Depression." *International Journal of Mental Health* 13 (1985): 148–177.

Kostrubula, T. *Joy of Running.* New York: J.P. Lippincott, 1976.

Leith, L. and A. Taylor. "Psychological Aspects of Exercise: A Decade Literature Review." *The Journal of Sport Behavior* 13 (1990): 1–22.

Lobstein, D. and C. Rasmussen. "Decreases in Resting Plasma Beta-endorphine and Depression Scores After Endurance Training." *Journal of Sports Medicine and Physical Fitness* 31, no. 4 (1991): 543–551.

Martinsen, E. W. "Therapeutic Implications of Exercise for Clinically Anxious and Depressed Patients: Exercise and Psychological Well Being." *International Journal of Sports Psychology* 24, no. 2 (1993): 185–199.

McAuley, E., K. Corneya, and J. Lettunich. "Effects of Acute and Long Term Exercise on Self-efficacy Responses in Sedentary Middle Aged Males and Females." *The Gerontologist* 31, no. 4 (1991): 534–542.

Mondin, G.; W. Morgan; P. Piering; A. Stegner; C. Stotesbery; M. Trine; and M. Wu. "Psychological Consequences of Exercise Deprivation in Habitual Exercisers." *Medicine and Science in Sports and Exercise* 42, no. 9 (1996): 1199–2003.

North, T. C., P. McCullaugh, and Z. V. Tran. "Effect of Exercise on Depression." *Exercise and Sports Sciences Review* 18 (1990): 379–415.

Norvell, N. and D. Belles. "Psychological and Physical Benefits of Circuit Weight Training and Law Enforcement Personnel." *Journal of Consultative Clinical Psychology* 61, no. 3 (1993): 520–527.

Pelham, T. W.; P. D. Campagna,; P. G. Ritvo; and W. A. Birnie. "The Effects of Exercise Therapy on Clients in a Psychiatric Rehabilitation Program." *The Psychosocial Rehabilitation Journal* 16, no. 4 (1993): 75–84.

Petruzzello, S.; D. Landers; P. Hatfield; K. Kubitz; and W. Salazer. "A Meta-analysis on the Anxiety-reducing Effects of Acute and Chronic Exercise: Outcomes and Mechanisms." *Sports Medicine* 11, no. 3 (1991): 143–182.

Rajala, U.; A. Uusimaki; F. Keinanen-Kiukaanniemi; and F. Kivela. "Prevalence of Depression in a 55-year-old Finnish Population." *Social Psychiatry and Psychiatric Epidemiology* 29, no. 3 (1994): 126–130.

Roth, D. L., S. D. Bachtler, and R. Fillingim. "Acute Emotional and Cardiovascular Effects of Stressful Mental Work During Aerobic Exercise." *Psychophysiology* 27 (1990): 694–701.

Sacks M. and G. Buffone. *Running as Therapy: An Integrated Approach.* Lincoln: University of Nebraska Press, 1984.

Sime, W. "Psychological Benefits of Exercise Training in the Healthy Adult. In *Behavioral Health: A Handbook of Health Enhancement and Disease Orientation,* edited by Mattazaro, et al., 488-508. New York: John Wiley and Sons, 1984.

Sime, W. E. "Discussion: Exercise, Fitness and Mental Health." In *Exercise, Fitness and Health*, edited by Bouchard, Shephard, Stephens, Sutton, MacPherson, 627–633. Champaign, IL: Human Kinetics, 1990.

Sime, W. E. "Exercise in the Prevention and Treatment of Depression." In *Exercise and Mental Health*, edited by W. P. Morgan and S. E. Goldstein, 145–152. Washington, DC: Hemisphere, l987.

Sime, W. "Guidelines for Clinical Applications of Exercise Therapy for Mental Health." In *Exploring Sport and Exercise Psychology*, edited by J. VanRaalte and B. Brewer, 159–187. Washington, DC: APA Press, 1996.

Sime, W. and K. Hellweg. "Stress and Coping: Challenge, Appraisal and Hardiness." In *Resource Manual for Guidelines for Exercise Testing and Prescription*, edited by J. Roitman and D. Southard, Philadelphia: Williams & Wilkens, In Press.

Sonstroem, R. and W. Morgan. "Exercise and Self-esteem: Rationale and Model." *Medicine, Science in Sports and Exercise* 21 (l989): 329–337.

Stein, P. and R. Motta. "Effects of Aerobic and Nonaerobic Exercise on Depression and Self Concept." *Perceptual and Motor Skills* 74, no. 1 (1992): 79–89.

Steptoe, A., M. Kearsley, and N. Walters. "Acute Mood Responses to Maximal and Sub-maximal Exercise in Active and Inactive Men." *Psychology and Health* 8, no. 1 (1993): 89–99.

Weyerer, S. "Physical Inactivity and Depression in the Community: Evidence from the Upper Baveria Field Study." *International Journal of Sports Medicine* 13, no. 6 (1992): 492–496.

ABOUT THE AUTHOR

Dr. Sime is both an exercise physiologist and a health psychologist who uses exercise therapy as an adjunct to counseling in the treatment of anxiety, depression, addiction, and pain disorders. He received a Ph.D. in exercise physiology from the University of Pittsburgh in 1975 and a second Ph.D. in counseling psychology from the University of Nebraska, 1991. Dr. Sime has authored or edited over 100 publications and numerous books or book chapters, including many on exercise therapy for mental health. He is a leading authority in the field, which uniquely requires a background in both exercise prescription and psychotherapy. Dr. Sime is a regular exerciser who alternates between jogging, stationary bicycle, rowing machine, and stair-stepper as part of his health

program. In addition, he enjoys skiing, recreational soccer, hiking, and rac-
quetball. Part of his penchant for exercise as therapy also is based upon the personal benefits he experiences in relief of muscle pain. Dr. Sime had suffered
numerous neck and back injuries and finds the exercise necessary to maintain
flexibility and strength while blocking the pain. He also says, somewhat jok-
ingly, that he must keep exercising to ward off the devastatingly depressive
effects of the long winters on the plains of Nebraska.

18 Flower Essence Therapy:
Integrating Body and Soul Wellness

WHAT IS FLOWER ESSENCE THERAPY?

Flower essences are subtle liquid extracts of flowering plants, generally taken in oral form, which are used to address profound issues of emotional well-being, soul development, and mind/body health. The flower essences are made from fresh flowers collected in pristine habitats at the precise moment of flowering. Solar extraction methods create a new form of medicine, which is uniquely capable of addressing very delicate and subtle aspects of the emotions and thoughts of human beings. They are used by a very broad range of professional health practitioners, as well as for self-care. The use of flower remedies is usually integrated with other therapeutic techniques, as a support for the holistic therapeutic process.

Flower essences are different from medicines such as Prozac or Valium, which directly alter brain chemistry in order to control or suppress human emotions; for instance, depression, fear, or anxiety. Nearly all psychopharmaceutical drugs can also be harmful if overused, or can produce unwanted side effects. On the other hand, flower essences work as catalysts. They do not suppress symptoms; rather they stimulate consciousness by introducing new information into the emotional and mental fields of the individual. Flower essences work in a way similar to our experience of music or art: through the vehicle of sound or light we perceive something that moves or inspires us. The essences operate through the medium of water, which holds an extraordinary imprint of the color, form, and beauty of the flower in a way that speaks to the feelings and thoughts of people. Thus, flower essences reveal rather than conceal aspects of the self, so that new choices can be made about life issues. Because they are potentized energetic medicines, they work in a manner which is gentle and life-affirming, without danger of overdose or long-term dependency.

Many cases have demonstrated the successful application of flower essences for a broad range of conditions and ailments including learning disorders, child abandonment and abuse, family systems and personal relationships, work performance and career goals and values, environmental sensitivities and allergies, depression and grief, body tension and general stress, nutritional and lifestyle choices, parenting, masculine and feminine identities, problems of artistic expression, sexuality, coping with terminal illness or chronic disease, psychosomatic illness involving prior emotional trauma, and overall immune response. Flower essences have also provided broad support for healing from a large number of specific diseases and physical dysfunctions.

HOW IT BEGAN

Healing with flowers is both ancient and universal. All cultures, including our present-day culture, intuitively sense that flowers express a soul language far more profound than words. Flowers are used to convey one's deepest feelings of joy, grief, love, or tribute at births, weddings, funerals, and numerous other celebrations and commemorations in human culture.

It was in England in the 1930s, however, that Dr. Edward Bach, a well-known medical doctor and homeopathic physician, formulated the first precise system of soul healing based on medicines extracted from the flowering parts of plants. Dr. Bach was an early advocate for the kind of holistic healing that is finally receiving more widespread attention in the latter part of our century. Bach completed his undergraduate training at Birmingham University and then graduated from University College Hospital in London in 1919. He immediately assumed a post as casualty medical officer for this same hospital and was in charge of over 400 beds during World War I. It was here that he clearly observed the effects of stress and trauma in relationship to the recovery potential of his patients. He believed that surgery and standard medicine did not hold all the answers for his patients, and he became deeply interested in the field of immunology, assuming the role of chief bacteriologist at the hospital.

Bach went on to develop a number of bacterial vaccines that were credited with saving many thousands of lives when he inoculated war troops during a virulent influenza epidemic. He felt, however, that these vaccines were still too crude in composition, and when he accepted a new post at the London Homeopathic Hospital he developed a series of seven bacterial nosodes (vaccines that are homeopathically diluted and potentized). More significantly, Bach was able to discern and document clear archetypal personality traits correlated with each nosode, and he began to diagnose and treat according to these mental and emotional aspects, rather than outer physical symptoms. These nosodes received wide recognition and were used by many homeopathic practitioners in both the United States and Europe. They are still included in the standard homeopathic pharmacopoeia.

As Bach became increasingly sensitized to the emotional and mental issues presented by his patients, he continued to seek remedies that could act with even greater depth and harmony than the homeopathic nosodes. By 1930, Bach completely abandoned his prominent Harley Street London career. He returned to the countryside of his Welsh ancestry to begin an intensive study of the native plants that he had esteemed so much in his youth. As he treated patients in the small villages of the Welsh and English countryside where he traveled, he developed entirely new remedies from the flowering parts of plants. He found these remedies could benefit the emotional and mental conditions that undermined the health and well-being of his patients. By the time he died in 1936, Bach had developed a collection of thirty-eight flower essences.

Since then, other practitioners from around the world have confirmed, through their own observation and research, the unique healing benefits of flower essence therapy. In 1979 the Flower Essence Society (FES) was founded by Richard Katz in Nevada City, California as a non-profit worldwide educational and research organization. The Society has investigated and collected empirical case studies, not only for the original thirty-eight English remedies, but also for significant new essences derived from medicinal herbs and North American wildflowers. The society conducts an annual certification program for practitioners and publishes research in regular editions of its *Repertory*, as well as a member newsletter. The Flower Essence Society has a worldwide network of over 60,000 practitioners, who serve hundreds of thousands of clients.

HOW IT WORKS

A model of wellness is now emerging that recognizes that the body and soul cannot be regarded as separate, but must be seen as one interwoven reality. We know that emotional responses affect the body. Especially since World War II, researchers have correlated distinct personality traits with specific diseases. One of the most famous of these studies was conducted by Drs. Meyer Reidman and Raymond Rosenman, who coined the term "Type A behavior" for the impatient, hostile attitude connected with the greater risk of heart disease. Since then, numerous studies have pinpointed the decisive role of emotional factors such as anger, grief, depression, or self-esteem on the outcome of specific diseases as well as overall immunity. A whole new field of medical research, called psychoneuroimmunology (PNI), has documented important changes in emotional and physical wellness by identifying biochemical messengers which transmit emotional responses to and from the glands in the body.

Definite scientific links between flower essences and these biochemical messengers have not yet been established. However, on a whole, PNI confirms a much broader picture of the human being, involving the complex interactions between feelings and bodily states. As we identify the larger energetic structures that comprise each human being, medicines like flower essences, which address these links, are becoming more prominent.

WHAT THE RESEARCH SHOWS

The Flower Essence Society has conducted research for the past two decades. This research consists of case studies collected from professional practitioners who are involved in its certification training program, as well as hundreds of other practitioners who regularly report significant cases or overall trends involving flower essence therapy. The society has also worked closely with approximately fifty practitioners who have now administered flower essences to clients for a number of years. These practitioners have been able to provide comprehensive information about flower essence therapy extending beyond the immediate cause-and-effect phenomena that may occur within the first several weeks. Instead, these practitioners are able to assess the results over time periods ranging from one to three years, during which the essences are used at various intervals to assist with unfolding life challenges. This research identifies seven major areas of change that flower essences appear to facilitate, either concurrently or sequentially, regardless of the initial symptoms or dysfunctions of the client. These "meta-levels" of change include: 1) greater range of emotional responses to typical life challenges; 2) ability to see relationships between body issues and emotions, along with the ability to achieve a greater sense of personal well-being; 3) ability to take risks and make changes that previously seemed out of reach to the individual; 4) ability to identify and create meaningful work or other contributions to one's family and community; 5) increased sensitivity and inner awareness, including dream recall, as well as various forms of artistic expression, and awareness of nature; 6) ability to take responsibility for one's life, including the ability to forgive, as well as to make amends for harm caused to others; and 7) increased awareness of spiritual and moral issues, including new or renewed choices of religious expression or spiritual discovery.

In addition to identifying these major benefits of flower essence therapy, the Flower Essence Society has also analyzed the case phenomena itself to better understand the therapeutic process. The preliminary results show that there are four basic stages that can be associated with flower essence therapy.

- Release or relaxation. If the remedy is well chosen, the initial experience is usually a sense of well-being or relaxation. The more obvious symptoms improve, sometimes dramatically. A tense stomach begins to relax. A depressed person might feel more cheerful. Insomniacs may sleep better. At times, the sensations of release or letting go may be more pronounced — some individuals may need more sleep, or there may be emotional release such as crying or laughter.

- Recognition or insight. This stage is the most pivotal in flower essence therapy, and also the area which distinguishes its truly unique and important benefits. Flower essences are not intended simply for symptom relief, and although they may provide initial clearing or calming, their true action is much deeper. As they are used, the connection between the bodily dysfunction and underlying emotions or attitudes becomes clearer. For example, one may become more aware of tension held in the stomach, but now also begin to identify when the emotional triggers occur. A sleep problem might now be seen as a failure to clear something that happened earlier in the day, rather than as an isolated symptom. These insights may be spontaneous or they may gradually emerge over a longer period of time. Professional counselors, who are also using other modalities to assist the mental and emotional developmental process, report that the flower essences make a definite and distinct impact on the therapy, providing deeper and quicker cognitive connections in the mind-body process.

- Resolution or reconciliation. Once insights have emerged about the emotional factors that are causing dysfunction, it is still necessary to bring the

conflicting parts of the self to resolution. Flower essences initiate a dynamic process within the individual that can best be described as an *integration
of opposites*. This characteristic distinguishes flower essence therapy from
the other two major streams of medicine: *allopathy*, which is based on the
Law of Contraries, and *homeopathy*, which is based on the Law of Similars.
Allopathic medicine, by far the predominant form of medicine in contemporary culture, treats symptoms by introducing an opposite, such as a
decongestant to unclog mucus membranes. On the other hand, homeopathic medicine uses potentized substances that parallel as closely as possible the presenting symptoms, thereby stimulating the immune system to
form its own response to the illness. Flower essence therapy most closely
follows the paradigm established by Carl Jung in Jungian archetypal psychology. This approach to healing involves the dynamic resolution of seemingly opposite tendencies in the self, and the integration of the so-called
shadow of disowned parts of the self.

This third, in-depth stage of flower essence therapy usually requires a
commitment to inner work, either through a program of self-development
or with the help of a trained counselor if the problem is deeply established.
Because the flower essences do not operate like drugs, which simply introduce a new behavior by altering brain chemistry, the change initially stimulated by the flower essences must also be met by conscious inner work for
the results to be in-depth and enduring. For example, an individual who
has a history of ulcers or other digestive upsets may begin to identify the
causal links — her stomach knots up whenever her employer enters the
room, and she begins to realize she is holding a great deal of anger and tension about her job and working conditions. However, at a deeper level, she
is invested in seeing herself as a good, "nice," or compliant person — the
angry part of herself is disowned or repressed. Yet this shadow aspect of
herself is not necessarily "bad"; instead, such an individual will need to
find a way to express anger or other dissatisfactions appropriately and positively. In the healing process facilitated by flower essence therapy, such an
individual will not simply return to being a "nice" person; instead, a developmental process of continuing depth and authenticity will be fostered.
The appropriate flower essences will help to stabilize and maintain this
developmental cycle until the individual has achieved true change. Again,
this method of healing differs greatly from psychiatric drugs, which are

often habit-forming and must be taken indefinitely to prevent dysfunctional behavior from recurring.

■ Regeneration of the self. Flower essence therapy is not simply about fixing personality problems or modifying behavior. It is about transforming the self. When taken to its ultimate conclusion, this therapeutic process actually introduces new potentials and creative possibilities. For example, an individual who has learned to recognize and transform previously repressed anger will often discover new sources of energy or creativity that had previously been blocked or dormant. An individual who comes to terms with her repressed anger at the workplace may now learn how to communicate more effectively and authentically. But ultimately such an individual may see that a completely new career or job situation is possible, one much more suited to her newly forming personality. Those flower essence therapists who are now tracking clients in the later stages of their therapy have consistently noted major biographical changes — leaving marriages or finding new life partners, changing careers, finding new places to live, or making other significant lifestyle changes.

Additional research on flower remedies has tended to focus primarily on stage one changes. Jeffrey Cram (unpublished) of The Sierra Health Institute in Nevada City, CA, reports that with Five Flower Formula (a special combination remedy for stress and trauma), people who were facing the stress of a timed math test or a loud noise recovered more quickly (as measured with biofeedback of galvanic skin response) than did people receiving a placebo. In Germany, Gudrun Rühle (1994) examined twenty-four women overdue to give birth. Those taking flower essences had better coping styles and required less medication when labor started.

Many other research projects involving standard test measurements or placebo controls are now in various stages of progress, both in the United States and abroad. As flower essence therapy becomes more visible and credible, more funding will be allocated for "hard" scientific research that can be added to the foundation of empirical research collected and analyzed by the Flower Essence Society.

REAL PEOPLE AND FLOWER ESSENCE THERAPY

Bleeding Heart

 An 8-year-old girl suddenly developed acute stomach pains and diarrhea. A gastrointestinal expert conducted a full battery of tests and could find nothing wrong with the child. Finally, her parents took her to a family counselor who also used flower essences. In the opening diagnostic session, the child drew a large picture of a heart that was broken. The counselor used bleeding heart to help her address what was sensed as a deep source of grief within the child. The young girl began to share her sense of loss for a playmate who had been killed suddenly several months prior to the onset of her symptoms. Her family had no idea that she had been so profoundly affected by the death of her friend. Within several days of taking the bleeding heart, the child's symptoms were drastically reduced and within several weeks, they completely disappeared and never returned again.

Impatiens, Zinnia, and Borage

 A 58-year-old executive salesman contended with a great deal of stress in his daily lifestyle. He was diagnosed by his physician as having chronic high blood pressure and in the early stages of coronary heart disease. The doctor asked him to make nutritional changes, and to incorporate exercise and stress reduction in his daily lifestyle. Despite enrolling in two different programs for reducing stress and learning relaxation techniques, the man made little progress. He still found himself anxious and irritable at the end of the day. A flower essence therapist recommended a combination of impatiens, zinnia, and borage. The man noticed an immediate effect using these remedies — he felt more calm and centered. The relaxation techniques that he had previously attempted seemed easier to incorporate. He noticed many situations at home and in the family that were changing due to his feeling of greater ease and self-control. When he went for his regular checkup six weeks later, the physician was amazed to discover that his blood pressure had dropped significantly and he wanted to know what had changed for his patient.

Mimulus

A woman in her seventies had gradually become a shut-in following the death of her husband. She was afraid to do household errands or go out alone, despite the fact that she was physically capable of doing so. Although she had a valid driver's license, she had depended on her husband to drive and was reluctant to use her car. As her fear grew more pronounced, she became hypersensitive to many noises in her house and began to become afraid that her house would be broken into. Due to these fears, she began to sleep very restlessly and became increasingly fretful and agitated. A flower essence counselor prescribed the single remedy of mimulus. No clear changes were noted until about the third week of use. The woman then reported that she felt calmer and was getting more sleep at night. A week later she remarked to her daughter, "I certainly have been acting like a frightful child, it's time for me to make some changes." Two weeks later, she reported to her counselor, "It's time for me to get another life. I can't pretend I'm dead just because my husband is." She made many incremental changes in her lifestyle, learning to drive her car and accepting many social invitations that she had previously declined.

California Wild Rose

This flower essence was used for a 16-year-old young woman who had become moody, began to dress in dark colors, and grew emotionally distant from her family. Her grades suddenly plunged from above average to barely passing. In a counseling session, the young girl stated she felt "bored" with life and didn't feel much interest or hope for her future. She had recently parted with a boyfriend and had also not been chosen for a part in a school play that she had wanted. Her mother noticed a change within two weeks of taking the California wild rose. She was more willing to talk about her feelings of pain and rejection, and she found a new friend at school. Within several months, her disposition was brighter and more cheerful and her grades at school had returned to their normal level.

Star of Bethlehem

 A young woman in her twenties had been violently attacked, raped, and robbed at gun point. She had received counseling for these incidents and seemed to be in recovery. Six months later, she developed a severe eating disorder along with food allergies. Despite nutritional and psychotherapeutic counseling, she continued to lose weight, and showed other signs of depression. She was given star of Bethlehem to address the shock and trauma of her violent attack. Through the use of the essence, she began to relive the original incident, but now she acknowledged the tremendous feelings of rage, grief, and shame she felt about her attack. As she worked through and resolved these emotions, her eating disorder also subsided.

Tiger Lily, Mariposa Lily, Alpine Lily

 A woman who had just turned forty went for her regular gynecological check-up. She was diagnosed with severe cervical dysplasia (CIN III), confirmed by tissue biopsies from five different areas of the cervical and vaginal tissue. Her physician recommended immediate surgical intervention, removing all of the affected tissue in the cervix and vagina, through a process called conization. This required hospitalization, general anesthesia, and a two-month recovery period. In his opinion, she was at high risk for cancer without these measures. Because this condition had developed so suddenly without any prior history, the woman sought psychotherapeutic counseling and nutritional counseling. She modified her diet to exclude foods that were irritating or difficult to digest. Her counselor suggested a trio of lily remedies including tiger lily, mariposa lily, and alpine lily to address her feminine identity and its connection with her gynecological issues. During the next several months, the woman did deep emotional work around her sense of grief about never having a child; she also realized she had many ambivalent feelings about motherhood due to her own traumatized relationship with her mother. Her dream journal and daily life journal, and sessions with her counselor, revealed much submerged emotional material that was now being revealed to her. After a period of six months, the woman returned to her gynecologist for another evaluation, intending to allow surgery if her cell tissue was still disturbed. Tissue biopsies were taken of the original sites — to the astonishment of her doctor, the new tests showed absolutely no areas of cervical dysplasia, even in mild form. Her tests were completely normal and have remained normal for five years.

Holly

A young boy of nine years of age was diagnosed as hyperactive. His parents sought help from a holistic doctor who also uses flower essences. In a diagnostic work-up for the boy, no significant nutritional or physiological problems were identified. However, the child showed clear emotional problems. His behavior was on edge; he was always irritated or hostile in his response to others. He seemed unable to be a part of his family system, or to receive warmth and affection from others. The single remedy of holly was chosen. The parents reported amazement at the changes in their son. They commented to their doctor, "We can't thank you enough, whatever was in those drops has been so transforming to his personality; he's reintegrated himself into the warmth of our family."

Elm

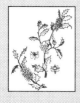

A middle-aged man visited his chiropractic/naturopathic doctor, presenting symptoms of severe, deep pain in his left shoulder joint. All typical protocols and tests were followed in evaluating this man's condition. After six visits for chiropractic adjustments and soft tissue therapy, the agonizing pain continued unabated. The doctor concluded that the cause of the pain was not of physical origin and prescribed elm flower essence. After eight days, the patient reported that his pain was completely gone. During this time, he gained the insight that his discomfort came from his overwhelming sense of responsibility and burden, which had manifested as a psychic "weight" on his left shoulder. With the help of the elm flower essence, this man made a permanent shift in his inner attitude about his life and work. The intense pain he felt in his left shoulder has never returned.

WHAT TO EXPECT

The key to successful use of flower essences is the ability to select appropriate remedies. An inappropriate remedy will not be harmful, but neither will it be helpful — it simply will not register a significant response. Flower essences work by a principle called resonance. This means that the character of the remedy must match a similar pattern within an individual in order to evoke a healing response. Not all remedies work in the same way on different people. There might be five different remedies for five different people with the same presenting symptoms. The practitioner must identify the patterns of emotional dysfunction that are unique to the person. This involves looking beyond the surface, on a number of different levels, and making an assessment of the unique emotional picture of the individual. Most people can perceive and describe physical aches and pains without difficulty, but in our culture, we tend not to fully develop our ability to identify and describe emotional or mental imbalances. Models of psychotherapy are helpful in looking at and conceptualizing these aspects of human life. In the last forty years, psychologists have gained a much deeper understanding of the dynamics of the human soul. For example, clinical research has substantiated that core beliefs from childhood significantly impact adult life. Much is now known, too, about the process of internalizing gender roles and cultural expectations, and how the stress of modern living and technological culture affects our general well-being.

For this reason, when first using flower essences, most individuals find it useful to visit a psychotherapist skilled in diagnosing personality dynamics. Some therapists specialize exclusively in flower essences, although most incorporate them within a range of options offered to the client. Flower remedy portraits involve the interweaving of both the mind and the body; therefore an effective practitioner is one who has developed the ability to see these relationships. This has more to do with the practitioner's skill in observing and asking questions than any particular healing modality; flower essences are successfully used by a broad range of practitioners including medical doctors and nurses, psychotherapists and other counselors, energetic practitioners such as acupuncturists and homeopaths, art therapists, teachers, nutritionists, and body workers.

As with any healing modality, practitioners must be objectively assessed according to their actual qualifications, skills, and experience. Some practitioners use pendulums, applied kinesiology testing, questionnaires, and other aids in determining the correct remedies. These methods can be helpful, but they cannot substitute for the essential knowledge of the practitioner, since the information gained through these methods is modified and colored by the practitioner's own beliefs and insights.

Flower remedies are used quite safely and successfully by many families for basic home care. When the remedies are used for self-care, it is important to do extensive reading about the remedies and to study the issues for which each is indicated. It is helpful to discuss the presenting concerns with somebody else, perhaps a trusted friend, in order to get past any blind spots. It is also very helpful to keep a journal while taking the remedies, in order to more accurately capture the process initiated by the flower essences. Most people find that there are one to three archetypal remedies that they need over a period of time, or during various intervals, as new challenges or destiny issues emerge. This is similar to the homeopathic concept of constitutional remedies.

Flower essences have outstanding and even astonishing success with children. Because the essences do not produce physical side effects, they are very safe at all ages. With children, the issues are usually less established in the psyche or conscious belief system; as a result, finding the right remedy is relatively more straightforward, with results that are more clear cut. The same is true when treating animals with flower remedies. Although the range of available flower essences is about 200 single remedies, there are about one dozen remedies commonly used for children and another dozen commonly used for animals — the selection process is simpler because the issues presented are usually much more basic.

Flower essences are generally taken orally in liquid form, several drops at a time, although some practitioners apply them directly to meridians or other

energy points on the body during a therapeutic session. They can also be added
to skin creams or bath water, or put in misting bottles to be sprayed around
the body and the environment. Although single remedies are quite effective,
flower essences can be skillfully combined to create synergistic formulas — a
typical formula involves up to five or six remedies. These "dosage bottles" are
used several times daily — just before and after sleep, and before meals. The
flower essence formulas are used in cycles of about one month. During this
period, the emotional body, like the moon itself, has usually "waxed and
waned" through a phase of inner development. Flower essence therapy usually
takes several months, with new applications of remedies as the individual moves
through successive stages or "layers" of change.

Typical response time for flower essence use is about one month, although
in many instances results may be noticed within days, or even hours. Even
though some change may have occurred, it is important to continue the flower
essences, perhaps with some modification to the formula, for about three
months in order to insure a deeper level of development. Typically, the response
to the remedies is more general in the beginning stages. Individuals report feeling calmer, clearer, better able to cope, or less fatigued. Through counseling,
working with dreams, keeping a journal, or other ways of learning to observe
and articulate levels of emotional and mental phenomena, much more specific
responses can be documented, and new issues may surface. For instance, the
following is an actual quotation from an individual who is being treated with
flower essences by a family therapist: "My usual reaction whenever my daughter starts whining and crying is that I get a knot in my stomach and feel quite
tense and irritable. Invariably, I then begin to yell or get angry with her. However, since using flower essences, I don't seem to react so strongly to her. Instead,
I understand why she's upset and gradually seem to be discovering more creative ways to address her discomfort."

If a remedy is entirely inappropriate it will not produce any significant
response. However, if an individual is extremely resistant or in very deep denial
about a particular issue, the remedy may not appear to produce an obvious
response. In such cases, the therapist is challenged to help the client uncover
the psychological material that is just below the surface. One such case involves
a woman who had pronounced issues with her mother. Mariposa lily, a remedy
that addresses the mother-child bond, was strongly indicated by applied kinesiology testing, as well as basic counseling assessment. However, no clear

changes were noted until this woman was asked to record her dreams. A major breakthrough occurred shortly after, when this woman woke up from an intense dream in which she was on a submarine with her mother, and tried to throw her mother overboard. The significance of this dream was so clear to the woman that she could not deny its importance; she then became willing to address the issue. Flower essences often stimulate deep areas of the subconscious that must be brought to the conscious mind for successful resolution.

HOW TO CHOOSE A PRACTITIONER

It is important to speak with a prospective practitioner about his or her credentials, training, and experience, in order to choose a therapist who has the right qualifications and demeanor for your particular needs. You should inquire about general training and experience, as well as specific knowledge of flower essences.

The Flower Essence Society offers various educational programs for practitioners, including an 80-hour program for in-depth training, followed by a six-month case study program, which leads to certification. These certified practitioners are registered with the Society. However, many other kinds of professional training are also valid, and other practitioners are also enrolled on the Flower Essence Society practitioner referral list.

You can call FES for referrals to qualified practitioners at (800) 736-9222; Fax: (916) 265-0584; E-mail: info@flowersociety.org. The mailing address is P.O. Box 459, Nevada City, CA, 95959. The FES also maintains an informative Web site at http://www.flowersociety.org.

HOW TO LEARN MORE

Bach, E. and F. J. Wheeler. *The Bach Flower Remedies*. New Canaan, CT: Keats Publishing, 1979.

Barnard, J. and M. Barnard. *The Healing Herbs of Edward Bach: An Illustrated Guide to the Flower Remedies*. Bath, England: Ashgrove Press, 1995.

Barnard, J. ed. *Collected Writings of Edward Bach*. Bath, England: Ashgrove Press, 1987.

Howard, J. *The Bach Flower Remedies: Step by Step*. Saffron Walden, England: The C. W. Daniel Company, Ltd., 1990.

Kaminski, P. and R. Katz. *Flower Essence Repertory*. Nevada City, CA: Flower Essence Society, 1994.

Kaminski, P. "Choosing Flower Essences: An Assessment Guide." Nevada City, CA: Flower Essence Society, 1994.

Kaslof, L. *Traditional Flower Remedies of Dr. Edward Bach: A Self-Help Guide.* New Canaan, CT: Keats Publishing, 1993.

McIntyre, A. *Flower Power.* New York: Henry Holt and Company, 1996.

Rühle, G. *A Pilot Study: The Use of Flower Essences with Primipara In Delayed Labor Onset.* A Psychological Thesis for the Psychological Institute in Tübingen, Germany, 1994.

Scheffer, M. *Bach Flower Therapy.* Rochester, VT: Healing Arts Press, 1988.

Weeks, N. *The Medical Discoveries of Edward Bach, Physician.* New Canaan, CT: Keats Publishing, Inc., 1979.

Wildwood, C. *Flower Remedies: Natural Healing with Flower Essences.* Rockport, MA: Element Books, 1992.

ABOUT THE AUTHOR

Patricia Kaminski is co-director of the Flower Essence Society in Nevada City, California. She has a B.A. from the University of Nebraska, and graduate education in counseling and education. She has additional training in herbalism, Goethean nature studies, and Waldorf education. She is co-author of the *Flower Essence Repertory* and has written and taught around the world on the subject of flower essences for over sixteen years. She has been instrumental in designing and administering the society's research and practitioner training programs, and also maintains a private flower essence therapy practice.

All artwork, courtesy of the Flower Essence Society, by resident artist Catalina O'Brien.

Larry Christensen, Ph.D.

19 Food and Mood:
The Sugar- and Caffeine-Free Diet for Depression

WHAT IS THE SUGAR- AND CAFFEINE-FREE DIET?

Food and mood is the practice of making changes in what you eat to improve your mood and general feeling of well-being. This enables many individuals to lead a more productive and happy life. This appears to have the most significance for individuals experiencing depression.

Changing your diet can eliminate symptoms of depression for some people, reduce symptoms for others, or in some cases, may have no effect. It is generally best to use a diet change in conjunction with other types of therapy, such as psychotherapy.

HOW IT BEGAN

If you look at recorded history, you will find that there has always been a belief that food contributed to an individual's health. Ancient documents and art work reveal that food, and beliefs about the effect of food, have always played an important role in medicine. The Bible makes repeated reference to various foods and provides detailed and specific information concerning the animals that could and could not be eaten. The ancient Greeks believed that both physical and psychological disorders could be treated by eating certain foods. Physicians during the Middle Ages believed that a good diet helped cure the body, and physicians that did not give adequate attention to diet when caring for their patient could be sued for malpractice. Hippocrates even went so far as to state that medicine would never have been discovered if sick individuals ate, drank, and lived the same type of lifestyle as healthy individuals. During the Egyptian period, various foods were used to treat a wide variety of both physical and mental disorders. Vegetables were supposed to nourish the libido, turnips to increase sperm, for example, and meat to increase sexual urges.

Over the years, crude studies demonstrated that various deficiency diseases such as scurvy and pellagra, caused by a lack of vitamin C and vitamin B_3, could be treated with diet. By the early 1900s, research had identified most of the vitamins. It had also revealed that if a person was deficient in one or more vitamins, he or she would not only experience physical symptoms, such as bleeding gums or diarrhea, but would also experience a variety of mental symptoms, such as depression, irritability, and memory loss. This research provided support for the belief that the food we eat contributes significantly to our mental and physical health. In the 1940s, a program to enrich bread and flour with various vitamins was begun. This program virtually wiped out diseases due to vitamin deficiencies in the developed world.

Although deficiency diseases were now under control, interest in the effect of food on our physical and psychological well-being persisted. Attention shifted to other avenues. For example, hypoglycemia, or low blood sugar, attracted the attention of a large segment of the population in the 1970s and became the fad disease of that decade. Also, during this period, Dr. Ben Feingold proposed that hyperactivity was caused by the dyes, colors, and preservatives in our food supply. The significance of most of these approaches was greatly overexaggerated and research demonstrated that they affected only a small segment of the population. This has not, however, had much effect on the general public's belief in the effect that food can have on our well-being. A belief in the healing power of food is promoted in many self-help books, magazine articles, and "nutritional therapies." Some of these books and magazines (as well as other essays in this book) claim that eating certain foods or changing your diet can cure a whole host of physical and psychological disorders. Others claim that eating the right food can increase your mental and physical prowess.

My research investigating the mood-altering effect of diet was stimulated by an acquaintance who read a lot of popular literature on the effect that food could have on one's emotional state. She applied some of it to herself and found that it helped relieve her depression. I became aware of this and, at her encouragement, read many of the books on this topic. The books I read were fascinating. The authors were good journalists and wrote fascinating accounts of how altering one's diet can eliminate all kinds of physical and psychological problems. After reading several of these books, I became convinced that there had to be an element of truth to what was being said and made a commitment to look into the concept.

Now I needed to decide where to start and what to investigate. In reading the various books and literature that had been thrust at me, I discovered that the common thread was the underlying assumption that hypoglycemia was the cause of many of the disorders. Although I didn't believe this, I decided to investigate hypoglycemia — which means low blood sugar.

For the next several months, I read the scientific literature on hypoglycemia and found, much to my surprise, that hypoglycemia could mimic many psychological, as well as physical, disorders. There were instances of people with undiagnosed cases of hypoglycemia, who had been treated for other disorders, such as schizophrenia. I also became aware that various professional organizations such as the American Medical Association were adamant about the fact that hypoglycemia was an infrequent disorder and that it did not account for many cases of misdiagnosis. This actually is true. Hypoglycemia occurs quite infrequently. However, it was a good place to start, so I identified individuals experiencing the symptoms of hypoglycemia who were also seeking psychological counseling from a University Counseling Center. These individuals completed a five-hour oral glucose tolerance test, which diagnoses hypoglycemia. Much to my chagrin, none of these individuals had hypoglycemia, so I realized that further investigation of hypoglycemia was useless.

Fortunately, I asked several of the individuals who took the test to try the diet I had prepared. Several of these people agreed and, much to my surprise, they reported that it made them feel better and eliminated many of their symptoms. This gave me the glimmer of hope I needed and encouraged me to continue investigating the effect of diet on one's emotional state.

Since that time, I have conducted over half a dozen studies in which I have tried to identify the type of person, called a dietary responder, that is sensitive to and would profit from a dietary change. In addition to identifying the dietary responder, I have focused a lot of attention on identifying the type of foods that can cause one to feel emotionally distraught. This research has revealed that individuals experiencing some degree of depression are most likely to be dietary responders and that the two substances that are most likely to contribute to the feelings of depression are added sugar and caffeine. As a result, when I conduct my studies, I focus on depressed individuals and have them eliminate anything that contains added sugar and caffeine from their diet.

HOW IT WORKS

Now you know that the essential ingredients of the dietary intervention are the elimination of sugar and caffeine. This sounds simple and it really is. But it is not quite as simple as it appears. There are many subtle issues to be considered and steps to be followed to ensure that you get maximum benefit.

The first question you must ask yourself is whether you are likely to respond to the diet. Even though this diet is very simple, you don't want to spend the time and effort to try it if you probably won't get any benefit from it. So let's assume that you have been experiencing some feelings of depression. You have been feeling down in the dumps, have a very low self-image, are moody and tired, and just feel terrible most of the time. Will the diet let you enjoy life again? There are several questions you can ask yourself that will help you make this decision. Go over each of the following questions and, if the answer to most of them is yes, then it's very possible that diet is partially or totally responsible for the way you feel.

1. When you feel low, down in the dumps, or depressed, is there a specific reason for it? Often, dietary responders report that they have these feelings of depression for unknown reasons. It is as though they climb into this deep dark hole at times and they can't control when or why it happens. If this situation describes you, it is one indication that you may be a dietary responder or that the depression you are experiencing is caused by diet. On the other hand, if this situation doesn't describe you, it does not necessarily mean you are not a dietary responder. Sometimes you may think you know what is causing your depression. For example, if you are going through a divorce or having a difficult time with one of your children or a spouse, you may think that is cause. Indeed it may contribute to, or be the total cause of, your depression. But you must ask yourself whether the depression existed prior to this presumed cause. If it did, diet may be the cause of much of your depression.

2. Do you feel as though you are very moody? Dietary responders frequently view themselves as being moody people. They get irritated and angry very

easily. They cry easily. Or, they feel fairly good one moment — and the next they can feel awful.

3. Are you tired and fatigued most of the time? Can you sleep eight or more hours a night yet wake up tired? Do you ever feel as though the energy is suddenly being drained out of you? This experience of fatigue and being sapped of energy is very characteristic of dietary responders. Individuals with this persistent fatigue seem to have little motivation. They will do virtually anything to get out of doing work. They appear lazy, which is very irritating to those around them. Others frequently feel as though this person needs a swift kick in the rear to motivate them. However, the real reason behind the apparent laziness and lack of motivation is extreme and persistent fatigue. These people don't have the energy to do anything.

4. Do you have frequent headaches? Although headaches are not one of the most dominant symptoms of dietary responders, they occur with sufficient frequency to be included as an indicator. Dietary responders often report experiencing headaches several times a week; some have them almost every day. The headaches range from a dull ache to something approaching a migraine. There is no consistent pattern. Frequent headaches are one indication that your depression may be due to diet. However, you should not use headaches as the primary indicator. You must have other symptoms such as the fatigue, moodiness, and depression along with the headache to qualify as a good candidate for being a dietary responder. These symptoms must be present most of the time, not just when you have a headache.

Now let's assume that you have read each of these questions and agree with most of them. You feel depressed, you are tired most of the time, moody, and frequently have a dull headache. This means you may be a dietary responder. I emphasize *may be* because a positive answer to these questions is only an indication. Try the diet. You have nothing to lose and everything to gain. The diet is definitely not going to harm you and may do you a world of good.

If you have decided to try the diet, you must adhere to the following guideline strictly. Eliminate any food or beverage that contains caffeine or added sugar. This means that you must read the label of the products you purchase to make sure that no caffeine or sugar is included. Also be alert to various other names that amount to the same thing as sugar. Some products will state that sucrose is included. This is just another term for sugar. Similarly, if a product states that it contains dextrose or glucose, this is basically stating that sugar has been added. You should avoid this product. On the other hand, you may be able to handle fructose or corn sweeteners. Fructose is metabolized more slowly than sugar and apparently is tolerated fairly well by most individuals sensitive to sugar. However, I suggest you avoid all sweeteners at first, including products such as honey, maple syrup, and molasses.

When checking products for caffeine and sugar, make sure that you don't forget to check medications. Many medications add caffeine or sugar for a variety of reasons. For example, some headache medications add caffeine, probably to treat headaches caused from withdrawal from caffeine. Also recognize that caffeine is in many beverages other than coffee, tea, and some cola drinks. For example, beverages such as Mountain Dew contain quite a bit of caffeine. When following this diet, remember that the important rule is to make sure you don't eat sugar or consume caffeine. You can have unlimited variety in your meals. Just make sure that they do not include sugar, dextrose, glucose, or caffeine. You must stick to the diet with absolutely no deviations, at least initially.

When you eliminate sugar and caffeine from your diet, make sure that you substitute other foods for them. Don't stop eating or dramatically reduce your food consumption. Reducing your calorie intake to the point that you are losing weight can also contribute to feelings of depression.

Be prepared to experience some withdrawal effects when you eliminate sugar and caffeine from your diet. The most common withdrawal effect is a headache, which is probably due to the lack of caffeine. These headaches can be very severe in some people, but in most they are tolerable and will last from about two to four days. For those that experience severe headaches, which can last up to two weeks, the best procedure is to gradually reduce your caffeine intake over about a one to two week period. In addition to headaches, some people report experiencing light-headedness or shakiness between meals. These symptoms are probably from eliminating sugar. If you experience these symptoms, eat something immediately. If these symptoms last more than several days, you should record when they occur and then eat something about half an hour prior to when you think they'll occur.

Most individuals can expect relief from their depression and moodiness within four to seven days, although some individuals have to be on the diet for two weeks to experience relief. If you don't experience relief within two weeks, you can be fairly sure that caffeine and sugar are not contributing to your depression. This assumes, of course, that you have totally eliminated these substances from your diet.

Now let's assume that you have totally eliminated these two substances from your diet and that your depression is gone or has dramatically improved. Does this mean that you're sensitive to both sugar and caffeine and have to completely eliminate them from your diet forever? Most people are sensitive to one or the other substance, rather than both. This is why it is important for you to test yourself to determine which of these substances is causing your mood problems. To do this, you must consume each of these substances and monitor your depression and mood state to see if the depression returns. I recommend starting with sugar because more people are sensitive to this substance. Eat things with sugar in them for breakfast, between meals, and for desserts. Do this for at least two to three weeks. If your depression and moodiness return, then you can be fairly confident that sugar is the cause. While doing this, make sure that you do not consume caffeine; remember, you are attempting to isolate the offending substance.

After you have tried the sugar challenge, you should challenge yourself with caffeine. Use the same procedure you used with sugar. Consume products with caffeine, but make sure that they do not contain sugar. Again, you want to see if your depression returns when you consume caffeine so you must limit yourself to caffeine consumption. Do this for up to two weeks. If your depression returns, caffeine is probably the problem and you must stay away from it. If it does not return, then caffeine is probably not the problem.

Now let's assume that you have found that you are sensitive to either caffeine or sugar. Do you have to stay off it the rest of your life? The answer is probably yes, but you may be able to consume small amounts and still avoid their negative effects. The longer you stay off these products, especially sugar, the less sensitive you become, up to a point. After avoiding these products for some time (months) you can probably consume some without harmful consequences. But don't let this lack of symptoms fool you into thinking that you no longer react to, say, sugar — if you continue to consume it, your depression will gradually return. However, at this stage you may be able to tolerate some sweet products like honey or maple syrup. If you want something sweet, I would recommend that you try it and see what happens. Remember, let your mood state be your guide.

WHAT THE RESEARCH SHOWS

A small contingent of researchers have demonstrated that the food we eat has an effect on biochemical substances in the brain. Dr. Richard Wurtman and his colleagues at Massachusetts Institute of Technology (MIT) have demonstrated that consumption of pure carbohydrate has the effect of stimulating the production of a brain neurochemical called serotonin. This substance is known to have an effect on mood, especially depression.

My research and dietary intervention program has, as mentioned, focused on the contribution of caffeine and sugar to depression. This intervention program developed as the results of years of research in my laboratory. However, others have conducted research that has provided support for these findings. For example, Dr. Fernstrom and her colleagues (1987) found that depressed individuals report changing their dietary preference for specific foods as they become depressed. Specifically, the depressed individuals in their study reported that they increase their consumption of carbohydrates as they become depressed, and that their preference is for sweet carbohydrates. Dr. Leibenluft and his colleagues (1996) found that individuals diagnosed with depression, seasonal affective disorder, and alcohol dependence all report consumption of carbohydrates and caffeine when experiencing depression. This is consistent with a study Sharla Somers and I conducted (Christensen and Somers, 1996). In this study we asked depressed and nondepressed individuals to record everything they ate or drank for three days and then we analyzed this data for the specific nutrients they consumed. Depressed and nondepressed individuals consumed similar amounts of all nutrients, except for carbohydrates. Depressed individuals consume a greater amount of carbohydrates than did the nondepressed and most of this increase came from increasing their intake of sugar.

Why do depressed individuals consume more sugar? Dr. Leibenluft (1996) and others have postulated that the consumption of a carbohydrate such as sugar has the effect of producing an improvement in a person's depressed state by, for example, decreasing their feelings of fatigue. There is some support for this proposition. Rosenthal and his colleagues (1989) found that individuals with seasonal affective disorder experienced a more positive mood than did nondepressed individuals two hours after consuming a carbohydrate rich snack. Thayer (1987) also found that consuming a carbohydrate snack increased a person's energy level. However, Thayer also found that this boost in energy was short-lived and that after this initial energy boost, energy level declined to a level below that of an individual who engages in a brisk walk instead of consuming a candy bar.

This suggests that the energy boost from carbohydrate consumption is only a temporary fix. My belief is that a vicious cycle possibly occurs in depressed individuals. Foods that contain a lot of simple carbohydrates (sugars) provide a temporary relief from feelings of dysphoria and fatigue. Following this temporary relief, feelings of depression and fatigue increase, not only creating a further desire for eating a food rich in sugar, but also contributing to the development and maintenance of mood states such as depression. While this hypothesis has not been tested in depressed people, it is similar to that which exists among alcoholics. Alcoholics remember the more immediate mood-elevating and energy-enhancing effect of alcohol consumption and not the negative effects that occur much later. I believe this is why my research has revealed that eliminating added sugar and caffeine from your diet will not only help you control your depression in the short term, but also that these beneficial effects will last over time.

My students and I have conducted several studies (e.g., Christensen, Krietsch, White, and Stagner, 1985; Krietsch, Christensen, and White, 1988; Christensen, and Burrows, 1990) in which we have demonstrated that individuals experiencing emotional distress profit from eliminating added sugar and caffeine from their diet. In the Christensen and Burrows (1990) study we demonstrated that individuals who stayed on the diet continued to be free of their depressive symptoms three months after they began the diet. However, it must be emphasized that this long-term benefit exists only if you continue to avoid caffeine and added sugar.

REAL PEOPLE: THE SUGAR AND CAFFEINE-FREE DIET

Ann was an attractive brunette in her mid-twenties, married, with one child. During the initial interview, Ann revealed that she felt depressed much of the time. She also reported she was quite intolerant of little things her husband did and that they frequently argued. Ann felt as though she was very moody and had a short fuse. She would fly off the handle and get mad at insignificant things. Her anger was so intense at times she felt as though she would get mad enough to kill.

After Ann had been on the diet for two weeks, her depression lifted and her moodiness and anger virtually disappeared. This is not to say she never got mad. Only now she was not as quick to anger. She was more tolerant and had a better marriage. Then I challenged Ann with caffeine. I gave her caffeine-filled gelatin capsules to see if she was sensitive to this substance. When I talked to her at the end of the sixth challenge day, she told me if she didn't get off this substance her husband was going to divorce her. Ann's moodiness, short fuse, and anger had returned. This was a case of caffeine causing the depression.

Linda represents a case where the diet helps but psychotherapy is also needed to treat the conditions causing the depression. When I first saw Linda, she stated that her son, daughter-in-law, and ex-husband were all living with her. She was providing food and shelter for them — yet they did little or nothing to help her clean the house, cook, or even do the dishes after she prepared the meal. To make matters worse, she paid most of the bills. Yet they would criticize her for being selfish and not thinking of them. They constantly asked more and more of her and she would never refuse them! Linda was unable to confront them and to demand that they help or leave. She felt worthless; nothing she did was good enough.

At the time I saw Linda, she was in counseling with another psychologist and taking antidepressant medication. I encouraged her to follow the dietary intervention closely, which she agreed to do. Within two weeks Linda's depression began to lift. As her despondent mood lifted, she decreased her antidepressant medication. (She didn't like taking it because it made her mouth and hair dry.) She eventually quit taking the antidepressant medication and her depression continued to improve as long as she stayed on the diet. Linda also found other benefits to the dietary intervention. As her mood improved, she became more assertive with her freeloading family and insisted they contribute their fair share. However, Linda was living in an unhealthy environment and no amount of dietary intervention could eliminate the unhealthy family interactions. She needed continued counseling to help her deal with her children and ex-husband.

HOW TO FIND A PRACTITIONER

The dietary treatment I have just described is quite new and does not currently have a group of committed practitioners. This is also a treatment program that you can easily attempt yourself. If you have any difficulties feel free to contact me at the following address:

Larry Christensen, Ph.D., Department of Psychology/University of South Alabama, Mobile, AL 36688.

You could also contact a former student of mine at the following address: Kelly Krietsch, Ph.D., Department of Psychology/University of Northern Arizona, Flagstaff, AZ, 86001.

HOW TO LEARN MORE

Christensen, L. *The Food-Mood Connection*. College Station: Pro-Health Publications, 1991. (To get a copy of this book please write me at the above address. The cost of the book is $9.95 plus $3.00 for shipping and handling.)

Christensen, L. *Diet-Behavior Relationships: Focus on Depression*. Washington, D.C.: American Psychological Association, 1996.

Christensen, L. and R. Burrows. "Dietary Treatment of Depression." *Behavior Therapy* 21 (1990): 183–193.

Christensen, L.; K. Krietsch; B. White; and R. Stagner. "Impact of a Dietary Change on Emotional Distress." *Journal of Abnormal Psychology* 94 (1985): 565–579.

Christensen, L. and S. Somers. "Comparison of Nutrient Intake Among Depressed and Non-Depressed Individuals." *International Journal of Eating Disorders* 20 (1996): 105–109.

Fernstrom, M. H., R. I. Krowinski, and D. J. Kupfer. "Appetite and Food Preference in Depression: Effects of Imipramine Treatment." *Biological Psychiatry* 22 (1987): 529–539.

Krietsch, K., L. Christensen, and B. White. "Prevalence, Presenting Symptoms, and Psychological Characteristics of Individuals with a Diet-related Mood-disturbance." *Behavior Therapy* 19 (1988): 593–604.

Leibenluft, E.; P. L. Fiero; J. J. Bartko; D. E. Moul; and N. E. Rosenthal. "Depressive Symptoms and the Self-reported Use of Alcohol, Caffeine, and Carbohydrates in Normal Volunteers and Four Groups of Psychiatric Outpatients." *American Journal of Psychiatry* 150 (1993): 294–301.

Rosenthal, N. E.; M. J. Genhart; B. Caballero; F. M. Jacobsen; R. G. Skwerer; R. D. Coursey; S. Rogers; and B. J. Spring. "Psychobiological Effects of Carbohydrate and Protein-rich Meals in Patients with Seasonal Affective Disorder and Normal Controls." *Biological Psychiatry* 25 (1989): 1029–1040

Thayer, R. E. "Energy, Tiredness, and Tension: Effects of a Sugar Snack Versus Moderate Exercise." *Journal of Personality and Social Psychology* 52 (1987): 119–125.

Wurtman, R. J. and J. J. Wurtman, eds. *Nutrition and the Brain.* New York: Raven Press, 1987.

RESOURCES

Nutrition Reviews, Volume 44 (Supplement), 1986. A supplement to the regular issue of Nutrition Reviews covering numerous topics ranging from the effect of food on brain neurochemicals to the effect of food on children's disorders as well as delinquency and adult mental disorders.

ABOUT THE AUTHOR

Larry Christensen, Ph.D. received his graduate degree from the University of Southern Mississippi and is a member of the American Psychological Association and the American Psychological Society. He advanced through the ranks of assistant, associate, and full professor at Texas A&M University and recently accepted a position as chair of the Psychology Department at the University of South Alabama. He has taught courses in research methods, psychological statistics, social psychology, and the psychology of nutrition. He is past president of the Southwestern Psychological Association and served as committee judge for the Gorden Allport Intergroup Relations Prize. Dr. Christensen has authored or co-authored more than fifty-five scientific articles. His books include *Experimental Methodology, Introduction to Statistics for the Social and Behavioral Sciences* (with Stoup), *The Food-Mood Connection: Eating Your Way to Happiness,* and *Diet-Behavior Relationships: Focus on Depression.*

Brent W. Davis, D.C.

20 Herbal Therapy I: *Medicinal Plants and the Mind*

WHAT IS HERBOLOGY?

Simply stated, herbology (also referred to as phytotherapy or medicinal plant therapy) consists of ingesting medicinal plants to obtain therapeutic benefit. However, if you believe, as did many ancient people, that all of creation is linked in a web of life that can be perceived on many levels (by the five senses and by more subtle, intuitive ways of knowing) then the subject of medicinal plants is more complex.

Plants have a way of getting along with one another; of surviving under the most difficult circumstances; of reliably bursting forth into the joyous gratitude of bloom and maturing to seed, ensuring that the marvelous process of life will continue. The many fine characteristics of plants and medicinal herbs seem to be bound around both their energetic and physiochemical makeup, and these can be transferred to humans under the right circumstances.

Herbs can be used in four different ways to influence the mind. Only the first two are generally recognized by the lay public or by health professionals of industrialized societies.

The first is the use of plant psychotropics such as marijuana, certain hallucinogenic mushrooms, and other "recreational drugs."

The second way is the use of herbs to influence the mind as natural chemical sedatives. An example is valerian, which is used for its natural sedative properties. A relative few master herbs, that is, plants which are unusually broad acting, can be used for therapy in the sweepingly general manner in which many pharmaceuticals are employed. For example, regardless of an individual's history and constitution, the herb echinacea can be successfully taken by most as preventive therapy to increase immune resistance and to avoid catching cold during flu season. However, many valuable herbs do not work as broadly as echinacea, and require deeper understanding to determine what and who they can heal.

The third way stems from the developing field of psychoneuroimmunology, which explores how the mind and the immune system interrelate. There have been findings in that field demonstrating that an impaired immune system exerts an adverse influence on mood states and behavior. Since it is established that the mind can be influenced by the immune system (A is related to C), and herbs definitely can influence the immune system (B is related to C), it is reasonable to suggest that herbs likely influence the mind (B is related to A) by other than sedative or psychotropic means.

The fourth way that herbs can influence the mind is when they are ingested and/or experienced as sacred matter. When this occurs, the consumer/participant can be the recipient of blessings and energizing that may have far reaching beneficial effects.

It is important to distinguish between the first and fourth ways of herbal use. In recent years, articulate and compelling writers and speakers have put forth the notion that the shamanic ritual use of plant hallucinogens represents the highest and most sacred form of herbal experience. I disagree. Ritualistically and chemically powerful hallucinogenic herbs such as ayahuasca (*Banisteriopsis caapi*) or mescaline often catapult the mind and the spirit into the dark places of the astral plane (a potential realm of evil), and without the guidance of a gifted and honestly benevolent shamanic guardian/interpreter, serious psychospiritual injury can occur. The astral plane is the plane of illusion. Unwittingly, an herbal hallucinogen voyager might ascribe significance to a vision that was actually quite irrelevant, or otherwise misinterpret a message out of the darkness.

The highest form of herbal experience, I believe, is achieved by recognizing the living character of herbs with a clear mind and intention, realizing the miracle of life they represent and maintaining an openness to the blessings they offer as pure healing agents.

In psychology, it is universally accepted that the dark or troubled places in the mind and personality must be brought to light before psychological maturity can manifest. Methods used to reveal and eradicate or transform the darkness, however, vary tremendously. Some therapists require patients to jump right into their most troubled areas to confront them and experience the pain of the encounter. Other therapists try carefully to knit together the positive pieces of personality they find to form a protective "housing" in the patient. From that safe place, those under therapy are gradually empowered to discover their own inadequacies and transform them by spiritual will. In the latter method, herbs of many kinds can be especially helpful support. Medicinal plants have an enormous capacity to strengthen spiritual will. And they seem to prefer working by gentle but persistent means. So herbs can be used as an adjunct to psychotherapy, or as part of an integrated approach to balancing the health of the body, mind, and spirit.

HOW IT BEGAN

Throughout history we can see that native peoples thrived as their cultures possessed the accumulated wisdom of centuries of experience with medicinal plants. The development of this knowledge depended on empirical observation, intuitive and mystico-religious perception, and balance and harmony with nature, rather than control over nature. The shaman and healer/priest knew herbs because they lived with them, used them, and understood them as friends and allies. They developed insights out of that special relationship, and they tested their insights by trial usage of the herbs.

For the past several millennia, until quite recently, many native peoples and their healers viewed disease as a teacher that encourages us to restore balance in our lives. Herbs were revered as beings — possessing a nonhuman collective body and consciousness — capable of helping to turn one's life toward harmony and health.

There were differences among civilizations, tribes, and clans in their ability to effect cures. Some were far more accomplished than others. And there was great possibility for variability among healers (and failure or chicanery by some), because healing was generally much more art than science. The most obvious failing of this kind of healing practice was that it generally did not include effective emergency medical care. The greatest accomplishment of many ancient medical systems was their understanding of the use of herbs for reversal of chronic illness, and for health maintenance, tonification, and related improvements in mood and psychic well-being.

Ancient methods of herbal preparation varied considerably, depending upon the state of advancement of the material culture in the society where the herbs were being prepared. For example, Egyptian healer priests at the temple of Ptah in 3000 B.C. had a vastly different intellectual framework and material culture than Australian aboriginals in the same time period. As a result, there were naturally differences in the herbal products each would make. Despite differences in material culture, however, most ancient peoples held a similar belief in the existence of living forces in nature, which should be preserved and concentrated into herbal medicines. The way in which "advanced" and "less advanced" peoples achieved concentration of vital energy into their medicines differed. Less materially advanced cultures used simple methods of herbal extraction that included hot water decoctions (teas). Tablets were sometimes made from dried herbs. Expressed juice of herbs was frequently used right from the fresh plant and, more often than not, was placed on the skin as a poultice rather than taken internally. To add the herb's vital energy to the preparation, "less advanced" cultures communicated with the nature spirits they saw, and asked for their cooperation in healing. They did not intellectually manipulate the herbal product to enhance its healing, but rather entrusted the complex task of healing to the superintelligences in nature — what we would call God or the Creator.

Ancient Polynesians extracted herbs by pounding them with cane juice and coconut, to increase the extraction of alcohol and fat soluble compounds from the plants — a rather ingenious, biologically compatible procedure! A Native American elder of the Iroquois nation told me that long before white men landed on these shores, Indians knew how to distill alcohol and used it only for the purpose of making extracts (tinctures) of herbs for healing.

Ancient peoples with more advanced intellectual and psychospiritual capacities developed more complex methods of herbal preparation. There were healer priests in Egyptian, Arabic, Tibetan, and other cultures. Due to rigorous spiritual disciplines and training they were able to intuitively and intellectually comprehend natural methods to enhance biological activity of herbal medicines. For example, natural ferments of herbs were prepared by complex processes developed long ago in what was formerly Sri Lanka. These processes, when measured by modern scientific means in the 1980s, increased the anti-inflammatory activity of specific herbs by several fold. Interestingly, the techniques called for preparation of products only at times when precise planetary configurations existed. When prepared and measured scientifically at other than the prescribed times, they were significantly less potent. Reducing herb to ash by sequential firing of the herbs in sealed earthenware vessels was developed in ancient India. This process produces a "dynamic energy" (similar to the process of homeopathic succussion and dilution) that makes strong medicine.

Modern science has largely rid medical practice of the mystico-religious experience and reality of older cultures, and has developed intellectual methods of experimental research that can rapidly yield physically useful findings. This approach has allowed great technological progress, and has contributed vastly to a higher material standard of living. We do not, however, live only in a material universe. Many earlier societies have, for millennia, been sustained in large measure by their religious beliefs, their metaphysical perceptions, and their reverence and honoring of nature. They regarded nature and its various life forms as the most tangible physical manifestation of God. To them, control of nature, validation of experimental hypotheses, and interoperator replicability (the watchwords of modern medical research) would have no useful meaning. They related to nature in a manner totally different from orthodox science and medicine. Their approach, which relied on empirical observation, intuitive perception, and balance and harmony, rather than control over nature, is the very thing that allowed them to master the use of medicinal plants, and to understand herbs' influence on the human psyche.

HOW IT WORKS

Herbal practice can take two forms, which I refer to as the sacred and the profane. The sacred deals with using our intuition and our attunement with plants to know how to choose them so that they can be of greatest service. Herbs chosen and used in this way most influence the spiritual heart and the mind. The profane deals with the chemical makeup of herbs, their material preparation, and the gross physical indications for their use. In some cases, the latter method uses herbs as pharmaceuticals (that is, recommending a particular herb for a named disease or a specific symptom). In my experience, using herbs in this way is only minimally effective. Such an approach ignores the wisdom of outstanding healers worldwide since antiquity. That wisdom advises us to treat the patient, not the disease. When treating people as individuals, their unique constitutional inheritance, individual history and state of health, and mental/emotional disposition, play an important role in guiding the knowledgeable physician/healer in the right choice of herbs.

Figure 1 explains some of what I have observed clinically about how herbs seem to affect cures. It represents the idea that, at one end of the therapeutic continuum, substances heal entirely in the subtle, nonphysical "energetic" realm. This is the domain that most influences the mind and emotions. At the other end of the continuum, substances heal by virtue of their gross chemical constituents. This is the domain that most influences the physical body. The center of the schematic represents the halfway point between "energy" and matter, partaking equally of both. A fresh plant extract, which is at the central or 50/50 point, in general represents the most broadly healing type of herbal product. It has a considerable concentration of therapeutic chemicals in it, and possesses, at the same time, a highly energized dynamic character similar to low-potency homeopathic medicines.

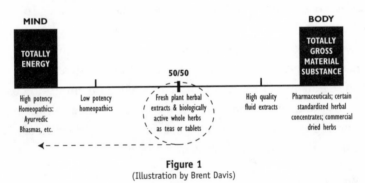

Figure 1
(Illustration by Brent Davis)

The effectiveness of herbs depends on their quality, the knowledge of the herbal prescriber (matching the appropriate herbs to the appropriately identified imbalance), and upon the belief systems of the healing participants. If the herbal healer attending his or her patient believes that herbs can support and heal the psyche, then simple herbal extracts can become more potent and dynamically healing. If a health problem is primarily physical (e.g., simple chemical toxicity), then the concentrated therapeutic chemical aspect of herbs may be most important. If the problem is heavily mental/emotional (psychosomatic), then the subtle nature of the herbal product is of utmost importance. If the problem is mixed in etiology, which so many are, herbs at the center of the continuum are often most helpful. It is worthwhile at this point to describe some of the many methods by which herbs are prepared, and the general character of each.

Commercial (nonorganic) herbal tablets and capsules fall toward the right side of the schematic. They are often relatively devoid of energy. Commercial quality tablets are generally made from dried, powdered herbs pressed together with binders, lubricating agents, and a coating that may comprise as much as 20 percent of the tablet weight. If the tablets are compressed too hard, they do not break down in the digestive tract and are relatively useless. It is possible to make tablets with a higher herb content, and with beneficial properties superior to capsules. In recent years, such beneficial tablets are not commonly found. Mass production of capsules seems to be easier, and that is what most vendors have opted to do. Herb capsules consist of dried, powdered herbs with flow agents in gelatin capsules. A relatively new development is nongelatin capsules, which I feel are superior. Tablets and capsules of dried herbs, if prepared correctly, can be very beneficial if the therapeutic part of the herbs is water soluble. If the therapeutic compounds are not water soluble, then they need to be extracted with alcohol so that they can be absorbed in the digestive tract.

Standardized extracts are herb isolates, which are occasionally made with water or grain alcohol, but which are also frequently made with unhealthy organic solvents and by other industrial chemical means. Such processing destroys the "vital energy" of herbs and renders them as pure chemical substances (like pharmaceuticals). This reduces their healing capability in the mental/emotional realm, but they are useful when concentrated herbal chemicals are all that is needed.

Fluid extracts are one of the older techniques used to concentrate herbs. They are made with grain spirits (and usually glycerin), and are a very good way to make a strong herbal product. Fluid extracts are five to ten times more concentrated than most liquid extracts found in the health food store marketplace. They are not made by most companies because they are costly to produce, and would elevate the retail cost of products. They are a very good way to administer concentrated material, and at the same time, preserve the subtle "energetic" nature of the herbs that benefits the human psyche. The highest quality fresh plant herbal extracts are prepared by crushing freshly picked (undried) medicinal plants, mixing them with an alcohol/water solution to extract therapeutic chemicals and to capture vital energy, letting them soak, pressing out the liquid herbal essence, and filtering the extract. Two companies that have long experience in making high-quality fresh plant herb extracts are listed at the end of the chapter. The benefit of this type of preparation is that it contains a good amount of healing plant chemicals that are highly absorbable, and it captures the vital essence of herbs, which can positively influence the mind and support our spiritual nature.

Homeopathic medicines are made in liquid and dry forms (tablets and pellets) and are prepared from herbs as well as from minerals, animal substances, and chemicals. Their particular healing character comes from the precise way they are dynamized, that is, diluted and shaken, or ground up (succussed or triturated.) As material becomes more dilute when it is dynamized, it gains in the amount of therapeutic energy stored in it, but it loses straight chemical concentration. Many cases call for energy and not for the chemical concentrates that one finds in pharmaceuticals and standardized extracts. Relatively speaking, low-potency homeopathic medicines have not been diluted very much. At very high potencies, there is no matter left in the product — only "energy." High-potency remedies essentially affect the mind and emotions.

Bhasmas are an ancient type of medicine from India (pre-dating homeopathy). They achieve a dynamic energy similar to homeopathics by being sequentially fired in clay vessels rather than by serial dilution.

WHAT THE RESEARCH SHOWS

The highest form of herbal treatment today involves a reverence for nature and an appreciation of the subtle qualities of the plants. It also involves consideration of a vast number of factors that influence the overall health of each individual patient. This kind of healing process does not yield to mainstream academic research methods, for there are too many variables to control in the experimental framework. Consequently, although much research exists on the use of medicinal plants as pharmaceuticals, there is little or no "scientific" research on the subtle, intuitive approach to treating mental illness with herbs, outside of thousands of years of accumulated experience and wisdom. Modern institutional medicine, which is by nature conservative, seems to have adopted the view that if healing procedures of former times are not experimentally measured by current means, they are dangerous to contemplate and irresponsible to employ. Though entrenched attitudes in health care are changing due to pressure from patients who are benefiting from unorthodox healing, institutional medicine and mainstream science have a powerful vested interest in maintaining the status quo.

REAL PEOPLE AND MEDICINAL PLANTS

Randolph Lowell was a giant of a man, just able to clear the six-foot-eight standard doorway entering my treating room. But the first time I saw him, he cleared quite easily, because he was bent over with a lower back injury. Superficially, this gentle, quiet fellow would have appeared to be standard fare for the average chiropractic or orthopedic physician. But in reality, his case was quite complex, as so many are. He had suffered low back disc herniation and strain/sprain to the spinal joints. In providing his medical history during his initial visit, Mr. Lowell revealed much about his life. He worked full-time in a machine shop turning out metal parts on a lathe. As that did not provide adequate income for his wife and children, he felt compelled to work extra hours as a part-time horse shoer. He was often exhausted. Over the last few years he noticed that he often felt listless. His children were often sick with flulike symptoms and middle ear infections.

His wife was weary and concerned about her children and about his long hours of work. There was a lot of love between him and his wife, but there was something wrong in their relationship. He did not want to go into detail in that area. I suspected more would be revealed later.

I explained to Mr. Lowell that based on his history and my physical examination of him, my plan was to reduce acute pain, restore normal mobility, and help him regain normal muscle strength in the low back, sides of the trunk, and abdomen. Strong, balanced muscles act like a splint that promotes healing and can prevent re-injury. That is the mechanical part of the equation. I then would investigate how his internal organs functioned, particularly the bowels. Congested, toxic, or otherwise irritated bowels (and depleted kidney meridian energy) often send out disturbed nervous signals that weaken support muscles, which can predispose the low back to injury. I explained that I would also use reflex analysis to discover how emotional distress might be causing muscle weakness and other body malfunctioning. I told him it would take a few visits to complete this treatment plan.

I made specific gentle structural corrections to Randolph's low back and skull (cranial therapy). I gave him a very high-quality fresh plant extract and flower remedy of the herb echinacea to be taken in small doses frequently, and told him to come back in two days.

When he returned, he stood straight and was obviously in less pain. He had a good response to the structural therapy. But another response was spectacular. His whole energy level was much higher. His face was clearer. Some burden had been lifted from him. I knew that a nurturing herbal force in nature had given him support. The echinacea had acted very well. He and I both knew he would recover nicely.

Echinacea is not normally given for back pain, but in Randolph's case it was indicated. His bowels were sluggish and toxic, which was one of the underlying causes of his back weakness. But his bowel malfunction was not due so much to intestinal dysfunction as it was to total body toxicity. I surmised that the ambient vaporized oil droplets, heavily concentrated in the air at the machine shop where Randolph worked, had built up in his blood and acted like a poison, eventually putting a strain on all eliminative organs.

Echinacea is outstanding in its ability to activate the immune system and increase phagocytosis (engulfment) of foreign matter by the white blood cells. Echinacea helped his whole body by clearing the blood of toxins. Echinacea is also a strongly benevolent plant and can donate vital energy to those who take it if the conditions/circumstances are correct. Many master herbs, both recognized and forgotten, have that wonderful ability.

Over another few visits, with the help of low-potency homeopathic Barberry (*Berberis aquifoliem*) and dietary changes, the structural complaints and pain that brought Randolph into the office had resolved. But he was still not well, and he knew it.

Mr. Lowell was truly a humble and kind man, and although I never mentioned that, he appreciated that I honored him for it. Each of us honored the other. He extended deep gratitude to me for my effort at diligence in his case and for my interest in his life. I appreciated him for learning from his illness and for recognizing the opportunity to reevaluate his life and make necessary changes. It was a privilege for me to treat him, because out of mutual respect a condition was created where he entrusted me to contribute to his spiritual well-being.

Gratitude, honor, gentleness, trust. Those are the characteristics of the transformative healing environment where quantum shifts can occur in a person's life. That is the milieu where the miraculous side of medicinal plants (and homeopathic remedies made from them) can optimally manifest.

As soon as Randolph's condition became stable, he asked me to treat his children — two boys, five and seven years old — and later his wife. When I had seen the whole family, I recognized that there was a pattern to the malaise that seemed to be gripping all of them. It contributed to varied structural and metabolic problems. I began to inquire into the water quality in his neighborhood. It turned out that the water supply had been contaminated with agricultural runoff. Mr. Lowell had avoided the water issue because he feared that this would make the planned sale of their home, and relocation out of state, impossible. In good conscience, he explained, he could not sell his house, for he would not pass his problem on to another. He would not want them to suffer the consequences. After hearing that, my esteem for him rose even higher. There would have to be a way, I thought, for Universal Intelligence to support this fine man and allow his decent hopes and fond dreams to be realized.

I advised Mr. Lowell to use water filtration devises on his drinking and bathing water, and to have his water analyzed. I also advised him to speak with the local health department, water quality assurance officials from the state, and also with his neighbors — in short, to become involved. That was quite a step for this meek, retiring fellow. It must have been what was needed because so much good came of it.

Eventually it was determined that the water was badly contaminated, and there were documented cases of health problems resulting from it. The local water district was closed by the state, and the activism of the area residents caused them to be adequately compensated for the costs of relocation.

One day, after his sons had been treated and had joined their mother in the waiting room, Lowell took me aside and asked if he could speak with me about his wife, JoAnne. He mentioned that she was often weary, noting, though, that she had improved since changes had been made to the family's water and diet. She had various sporadic structural and muscular complaints. A small list of other problems followed. It took him a while to get to the real issue at hand, which was difficult and painful for him to describe. His wife had been the victim of incest by her father, although she never spoke about it. Nor would she seek normal avenues of care such as special counseling or psychotherapy. She loved Randolph very much, he was sure, but she had sexual phobias and ambivalence about receiving and expressing affection. He felt her unresolved experience of violation was responsible for a high background level of nervousness. He asked me to treat her.

I treated JoAnne with techniques based upon the physical complaints she described when I took her history, and upon her physical exam findings. I used eclectic chiropractic therapies, including craniopathy. I saw her perhaps once every four to six weeks over the next year.

Each visit, I changed the vital herbs she received and occasionally applied specific single homeopathic remedies. Initially she responded very well to *Passiflora* (passionflower), first in the herb extract strength, and then in homeopathic preparations. It stopped her nervous tremors. I used other carefully chosen remedies as well. Even though they were very important, there was another force at work. As with her husband, JoAnne had a sense of gratitude when she was being treated. I was heartened that the necessary state of thanksgiving and surrender to the divine had taken place within her heart to foster deep healing.

Six months later Mr. Lowell returned. He was reserved and quiet as usual, but was energetically much richer as a person than when I first met him. He was full of good news about his life. As I treated his minor structural complaints, we chatted. He had found a small farm out of state where he was intending to move with his family. As he rose from the table and stood, preparing to leave, he expressed appreciation for the care he had received and for the improvement in the health of his family. It looked as though he wanted to give me a hug, but he restrained himself. I could see a glistening tear on his cheek. He said quietly, "My wife is all well."

By the look of profound thanksgiving in his eyes, I knew what he meant. JoAnne had been transformed by herbal grace and compassion, and was whole again.

Rose McGuiness always made me laugh, regardless of how terrible the condition of her health. She had a booming voice, a bawdy sense of humor, and a massive, overweight body. She smoke, drank, and ate to excess. When she first saw me, several of her liver function tests were as much as fifteen times higher than normal. Her eyes were jaundice yellow and her skin was yellowish gray. Despite her normally ebullient nature, she was subclinically depressed as a result of her dire medical condition.

She recounted that her whole problem began a few months earlier, after her medical physician prescribed a drug called Tegretal. She took it for two weeks to treat severe facial pain (trigeminal neuralgia), developed a critical liver problem, and was hospitalized. After one month in the hospital and a tremendous number of tests including liver scans and a biopsy, she was sent home with the expectation of liver failure and death within the next few months. Being too ornery to die, she managed to survive by making some essential changes on her own. Basically, she fasted, with occasional chicken and vegetable soups, and lots of water. That pulled her out of the immediate crisis, but she was still in a pitiful state of health.

Rose's case was a classical example of the need for dandelion, a very cooling herb, to quench the "heat" (inflammation/infection) in her liver, and to increase excretion of toxins through the kidneys. She looked at me quizzically when I questioned her about the condition of her back yard. "Of course it has weeds," she boomed out, "what do you think!" Good. I told her husband to dig a quantity of dandelions, and to chop the washed roots and greens into a salad to be thoroughly chewed three times a day. I saw her three days after she began that regimen and the yellow in the sclera of her eyes had diminished by half. She used colorful language to describe both the increased quantity of urine she was passing and its odor. She was utterly amazed at how much better she felt. Within three weeks,

Rose was slowly crawling in her garden, digging her own dandelions and enjoying the process. In addition to herbs, I used all therapies at my disposal, including diverse chiropractic modalities, cranial/sacral treatment, homeopathy, and specific dietary recommendations. The combination of integrated therapies is essential for efficient management of all complex health problems. Historically, herbs were always used as part of a total health system, including diet, spiritual or ritual practices, and some form of manipulation or massage.

In Mrs. McGuiness's case, dandelion was discontinued after six weeks and replaced with herbal combinations and homeopathics. But its initial use made quite an impact upon her. In her own rough way, she described her spiritual joy and renewed faith in the Creator for the grace and mercy of having created healing plants for the benefit of humanity and the earth's creatures.

Because herbs and the allied forces of nature have entered into the healing environment of my office and my life, I have had the privilege of seeing resolution of many different complex health conditions. Herbs are exemplars which aid us along the path. Yes, they have therapeutically active chemicals within them, but that is only a part of their character. And I believe it is an effect of their divine nature, not their principle identity. The most important part of herbs, which can be transferred by consumption, is the love that is embedded in them, distinct in each one, as each human is distinct.

HOW TO FIND A PRACTITIONER

Relatively few practitioners share my herbal methodologies to foster healing and mental health. Those that do have diverse kinds of training. To find a specially qualified person to help you may take time. With that in mind, I suggest the following.

1. Develop an understanding of the two sides of healing: diagnosis and treatment. Dedicated and competent orthodox medical physicians can provide a great service in the area of conventional modern diagnosis, especially if

they can non-invasively pinpoint which of your parts are failing, and how much they have deteriorated. If you have a serious health condition, avail yourself of that information. Save the therapy and unorthodox diagnosis part of healing for someone trained in natural medicine, and avoid using any drugs unless you are in the midst of a medical emergency. If you are already on medication, you will need professional assistance to try to reduce or eliminate its necessity.

2. As you are searching for a qualified natural practitioner, make essential dietary changes on your own. A simple guide to help you in that area is available from Forest Center Herbs. Call (800) 274-3727 for your copy of it.

3. If you have a serious medical condition, find a medical physician who will support you in pursuing natural healing with so-called alternative therapies. You can get a listing of physicians with an open mind to alternative therapies by contacting:

AMERICAN COLLEGE OF
ADVANCEMENT IN MEDICINE
(ACAM)
P. O. Box 3427
Laguna Hills, CA 92654
Tel: (714) 583-7666

AMERICAN PREVENTIVE MEDICAL
ASSOCIATION (APMA)
P. O. Box 211,
Tacoma, WA, 98401-2111
Tel: (800) 230-APMA

4. Herbal Practitioners who have a good appreciation of the subtle, living quality of medicinal plants may be found in the membership of the American Herbalists Guild. These practitioners often work in association with primary health care providers licensed to diagnose.

AMERICAN HERBALISTS GUILD
Box 746555
Arvada, CO 80006
Tel: (303) 423-8800; Fax: (303) 423-8828

5. Your alternative practitioner should be widely trained with a primary background in either chiropractic, naturopathic medicine, or acupuncture. Additionally, it is helpful if he/she is trained in craniosacral therapy, applied kinesiology, and homeopathy. The best herbal healers I know have these qualifications and often one more: they have traveled to other countries to study alternative healing practices firsthand.

For a possible listing of qualified health professionals in your area who share some of my views and who use quality herbs, you may write Phytotherapy Research Laboratories at:

PHYTOTHERAPY RESEARCH LABORATORIES
P. O. Box 627
Lobelville, TN 37097 (Mention this publication.)

To locate health professionals with advanced training in structural therapies (including chiropractic), contact:

INTERNATIONAL COLLEGE
OF APPLIED KINESIOLOGY
P. O. Box 905
Lawrence, KS 66044-0905
Tel: (913) 542-1801

UPLEDGER INSTITUTE
11211 Prosperity Farms Rd.
Palm Beach Gardens, FL 33410
Tel: (407) 622-4706

SACRO OCCIPITAL RESEARCH
SOCIETY INTERNATIONAL, INC.
(SORSI)
P. O. Box 8245
Prairie Village, KS 66208
Tel: (913) 649-3475

For acupuncture practitioners contact:

AMERICAN ASSOCIATION OF ACU-
PUNCTURE AND ORIENTAL MEDICINE
4101 Lake Boone Trail, Suite 201
Raleigh, NC 27607
Tel: (919) 787-5181

NATIONAL COMMISSION FOR
CERTIFICATION OF ACUPUNCTURISTS
1424 16th St. NW, Suite 601
Washington, DC 20036
Tel: (202) 232-1404

For naturopathic practitioners contact:

BASTYR UNIVERSITY
14500 Juanita Dr. NE
Bothell, WA 98011
Tel: (206) 823-1300

For homeopathic practitioners contact:

INTERNATIONAL FOUNDATION FOR
HOMEOPATHY
P. O. Box 7
Edmond, WA 98020
Tel: (206) 776-4147

NATIONAL CENTER FOR
HOMEOPATHY
801 N. Fairfax, Suite 306
Alexandria, VA 22314
Tel: (703) 548-7790

SOURCES OF QUALITY HERBS

In the rural areas of every state there are small organic herb farms that produce lovely quality herbs. It is certainly worthwhile to get to know such establishments. Frequently, however, these farms specialize in culinary herbs and have only a limited supply of medicinal plants. The three sources following specialize in herbal medicines. Their products have been used by leading health professionals for years, and are excellent.

DOLISOS HOMEOPATHIC MEDICINES.
Tel: (800) DOL-ISOS
High quality homeopathic medicines and homeopathic texts are available from this company.

HERB PHARM
P. O. Box 116
Williams, OR 97544.
Tel: (503) 846-7178

FOREST CENTER HERBS
All Saints Hollow
P. O. Box 307
Lobelville, TN 37097
Tel: (800) 274 3727

HOW TO LEARN MORE

Burton Goldberg Group, The. *Alternative Medicine: The Definitive Guide.* Fife, WA: Future Medicine Publishing, 1994.

Bremness, L. *Herbs.* London: Dorling Kindersley, Ltd., 1994.

ABOUT THE AUTHOR

Since 1980, Brent Davis has had a compelling interest in the world of medicinal plants. He has focused especially on bringing to light both forgotten and *de novo* applications of master herbs as they relate to use in everyday clinical practice. In the field of applied kinesiology, he has been the principal voice on herbs for over a decade.

Dr. Davis is internationally distinguished in the ability to create and implement an expansive model for herbal research and practice. He has collected and prepared herbs in the wild from around the world, clinically validated their usefulness, brought lost herbs to the attention of the academic research community, and has co-authored articles in peer-reviewed scientific journals.

In addition to his part-time clinical practice, he creates herbal products for health professionals at PRL-Phytotherapy Research Laboratories, and for the health food store product line of Forest Center Herbs.

Brett D. Jacques, N.D.
Jacqueline Jacques, N.D.

21 Herbal Therapy II:
Herbal Self-Care

WHAT IS HERBAL SELF-CARE?

Botanical medicine, which has enjoyed varying levels of popularity throughout time, is experiencing a true revival in the current decade. This form of medicine is a rich art, blending lore and science, ethnobotany, and double-blind studies. Herbs are good medicine and you can maintain your health with judicious use of them. Plants can be effective allies when addressing mental health issues. More and more research is backing the clinical success of many herbs and providing new ways to use herbs that have had a long and storied use.

Herbal self-care is an important step in taking responsibility for your health and well-being. It is best used for problems that are mild and haven't had a dramatic onset. We recommend that you use herbal self-care for cases of mild depression and anxiety, and occasional irritability. It is also useful in post-recovery phases of eating disorders and addictions. Herbal self-care can be appropriate for other mental disorders such as confusion and memory loss, behavioral disorders, and when used as an adjunctive therapy with more severe depression or anxiety. However, it is important to understand that self-care of any kind is no substitute for the guidance of a trained health care practitioner. The use of herbs should only be combined with prescription medication under the care of an appropriately trained physician.

HOW IT BEGAN

Traditionally, all of the basic maladies afflicting people were treated by herbal self-care. If there was a disease that simple measures didn't cure, the patient was then treated by the person in the village with the most experience. This was usually a woman, who had learned her understanding of plant medicine from her mother and her grandmother. There were also men entrusted to this work who were spiritual healers or shamans, and learned their craft as part of an apprenticeship. Today's botanical medicine owes a great debt to the women and men who preserved the traditions of plant medicines in the face of persecution and adversity. This persecution and adversity continues today, though on different levels.

The new herbal renaissance is built on a scientific foundation. Many studies are being done to verify the effectiveness of plants and their constituents. That we have truly come full circle is illustrated by the following anecdotal time line (from the website of Dr. Peter D'Adamo, N.D., http://www.dadamo.com):

2000 B.C. — Here, eat this root.

1000 A.D. — That root is heathen. Here, say this prayer.

1850 A.D. — That prayer is superstition. Here, drink this potion.

1940 A.D. — That potion is snake oil. Here, take this antibiotic.

2000 A.D. — That antibiotic is artificial. Here, eat this root.

HOW IT WORKS

There are many approaches to botanical medicine. We shall describe some of the more common schools of thought regarding the use of herbs.

In the allopathic approach to botanical medicine, herbs are prescribed based on symptoms and the diagnosis of disease. Allopathic medicine is what most people call traditional medicine, practiced primarily by M.D.'s, but a more accurate term would be conventional medicine. Most allopaths are accustomed to practicing medicine based on following certain protocols — they always use substance "*x*" for disease "*y*." Though the majority of allopaths would probably not use herbs at all, if they do, they are likely to approach herbal medicine in the same way as they prescribe drugs. This method can be very effective and simple to use, and is used by other health care practitioners as well. The good thing about this approach is that research can generally be found to support the herbs and protocols that are used. This may make patients feel more comfortable because the doctor can show them studies and data to back up their treatment. The downside is that, like drugs, not all herbs work for the same problem in different people.

The physio-medicalists, also known as Thomsonians, practiced a method of herbal prescription that involved finding excesses and deficiencies. This system of herbal medicine was developed by a self-trained, lay herbalist named Samuel Thomson, who didn't like medical doctors of the day (Wood, 1992). The physio-medicalists were M.D.'s who shunned the drugs of their day (early 1800s) in favor of plants. This system is still practiced today, primarily by trained herbalists and some naturopathic physicians in America, Australia, and England. Herbalists with the physio-medicalist orientation treat organ systems; they evaluate the status of organ systems by considering nervous system input to that organ and looking at circulation, elimination, and nutrition. Several organ systems may be involved in the diagnosis, and excesses and deficiencies can exist simultaneously. The herbs are chosen based on how they effect the nerve supply, circulation, elimination, and nutrition of an organ system. This approach can be extremely complicated, requiring both art and science.

A third approach is the eclectic system. The eclectics, who flourished in the late 1800s through the early 1900s, rely on physical diagnosis as well as key symptoms — this is an empirical approach similar to prescribing a homeopathic remedy. These doctors were, again, mostly M.D.'s who used whatever worked. They made extensive use of the so-called toxic botanicals in small doses. The eclectics helped to create the understanding that most plants had the potential to be a medicine or a poison depending on the administered dosage. Eclectic herbalism is practiced by many trained herbalist and naturopathic physicians. There are also some medical doctors who use this approach.

There are many other schools or approaches to herbal medicine, and their exclusion from this discussion isn't meant to invalidate them — they are just less relevant to our particular discussion of the topic. When discussing the treatment of various mental health concerns, an integrated approach will probably work best for choosing the botanicals you will use. Please also see the chapter on herbs by Brent Davis for additional insights.

WHAT THE RESEARCH SHOWS

It is common practice in the established U.S. medical community to say there is no scientific evidence for the safe and reliable use of herbal medicine. This is simply not so, and most doctors who say this don't take the time to validate their statements. There is a lot of good research on the safety and effectiveness of phytotherapy. The journals listed at the end of this chapter are just a sampling of the available research reports. Medline, the online computer database of medical journals, can steer you to more studies. Many of these findings are detailed later in this chapter under "What to Expect." The scientific and clinical analysis of phytotherapy (*phyto* means plant) is done in many countries, notably Germany, France, Great Britain, Japan, China, and the U.S. Germany, where phytomedicines are highly-regulated, is the clear leader in the research and classification of herbs. Likewise, in France, most botanicals can only be found in pharmacies. The regulation in Europe has led to safer use of plants and this may follow in the U.S.

However, research isn't everything. A long traditional use of herbs in a clinical setting can also be a valid method to determine the effectiveness and safety of a substance. Medicinal herbs work on many different levels. Some herbs work and no one is sure why, particularly since each health problem usually has many causes. Naturopathic physicians understand and work with this idea, but research is a reductionistic science (meaning that everything is reduced to a simple cause-and-effect formula) and has yet to accept this. Even with growing research, there are few herbs for which the exact mechanism of action is known. When the mechanism is known, certain successes and failures cannot always be explained based on the mechanisms. As a result, the reductionistic approach is hard to apply to plants, as they are complex entities that can work on many levels and are not yet understood in many ways. If they are safe and they work, why not make use of medicinal plants? Many aboriginal peoples understood this, modern naturopathic doctors understand this, but many other health care practitioners do not.

Another unfortunate side of current research, in our opinion, is that it has led to an emphasis on the extraction of individual active components from herbs or on drug development. There can be value in this for the purpose of standardization and reproducible research studies. However, the reduction of a plant to a single active constituent may also limit its application — it doesn't validate the complexity of the many levels on which a whole plant can work. The whole is always greater than the sum of its individual parts. Herbs generally contain multiple active compounds and nutrients. These compounds and/or nutrients can have effects which are systemic or local, long-term or short-term, immediate or delayed.

Still, science is providing new directions for botanical medicines. The discovery of chemical constituents of plants, and the knowledge of the biochemical pathways on which the constituents work, is leading to new uses for old herbs. It is also leading the way for the use of plants that, for whatever reason, had no extensive traditional use. *Gingko biloba* is one such example. The knowledge of its constituents and their biochemical effects has allowed millions of people to benefit from this ancient herb. Gingko wasn't very popular in traditional medicines but, due to science and research, it can now be used with confidence for a number of different health problems.

REAL PEOPLE AND HERBS

Michael was a 39-year-old divorced male who had a long history of anxiety and panic attacks. In the past, he had self-medicated with alcohol. Now a recovering alcoholic, he was turning to naturopathic medicine because, no longer putting harmful substances into his body, he wished to address his anxiety in as natural a way as possible. Michael's symptoms primarily occurred in the evenings after supper. Alone in his apartment, he would work himself into a very anxious state thinking about his children, ex-wife, finances, and job. Since he was no longer drinking to put himself to sleep, he had a lot of trouble falling asleep. He would regularly fall asleep in front of the television well after midnight. After dozing off, he would frequently wake — sometimes many times a night — in a state of great panic.

Because of this pattern, Michael was extremely fatigued when he first approached to the clinic. He was caught in a vicious cycle of anxiety and insomnia, and the resulting exhaustion only served to worsen his symptoms. We treated Michael with two formulas — one for day and one for night. The daytime formula consisted of kava, passiflora, and avena. All three of the herbs address anxiety, the passiflora and avena are good for exhaustion and have the added indication of being specific for people who have had an alcohol or drug dependency. At night we replaced the kava with valerian to help with the insomnia.

Michael's treatment plan also included a number of other naturopathic protocols, including a form of hydrotherapy (see Boyle and Saine, 1988). We addressed his nutrition, provided him with counseling, and eventually prescribed a homeopathic remedy. At his one week follow up, Michael reported that he was now able to fall asleep at around 11 P.M., within an hour of taking his nighttime herbs. He was still waking one to two times a night, but with much less anxiety, and he felt that the quality of his sleep was greatly improved. Between his daytime herbs and the fact that he was now sleeping, he felt that he could get through his daily activities with greater ease and productivity. We adjusted his medications somewhat after the first visit — primarily instructing him to take another dose of his P.M. formula the first time he woke from sleep. Eventually, however, as his anxiety lessened and his sleep continued to improve, he ceased to wake at night, except on rare occasions, and this second dose became unnecessary.

As of our last visit five months after starting treatment, Michael was virtually off his daytime herbs — reserving them for times of increased stress, or if he had not slept long enough the previous night. He was still taking the nighttime herbs, but at a decreased dose, and the second dose was rarely necessary.

Brenda was a 52-year-old female who came to the clinic reporting that she suffered from mild lifelong depression. She had been treated on and off with various medications, but had experienced side effects with the majority of them. Primarily, she had addressed her depression with counseling, a good diet, and regular exercise, which had been fairly effective for her until now. About a year before she came to see us, Brenda had begun to have mild menopausal symptoms — hot flashes, diminished menses, and mild headaches. She had discussed this with her gynecologist, who evaluated her and recommended hormone replacement therapy (HRT), but she declined, not wishing to take the hormones. Brenda came to see us because, while the hot flashes had stopped, she noticed that she was becoming increasingly depressed.

We began by addressing Brenda's menopause symptoms more completely. We evaluated all her hormones (estrogens, progesterone, DHEA, testosterone, and thyroid) via blood and salivary tests, and assessed her cardiac and osteoporosis risks with blood tests, bone density evaluation, and patient history. Based on this work-up and a thorough physical, we determined that Brenda was at very low risk for osteoporosis and heart disease (due to her dedication to exercise, good diet, and minimal family history), and so could be responsibly treated without HRT. We did find that her DHEA was somewhat low, but decided to try other treatments before supplementing this adrenal hormone.

The two herbs that we gave Brenda were black cohosh (*Cimicifuga racemosa*) and St. John's wort (*Hypericum perforatum*) — both in standardized extracts at a dose of one capsule three times a day. We also gave her a high-quality multivitamin/mineral supplement, and encouraged her to continue exercising regularly. At a one-month follow-up visit, Brenda reported that not only was her depression "all but gone" but that her headaches had ceased after one week on the herbs. At this time, we offered her the DHEA again, but she declined, feeling that would rather avoid taking the hormone, especially since she felt so good.

Dean is a 27-year-old male who came to us with mild to moderate depression. When he was younger, Dean had a history of stimulant use, and his depression had essentially begun when he ceased this use. The major symptoms of Dean's depression were low moods and extreme apathy — he didn't want to get out of bed, he didn't want to go to work, then he didn't want to come home from work or get into bed at night. He found these basic decisions were too difficult and stressful.

When he came to the clinic, Dean had been self-medicating with St. John's wort at an adequate therapeutic dose for over three months. He had seen no change in his symptoms and was now seeking guidance with his treatment. Based on the failure of the St. John's wort and the presenting symptoms of apathy, stress, and history of drug use, Dean was given Siberian ginseng — an excellent adaptogen for stress, enhanced energy, and mild depression — at a dose of two grams per day of dried encapsulated herb.

At a two-week follow-up visit, Dean reported that his symptoms were greatly improved. He was performing his daily tasks with much greater ease. He found that he only had apathy about going to bed at night, although he would eventually sleep. At this time, Dean was instructed to take a five-day rest from the ginseng and then resume taking it at a reduced dose of one gram per day.

A month later, Dean returned to the clinic for an unrelated issue. At that time he was questioned about his depression. He reported that he was still taking the ginseng — though not daily — and that he had all but forgotten that the problem had existed so recently.

WHAT TO EXPECT

Herbal self-care should be practiced with an allopathic foundation, adding bits and pieces of physio-medicalism and eclecticism. This chapter will provide you with the basic information needed to get started: The classifications of the herbs, the conditions that they can treat, and detailed descriptions of the herbs themselves. If you're using herbs and something doesn't feel right, stop taking the herb and see your alternative health care practitioner. People are unique. One person's food can be another's poison.

We have chosen eleven categories in which the botanicals available might be appropriate for over the counter use, based on their safety, availability, and usefulness. The indications came from research and from empirical data. We have left most of the hard science out, but have provided references at the end of this chapter for the curious.

One of our major goals here is to keep this information simple. This has led us to discuss only single herbs and not discuss formulas. The reasoning behind the making of a formula can be complex, and some herbs may be compatible together as a formula while others aren't. Single herbs, when used properly, are usually equally if not more effective than a mixture. Also, with few exceptions, most formulas have not been studied. You may wish to experiment with your own combinations, but remember: Keep it simple.

The length of time that you should take an herb can vary, but you need to take it long enough to give it a chance. We recommend taking an herb for about two to eight weeks, then taking a brief "drug holiday" (a few days to a few weeks), and taking it again. Cycling the dosages in this manner works better in the long run.

There are many forms in which plant medicines may be administered. First, one should consider the environment in which the herb was grown. Plants can be cultivated, organically grown, or wild crafted. Cultivated herbs are usually grown with pesticides and other less desirable farming methods. Wild crafted means that the plants are found in their natural habitat, which could be a good thing in northern Maine, but some unscrupulous plant gatherers seem to think the same term applies to plants found in median strips on the L.A. freeways. Organically grown is the best. Think about it — if you want to ingest something natural to improve your health and well-being, shouldn't it be something that you know isn't contaminated with pesticides and exhaust fumes?

When you shop for herbs, you may be overwhelmed by the multitude of forms in which they can be purchased. You may first want to consider what you are willing to ingest. If you don't like to take pills, you may want a tincture or a tea; if you don't care for peculiar tastes, you'll probably want a capsule or tablet. You will find herbal medicines in the following forms: teas/dried herbs, tinctures (alcohol, glycerin, or vinegar), fluid extracts, solid extracts, capsules, standardized extracts, and tablets. There are advantages and disadvantages to all of these forms depending on the herb, its constituents, and the nature of the drying or extracting process.

Classes of Herbs in Mental Health

Phytotherapeutic classification of herbs is based on the particular action that herb has on the body. Many herbs fall into more than one category, based on the fact that they have actions on a variety of systems. Also, different schools of herbalism may put different herbs into different classes. We have outlined here the most common Western classes of herbs that pertain to our discussion.

Adaptogens. This is a relatively new classification of herbal action. It was a term coined by two Russian scientists, and it refers to a plant's ability to balance or enhance the body's ability to deal with stress. Adaptogens usually simultaneously support the adrenal glands, and the nervous and immune systems. For this reason, adaptogens are very important in the treatment of mental health problems. The only real caution with these herbs is that they can be too stimulating. Siberian, American, and Asian ginsengs are the most popular and studied herbs of this category.

Nervines. Nervines are herbs that help nourish and modulate the nervous system. They are usually considered tonics and are needed in many mental health conditions. Nervines include the now popular St. John's wort (*Hypericum perforatum*), and other less famous herbs such as hops, scutelleria, and avena.

Sedatives. These are herbs that have a calming, "depressant" action on the nervous system. We have put quotes around the word "depressant" here because we don't want you to believe that these herbs can cause depression. In fact, many of them are very useful in the treatment of depression, especially if it has a component of anxiety or insomnia. Some herbs in the category are passiflora, kava kava, and valerian. There also is a fair amount of overlap between nervines and sedatives, with many of these herbs possessing both properties.

Stimulants. These are herbs that are considered to have an "upper-like" action on the body. Herbs in this class include coffee, black tea, ephedra, and ginger. Stimulants can be confusing because many plants in this category can also be nervines and/or sedatives. This may be in part related to the dose that is administered, but more likely it relates back to our concept of single herbs having multiple actions. The body usually seems to know what it needs from a particular herb, and that becomes the overall effect. Another way to think of this is that the herbs are acting to normalize function and restore balance. So if the imbalance is in the direction of anxiety, an herb might be more sedating, but if the imbalance is in the direction of lethargy, the same herb might be a mood elevator.

Emotional Conditions Herbs Can Help

Addictions. Addictions and addictive behavior are widespread, and almost everyone has been close to a situation involving addictions. Recovery requires support from friends and family. Herbs may offer some support as well. The cravings and withdrawal symptoms can be difficult to deal with. The side effects of years of substance abuse can also present significant health problems. It is probably good to start with the liver herbs in this case. Several well-studied herbs include milk thistle (*Silybum marianum*), licorice (*Glycerrhiza glabra*), and curcumin (*Curcuma longa*). Kudzu (*Pueraria lobata*) has been shown to reduce alcohol cravings (Keung and Valle, 1993). This vine also has been shown to decrease blood alcohol levels (Xie et al., 1994). Lobelia (*Lobelia inflata*) has been studied for nicotine cravings. Nicotine and lobelia are thought to have the same pharmacological actions, but lobelia is less potent (Murray, 1995). This herb has a long history of use in the United States by Native peoples and the European settlers. It is a much maligned plant, due to its potential toxicity, but can be very effective to aid in nicotine withdrawal. Valerian can be a valuable aid for withdrawal from benzodiazepine drugs like Valium. The active constituents in valerian bind to the same receptors in the body as this class of drug (Mennini, 1993). This should ease the symptoms, but we recommend that this be done under the supervision of a qualified health professional. Other herbs recommended include the green milky sap of oats (*Avena sativa*) to aid the nerves (nervine), and if there is insomnia from alcohol addiction, try passion flower.

Anxiety and panic attacks. Anxiety and panic attacks associated with anxiety limit a person's ability to participate in life. Many plants are useful for anxiety, and these usually fall into the sedative and/or nervine category. Chamomile is familiar for this but has not been backed up by research. The herbs that have been shown to have some benefit with anxiety are kava kava (*Piper methysticum*), ginseng (*Panax spp.*) and ashagawanda (*Withania somnifera*). Kava has significantly reduced anxiety levels in a double-blind study (Kinsler, Kromer, and Lehmann, 1981). Kava does not impair cognitive and mental function but actually improves it (Munte et al., 1993). Panax ginseng is especially effective if the anxiety is due to stress (Bhatta Charya and Mitra, 1991). Ashagwanda is known as Indian ginseng and has been very effective in studies (Werbach and Murray, 1994). Other herbs to consider are listed next with their primary indicators: Passion flower is indicated if the anxiety is accompanied by exhaustion and drug abuse; oats (*Avena sativa*) if there is exhaustion; skullcap (*Scutellaria lateriflora*) if there is oversensitivity; valerian (*Valeriana officianalis*) if there is depression and/or insomnia; and finally, St. John's wort is used if there is accompanying aggressive behavior.

Confusion. Confusion and "brain fog" are vague symptoms that come and go in all of us. There are botanicals that can help reduce these symptoms and the frequency of their occurrence. Mild stimulants, antioxidants, and nervines are the categories usually drawn from. Ginger, which is a mild stimulant, may be helpful. Kava kava (*Piper methysticum*) has been shown to improve mental function (see Munte, 1993). Stinging nettle (*Urtica dioica*) may alleviate confusion that is accompanied by congestion in the head. Gingko improves circulation in the cerebral area (Kleijnen and Knipschild, 1992) as well as having an antioxidant effect in the brain. This second action of gingko may be important because the damage done by free radicals in the brain has been implicated with many disorders of aging including confusion (Brown, 1996). Gotu kola has been used for centuries to improve cognitive function. A study in developmentally disabled children demonstrated improved mental ability (Murray, 1995). Siberian (*Eleuthrococcus senticosus*) and Chinese (*Panax spp.*) ginsengs have been studied and confirmed to help with confusion and brain fog. In another study, Siberian ginseng enhanced mental acuity (Fransworth, Kinghorn, Soejarto, and Waller, 1985). These adaptogens also help the body cope with stress and are good choices.

Depression. Depression is an epidemic in today's society. Many causes have not been studied or explored. The two herbs indicated by research to be most helpful with depression are gingko and St. John's wort. St. John's wort seems to work best in mild, unipolar depression. The actions of this plant are very similar to antidepressant drugs; the active constituents block an enzyme (MAO) that breaks down brain chemicals that act to maintain good moods and emotional stability. St. John's wort is virtually nontoxic. There are many well-done studies demonstrating *Hypericum's* efficacy. Gingko is best if the depression is due to vascular insufficiency or lack of blood flow (Murray, 1995, and Werbach and Murray, 1994). There are many other herbs that have been studied and/or have shown clinical benefits as well. There is research behind the use of Siberian ginseng indicating its effectiveness in depression, which might be due to a balancing of brain chemicals (neurotransmitters). Lemon balm (*Melissa officianalis*) is best for children with mild depression and is probably the best choice for seasonal affective disorder (SAD) depression. Black cohosh has been researched for menopausal depression (Duker et. al., 1991). If there is congestion, try passion flower. For sluggishness and depression use valerian. For someone who is oversensitive and depressed, use skullcap. Cactus (*Selenicereus grandiflora*) is used for depression with fear; oats when there is irritation. For depression after a long illness, try vervain (*Verbena officianalis*). Other herbs used with clinical success are damiana (*Turnera diffusa*) and gotu kola.

Eating disorders. There are three basic categories of eating disorder: starvation (anorexia), overeating (bingeing), and binge-purge eating (bulimia).

Herbal therapeutics for anorexia focus on four classes of plants. Sedatives such as hops and kava help to deal with anxiety around food. Appetite stimulants such as ginger or the bitter herbs including gentian (*Gentian lutea*) and goldenseal (*Hydrastis canadensis*) can be helpful to increase desire for food and to restart a digestive system that has become sluggish from lack of use. Adaptogens can help the body deal with stress better; these include Siberian ginseng and Asian ginseng. Finally, nutritive herbs, such as alfalfa (*Medicago sativa*) and kelp (*Laminaria spp.*) help correct nutritional deficiencies. For excessive eating, appetite suppressants are used, the safety of which are questionable. Green tea (*Camellia sinensis*) is the safest but contains caffeine — about four milligrams per cup (Murray, 1995). Fibers such as guar gum may help to induce the sensation of fullness, but eating a balanced meal containing lots of vegetables would be better. Sedatives and adaptogens are appropriate for bulimia as well, but the choice of herbs for this may depend more on presenting symptoms.

Irritability. The most effective herbs for dealing with irritability will come from three classifications: sedatives to calm the nerves; nervines to help the nerves function better; and adaptogens to help the body respond better to stress. Kava, again, is a good choice for its calming properties. If there is pain, then consider Jamaican dogwood (*Piscidia erythina*). Restless irritability calls for skullcap. If the irritability is from overwork or insomnia, try passion flower. Hops is another good sedative to consider, while a good nervine is oats. The Siberian ginseng, Asian ginsengs, or ashagawanda are all good choices as adaptogens.

Memory. Learning and memory share a lot of the same botanicals with the confusion/brain fog symptoms. The plants listed for those also have research related to learning and memory. Gingko has repeatedly proven effective for memory and learning because it improves blood flow to the brain (Werbach and Murray, 1994). Gotu kola exhibits antistress mechanisms that seem to improve cognitive function. All of the ginsengs have data indicating improvement in memory and learning, and it appears the Siberian ginseng may be the best.

Other conditions. Attention deficit disorder (ADD, ADHD) has been steadily increasing in the population. Treatment with herbs hasn't been studied much, but some clinicians have had success with oats, motherwort (*Leonurus cardiaca*), vervain, and ginseng. Personality disorders are usually treated as part of an overall symptom picture and they have not been clearly defined in botanical literature. The use of sedatives, nervines, and adaptogens might be a good place to start. Treating schizophrenia/psychosis has not been common for practitioners of plant medicine, and ginseng appears to be the only herb mentioned for such use (Sherman, 1979). Most people who are plagued by this affliction are on some kind of medication, so herbal self-care would be contraindicated unless under supervision of an appropriate practitioner.

Detailed Descriptions of Selected Herbs

Following is a list of some herbs commonly used for mental health concerns, along with the indications for their use, the best form to choose, dosages for *adults* and contraindications. Any good herbal reference book such as Francis Brinker's *Formulas for Healthy Living* can provide you with a formula (usually based on body weight and age) for calculating children's dosages. Some herbal products may also list a safe dose for children on the label.

Alfalfa (Medicago sativa): Nutritive for anorexia, many other uses.
Best forms: Freeze-dried capsules or the solid extract.
Dosage: Two to four capsules three times daily or 1/4 teaspoon of the solid extract, three times daily.
Contraindications: Pregnancy (uterine stimulant).

Ashagawanda (Withania somnifera): Adaptogen, for use in anxiety, confusion/brain fog, depression, eating disorders, learning/memory and personality disorders.
Best form: Alcohol extract.
Dosage: 15–30 drops twice daily.
Contraindications: None.

Black Cohosh (Cimicifuga racemosa): Antispasmodic, nervine and sedative for depression associated with menopause.
Best forms: Freeze-dried capsules or alcohol extract.
Dosage: Two capsules three times daily or 15–30 drops, three times daily, of the extract.
Contraindications: Pregnancy (emmenogogue).

Cactus (Selenicereus grandiflora): Cardiotonic that is used for depression associated with fear.
Best forms: Freeze-dried capsules or alcohol extract.
Dosage: Two capsules three times a day or 30 drops of extract three times a day.
Contraindications: People with heart conditions should not use without appropriate health care provider supervision.

Damiana (Turnera diffusa): Nervine and stimulant used for depression.
Best form: Alcohol extract.
Dosage: 15 to 30 drops twice daily.
Contraindications: Pregnancy (uterine stimulant).

Gentian (Gentian lutea): Bitter tonic herb to stimulate and improve
appetite in anorexia.
Best form: Dried powder in capsules.
Dosage: One capsule before meals.
Contraindications: Gastrointestinal inflammation.

Ginger (Zingiber officianalis): Stimulant that is used for brain fog and
depression.
Best forms: Freeze-dried capsules or as a tea.
Dosage: One capsule twice daily or 1/4 tsp. to make a cup of tea twice daily.
Contraindications: Gall stones (cholegogue) and pregnancy (abortifacent,
    though somewhat controversial).

Gingko (Gingko biloba): A mild stimulant that is useful for
confusion/brain fog, depression, and learning/memory problems.
Best forms: Standardized extract powder in capsules (24 percent gingko-
    sides), three times daily.
Dosage: 40-120 mg per day of standardized extract.
Contraindications: None.

Ginseng, Asian (Panax spp.): Adaptogen for addictions, anxiety, confu-
sion/brain fog, eating disorders, irritability, learning and memory difficul-
ties, and schizophrenia.
Best forms: Alcohol extract or powdered capsules.
Dosage: 30 drops three times daily, 100 mg of standardized powdered cap-
    sules, twice daily, or 1.5 grams per day of dried root capsules.
Contraindications: Pregnancy and while on the drug phenelzine.

Ginseng, Siberian (Eleuthrococcus senticosus): Adaptogen for addictions,
anxiety, confusion/brain fog, eating disorders, irritability, learning and
memory disorders.
Best forms: Solid extract, standardized extract (one to three percent
    eleuthrocides) alcohol extract, and powdered dried root capsules.
Dosage: One-half teaspoon twice daily of the solid extract; 100 mg of stan-
    dardized extract three times daily; 30–45 drops of the alcohol extract three
    times daily; one to two grams of the powdered root capsules twice daily.
Contraindications: High blood pressure, and with the use of phenobarbital.

Goldenseal (Hydrastis canadensis): Bitter digestive to stimulate appetite in anorexia.
Best forms: Freeze-dried capsules and alcohol or glycerin extract.
Dosage: One capsule before meals or 10–25 drops of extract before meals.
Contraindications: Pregnancy (uterine stimulant).

Gotu kola (Centella asiatica): A mild stimulant that is used in depression, confusion/brain fog, and learning/memory problems.
Best forms: Standardized extract and alcohol extract.
Dosage: 20 to 30 drops of standardized extract or 45–60 drops twice daily for alcohol extract.
Contraindications: Pregnancy (emmenagogue and abortifacent).

Green tea (Camellia sinensis): A mild stimulant that can be used as an appetite suppressant but has many other uses.
Best form: As a tea.
Dosage: One to three cups daily.
Contraindications: None.

Hops (Humulus lupulus): Sedative and nervine that is used in anxiety, anorexia and irritability.
Best forms: Alcohol extract and freeze-dried capsule.
Dosage: 25 to 50 drops of the extract twice daily or 2 capsules twice daily.
Contraindications: With use of phenobarbital.

Jamaican dogwood (Piscidia erythina): Sedative for irritability with pain.
Best forms: Solid extract and alcohol extract.
Dosage: One half teaspoon twice daily or 30–45 drops of the extract twice daily.
Contraindications: Not for use in the elderly and in children.

Kava kava (Piper methysticum): A sedative used for anxiety and confusion/brain fog. Best forms: Standardized extract (70 percent kava lactones).
Dosage: 100 mg twice daily.
Contraindications: Pregnancy, lactation, depression, and with use of CNS depressants including alcohol.

Kelp (Laminaria spp.): A nutritive herb used in anorexia.
Best forms: Dried powder in capsules.
Dosage: Two 500 mg capsules three times daily.
Contraindications: None.

Kudzu (Pueraria lobata): An herb that is effective in the treatment of alcohol dependence.
Best form: Standardized concentrated extract (5:1 concentration).
Dosage: 250–500 mg per day.
Contraindications: None.

Lemon balm (Melissa officianalis): A good herb for children when they are depressed; it has been clinically effective in seasonal affective disorder.
Best form: As a tea or extract (alcohol or glycerin).
Dosage: Two cups per day of the tea or 15–25 drops of the extract.
Contraindications: Pregnancy (emmenogogue).

Lobelia (Lobelia inflata): Antispasmodic that is effective for nicotine withdrawal.
Best form: Alcohol extract.
Dosage: 15 to 30 drops two to three times daily.
Contraindications: Heart disease, pneumonia, high blood pressure, and pregnancy.

Motherwort (Leonurus cardiaca): Nervine used with some clinical success with attention deficit disorder.
Best form: Extract (alcohol or glycerin).
Dosage: 30 to 40 drops three times daily.
Contraindications: Pregnancy (emmenagogue).

Oats (Avena sativa): A nutritive and nervine used for alcohol and drug addictions, anxiety with exhaustion, confusion/brain fog, and irritability.
Best form: Freeze-dried.
Dosage: Two to four capsules two or three times a day.
Contraindications: None.

Passion flower (passiflora incarnata): A nervine and sedative that is indicated in addictions if there is insomnia. Anxiety when it is accompanied by drug use and or exhaustion, and with depression when there is congestion.
Best forms: Solid extract, extract (alcohol or glycerin), and freeze dried capsules.
Dosage: One-quarter teaspoon twice daily of solid extract; 15–45 drops of extract or two to four capsules twice daily.
Contraindications: Pregnancy (uterine stimulant) and with barbiturate use.

St. John's wort (Hypericum perforatum): A nervine and sedative that is the herb of choice in mild, unipolar depression, and anxiety with aggressive behavior.
Best form: Standardized extract (.3 percent hypericin).
Dosage: 30 mg two or three times daily.
Contraindications: Pregnancy (emmenagogue and abortifacent).

Skullcap (Scutellaria lateriflora): A nervine that is used in anxiety and depression if the person is oversensitive, and for irritability with restlessness.
Best forms: Freeze-dried capsules and extract (alcohol and glycerin).
Dosage: Two freeze-dried capsules three times daily or 15–45 drops of the extract three times daily.
Contraindications: None.

Stinging nettles (Urtica dioica): A nutritive that aids in confusion/brain fog and learning and memory problems, if there is congestion.
Best form: Freeze-dried.
Dosage: Two capsules two to four times daily.
Contraindications: Pregnancy (emmenagogue and abortifacent).

Valerian (Valeriana officianalis): A nervine and sedative that is recommended for withdrawal from benzodiazepines, for anxiety when it is accompanied by depression and/or insomnia, and finally for depression when sluggishness is also present.
Best forms: Solid extract, freeze-dried capsules and extracts (alcohol or glycerin).
Dosage: One-quarter teaspoon twice daily of the solid extract, two to three freeze-dried capsules, or 30–45 drops of the extract.
Contraindications: None.

Verbena (Verbena officianalis): A mild stimulant used with clinical success in depression after a long illness and in attention deficit disorder.
Best form: Extract (alcohol or glycerin).
Dosage: 15 to 30 drops three times daily.
Contraindications: None.

HOW TO FIND A PRACTITIONER

Guidance from an alternative health care practitioner is very valuable and can provide insights worthy of consideration. Finding the right practitioner for you can be difficult. There are many types of alternative health care practitioners; all may be of some use and some are better than others. There aren't many qualified health care professionals trained in the use of botanical medicine. Naturopathic doctors study botanical medicine at a postgraduate medical school for four years under many clinical settings. Naturopaths also receive solid training in diagnostics and therapeutics. There are four accredited schools in North America that train Naturopathic physicians properly. There are a number of mail-order schools that attempt to provide naturopathic degrees, but they simply don't provide quality education and their graduates do not have the clinical training that we believe to be essential. The topic of Naturopathic medicine has been covered in detail in this book by Dr. Jamison Starbuck. We refer you to her chapter for a greater understanding of our practice of medicine, and for information about finding a Naturopath in your area.

There are many herbal schools in the U.S. and hopefully accreditation is forthcoming for these schools because some of these institutions offer outstanding training. Medical doctors and chiropractors do not routinely receive training in the use of herbal medicines and if they do, it is very limited. They do, however, have an understanding of pathology and biochemistry. This allows them to use herbs on a purely allopathic basis with reasonable safety. Some may seek postgraduate training in the use of herbs.

HOW TO LEARN MORE

Alstat, ed. *Eclectic Dispensatory of Botanical Therapeutics, Vol. I.* Portland, OR: Eclectic Medical Publications, 1989.

Bhattacharya, S. K. and S. K. Mitra. "Anxiolytic Activity of Panax Ginseng Roots: An Experimental Study." *Journal of Ethnopharmacology* 34 (1991): 87–92.

Boyle, W. and A. Saine. *Lectures in Naturopathic Hydrotherapy.* East Palestine, OH: Buckeye Press, 1988.

Brinker, F. *Formulas for Healthy Living.* Sandy, OR: Eclectic Medical Press, 1995.

Brinker, F. *Herb Contraindications and Drug Interactions.* Unpublished manuscript 1996.

Brown, D. *Herbal Prescriptions for Better Health.* Rocklin, CA: Prima Publishing, 1996.

Duker, E.M., et. al., "Effects of Extracts from Cimicifuga Racemosa on Gonadatropin Release in Menopausal Women and Ovariectomized Rats." *Planta Medica* 57 (1991): 420–424.

Farnsworth, N. R.; A. D. Kinghorn; D. D. Soejarto; and D. P. Waller. "Siberian Ginseng (Eleuthrococcus Senticosus): Current Status as an Adaptogen." In *Economic and Medicinal Plant Research, Vol. 1*, London: Academic Press, 1985.

Felter, H.W. and J. U. Lloyd. *King's American Dispensatory*. Portland, OR: Eclectic Medical Publications, 1983.

Keung, W. M. and B. L. Valle. "Daidzin and Daidzein Suppress Free-choice Ethanol Intake by Syrian Golden Hamsters." *Proceedings of the National Academy of Science U.S.A.* # 90, no. 21 (1993): 10008–12.

Kinzler E., J. Kromer, and E. Lehmann. "Effect of a Special Kava Extract in Patients with Anxiety-, Tension-, and Excitation States of Non-psychotic Genesis." *Arzneim Forsch* 41, no. 6 (1991): 584–588.

Kleijnen, J. and P. Knipschild. "Gingko Biloba for Cerebral Insufficiency." *Br. Journal of Clinical Pharmacology* 34 (1992): 352–358.

Mennini, T., et al., "In Vitro Study on the Interaction of Extracts and Pure Compounds from Valeriana Officianalis Roots with GABA, Benzodiazepine and Barbiturate Receptors in Rat Brain." *Fitoterapia* 54 (1993): 291–300.

Mitchell, W. *Naturopathic Applications of Botanical Remedies*. Seattle, WA: Self-published, 1983.

Moore, M. *Herbal Repertory in Clinical Practice*. Albuquerque, NM: Self-published, 1990.

Munte, T. F., et al., "Effects of Oxazepam and an Extract of Kava Root on Event Related Potentials in a Word Recognition Task." *Neurophysiology* 27 (1993): 46–53.

Murray, M. *Healing Power of Herbs*. Rocklin, CA: Prima Publishing, 1992.

Murray, M. *The Getting Well Naturally Series: Stress, Anxiety, and Insomnia*. Rocklin, CA: Prima Publishing, 1995.

Sherman, J. *The Complete Botanical Prescriber*. Portland, OR: Self published, 1993.

Weiss, R. *Herbal Medicine*. Gothenburg, Sweden: AB Arcanum, 1988.

Werbach, M. and M. Murray. *Botanical Influences on Illness*. Tarzana, CA: Third Line Press, 1994.

Wood, M. *The Magical Staff*. Berkeley, CA: North Atlantic Books, 1992.

Xie, Chang-I et. al., "Daidzin, an Antioxidant Isoflavonoid, Decreases Blood Alcohol Levels and Shortens Sleep Time Induce by Ethanol Intoxication." *Alcoholism: Clinical and Experimental Research* 18, no. 6 (1994): 1443–1447.

RESOURCES
Journals and Periodicals

Journal of Ethnopharmacology
Journal of Naturopathic Medicine
Medical Herbalism
Planta Medica
Australian Journal of Medical Herbalism

ABOUT THE AUTHORS

Dr. Brett D. Jacques holds a Bachelor of Science in Health and Fitness from Springfield College in Massachusetts and a Doctorate of Naturopathic Medicine from National College of Naturopathic Medicine in Oregon. He currently practices naturopathic medicine in Portland, OR, with an emphasis on the use of botanical medicine. He is also a frequent lecturer and a consultant to the natural health field.

Dr. Jacqueline Jacques holds a Doctorate of Naturopathic Medicine from National College of Naturopathic Medicine in Portland, Oregon. She is currently completing a residency in Naturopathic Family Practice with an emphasis on Physiatry and Neurology.

George Vithoulkas, M.I.H.
Vangelis Zafiriou, M.D.

22 Homeopathy

WHAT IS HOMEOPATHY?

Homeopathy is a holistic therapy. Sometimes called energy medicine, it is based on the idea that disease can be cured by strengthening the body's defenses with substances selected for their energy-giving properties. These substances, which may be herbs, minerals, or of animal origin, are diluted and purified beyond the point of harm to their quintessential energy state. Conventional medicine, on the other hand, treats the separate parts of the body separately, using nuclear instruments, doses of poisons, and surgery to repair the part that is believed to be "sick."

If this so-called conventional medicine — and especially conventional psychiatry — were satisfactory, there would be no need for any alternative. It does not, however, appear to be satisfactory for the following reasons:

1. There is no therapy for chronic diseases (if there were, such diseases would not be called "chronic" but "acute"!). There is only temporary relief of the symptoms, as long as the chemical action of the medicines lasts.

2. Even this symptom relief is not without cost. There is always some damage to other parts or functions of the organism, scientifically called side effect. These side effects may sometimes prove fatal, while the disease that was under treatment was not! The recall of previously widely used medicines because they "suddenly" prove to be dangerous is a well-known phenomenon.

The dominant medical practice often causes more harm than good. Its economic cost is one of the major problems of all Western governments.

No human being has ever been built by joining together eyes, liver, blood vessels, brain, and so on. What we all know is that we are *one* being, not manufactured, not made up of parts that someone has joined together, but born from one cell that evolved into many cells in order to reveal its inherent potential for life. This one cell develops into one complete organism with many functions. The stronger the organism, the more satisfactory the functions (in terms of life expectancy). The weaker the organism, the less satisfactory the functions (what we call "diseases"). Homeopathy aims to strengthen the entire organism so that all of its functions will be improved. If it is possible to change a weak organism to a stronger one, isn't it rational that this organism's functions should also improve? This simple reasoning is the basis for homeopathy. This explains why, for a patient suffering from different diseases, a homeopath will prescribe one remedy for all. The remedy is not for the so-called diseases but for the one weak organism. By making the weak organism stronger, the diseases improve or disappear (unless there is irreversible and permanent damage of the tissues), no matter how many there may be.

HOW IT BEGAN

In 1790, while translating a textbook of pharmacology, Samuel Hahnemann found himself disagreeing with the writer's explanation for quinine's ability to cure malaria. The writer maintained that the plant's bitter taste was the key. Hahnemann decided to test quinine's properties on himself by eating a certain amount of it every day and watching the effects. To his surprise, he noticed that malaria-like symptoms were appearing! After his first surprise, he started to test other natural substances on himself and on the students who began to gather around him. He noticed and wrote down the totality of symptoms that each substance produced, a totality that invariably imitated a natural disease. Hahnemann stated that this phenomenon has the value of a law, and called it the therapeutic Law of Similars. This was the origin of homeopathy as a system of therapeutics and as a medical science.

In his book *The Organon*, Hahnemann states that it is likely that the idea of "cure by similars" was used in ancient times. Cases with hints of cure using similars are mentioned in the Indian Vedas (written in the fifteenth century

B.C.), in ancient Chinese scripts, on ancient Egyptian papyrus, and in ancient Mesopotamian scripts.

Crude forms of homeopathy (cure with similars) are still used in many traditional medicines: chillblains are benefited if rubbed with snow (also mentioned by the ancient Greek historian Xenophon), and burns by warmth. Scorpion's extract relieves the pain of its bite. Covering a jaundiced baby with a yellow cloth may relieve it. "Similar suffering" is the English translation of the Greek word "homeopathy."

Hahnemann presented his integrated work on the foundation of homeopathy in 1810, with his book *Organon of the Rational Art of Healing*, and completed it in 1828 with the book *Chronic Diseases*. In the 1840s, almost half of all physicians in the U.S. were homeopaths, and many large homeopathic hospitals were established to serve the health needs of the population.

HOW IT WORKS

All homeopathic remedies derive from natural sources: animal, vegetable, and mineral. They undergo special production methods and are administered in very minute doses. These doses are so small that they never produce any side effects or have any interaction with conventional or other therapy (although coffee, antibiotics, and medicines containing certain hormones may neutralize the action and the result of homeopathy, if they are used for long). The basis of action of homeopathic remedies is found in their electrochemical nature. Each homeopathic substance, as all elements in the universe, resonates with a certain natural frequency or electromagnetic wave field. When the remedy is prepared, it is first diluted and then succussed, meaning that it is vigorously shaken many times. This apparently causes the water molecules and the primary substance in the formula to hit or bounce against each other, causing friction, and beginning an electrochemical reaction throughout the dilution. This process is repeated several times. With each repetition, the electrical charge becomes stronger. People, too, produce current or electricity, and around our cells we have an electromagnetic wave field that is representative of the cell's present state. When a person ingests the remedy, we believe that the charge in the cells of the body is subtly affected by the charge in the remedy. This can likely affect every cell in the body. This is probably why homeopathic remedies can affect the physical, emotional, and mental aspects of the person. For more information about the remedies themselves, please see *The Science of Homeopathy*, chapters 14 and 15 (Vithoulkas, 1980).

The action of homeopathic remedies is not based on quantity, but solely on the correct match between the person and the remedy. Finding the correct remedy for each patient is a complex process, and it is the main work of the homeopath. The remedy has to correspond to the totality of all mental and physical symptoms, ailments, and disturbances of each patient, with all the peculiarities each symptom appears to have, and all the factors that change it or bring it on. The following is an example of details needed for each symptom of the patient: headache that appears only before the menstrual period for five days, comes at 11 P.M. and leaves at 3 A.M., is ameliorated by external pressure, felt only on the right side of the head, and is pulsating in nature.

A patient who suffers from fear of death and anxiety about her health, is introverted and shy, and has intolerance to the sun, will need a different remedy if she also suffers from the above-described headaches; and yet a different remedy if she is very extroverted and "warm" to everyone, very social, suffers from nose bleed, cannot tolerate cold weather, and her headaches disappear after a little sleep. The difficulty in finding the recommended remedy is more than obvious, as there is only one remedy for each patient, each time.

Another important concept in homeopathy is that chronic diseases, both mental and physical, exist due to the predisposition of each organism for them to appear. This predisposition exists from birth and is due to the parents' general (mental and physical) condition of health, to their health at the time of conception, and to the mother's physical and mental condition during pregnancy. This predisposition includes phenomena that are not known as diseases according to conventional medicine, such as emotional vulnerability (oversensitive or easily hurt or easily offended), or lack of endurance to sleep deprivation or to physical exertion, cold or wet weather, etc. If the individual is exposed to normal environmental stresses, which he himself experiences as excessive and above his abilities because he is constitutionally vulnerable to them, this will weaken the whole organism, and the result is the appearance (or the aggravation) of the illness that was innate in the organism from birth. This concept is related to the conventional medical concept of psychosomatic disease.

The predisposition includes not only the chronic diseases from which the organism will suffer, but also a vulnerability to certain factors which vary from person to person and which will act as a result as exciting causes for the appearance of the chronic diseases. It is our personal belief that each individual's predisposition includes also the age at which each chronic disease will first appear if the patient lives a natural life. The more stressful and unnatural a life he or she leads, the earlier the onset of the diseases.

Modern medical investigations of the last few decades tend more and more to confirm this 200-year-old homeopathic concept of the predispositions as the real cause of chronic disturbances: "the genetic factor" and "the familial trait" are referred to as underlying most long-standing health problems, either mental or physical. Homeopathy decreases the effect of the predisposition, which is absolutely unique and peculiar to each one of us, so it is not only the real psychosomatic medicine, but also a true preventive medicine: by changing the whole organism to a healthier one, the possibility and the potential severity of a future illness under any circumstances is reduced.

WHAT THE RESEARCH SHOWS

The effectiveness of homeopathy on neurological or any other physical disturbances (which by their nature are not susceptible to placebo effect explanations); its positive results in many different diseases, on children, babies and even animals; and its immediate effect on insect and snake bites, and on bruises and sprains, prove its reliability beyond a doubt. Any physician can be persuaded of the efficacy of homeopathy, if he or she cares to spend ten hours of their time in the office of a homeopath, listening to patients' reports. This is exactly the way all homeopaths were initially convinced, from Hahnemann's first students to the authors of this chapter.

Conventional medicine demands the kind of proof that is compatible with its own needs and peculiarities, proof that focuses attention solely on the body part, and that can be demonstrated using so-called double-blind experiments. When it comes to testing homeopathy, the great difficulty with this form of experiment arises in three main areas:

1. There is no remedy-illness correspondence. Three patients suffering from panic disorder will need three different remedies respectively, depending on the whole mental/physical condition of their organism. Accordingly, it seems impossible to evaluate the effectiveness of homeopathy using a double-blind method, which requires the same therapy for all patients.

2. In the case of a patient who asks for homeopathic treatment for a skin problem, while she also suffers from asthma and phobias, we expect that during

treatment her skin problem will remain the same or even become worse, while at the same time her deeper and more serious problems of phobias and asthma will improve considerably or impressively. This means that the patient herself will become much healthier, although her skin disease remains the same or even grows worse. How can this skin disease ever be addressed in a double-blind experiment to examine the effectiveness of homeopathy?

3. There is no double-blind method able to test the total modification of health during or after the action of a remedy, because a) the factors that would have to be measured and evaluated are so numerous that the experiment would become impossible, and b) no conventional therapy has ever been made (or even planned) to act on improving the total health of a patient.

Researchers (Delinick, Bourkas, and Karagiannopoulos, 1994) have, however, developed a machine that can measure the electrical properties of homeopathic remedies. This shows promise as a useful research technique.

REAL PEOPLE AND HOMEOPATHY

In September 1994, a 35-year-old man came to the clinic, suffering from intense fear of people — a fear he had ever since his early childhood. He also had a mild stammer. After forty-five days of homeopathic treatment, he referred to a 70 percent improvement of his social phobia (he described it as "social cowardice") and his introversion. He felt that his self-confidence was much better, and the quality of his sleep and vitality had improved a lot. His stammering remained the same. On completing three and a half months of therapy, all the above became even better, while he mentioned a reduction of his "sexual weakness" and a diminished tendency to bite his nails. No improvement of the stammering has occurred to date.

A 13-year-old boy was brought to us in June 1992 by his parents for a strong fear of death and heart diseases. He was also very afraid of chickens

("I feel chills on seeing them") and a little less of other birds. He was scared of any height, worried a great deal about his parents, while he remembered that "even as a baby I was very anxious about everything." As far as he could remember, he had always had a fear of death, but it had become worse during the last three years, after his uncle's death. No doctor's assertions had any effect on his fears and anxieties. Even his dreams were often about death. After twenty-five days of treatment, his father referred to an improvement of 50 percent in his fear of death and of being alone. After four months of treatment, the father evaluated the result of homeopathy as "unbelievable": almost no fear of death or heart disease; he had started eating meat and all kinds of food, which he had previously avoided as hazardous for his health; his fear of chickens and birds had diminished considerably; he seemed and felt much less anxious. The dreams about death never appeared again. There has been no relapse as of February 1995.

∞

A 23-year-old woman with Down's syndrome (mongolism) came to us in 1983, escorted by her mother. For the last three years she had been "saying irrational things, she talks alone as if conversing with someone, she has become very irritable and quarrelsome. While before she was a calm character, now she gives the impression of not realizing where she is, she doesn't recognize voices when answering the telephone, she does not permit us to go very near her, and she reacts very violently." During the last three months, she had asked for a man and had masturbated in the presence of others. She needed thirty-two days of homeopathic treatment for a 70–100 percent improvement to all the above symptoms, plus the reduction of her extreme thirst and menstrual problems.

∞

In September 1990, a 46-year-old woman was visited at home. Her eyes looked vacant. She heard voices: "a female one from near, and another female one from far away. They are trying to confuse me." She said that the voices were having discussions, giving her suggestions and orders, and trying to tease or frighten her by planning to do harm to her relatives. Sometimes "they" joked and she laughed a lot. Her relatives often saw her swearing at invisible people, or making grimaces at them. It was very difficult to make her talk in detail about what was happening inside her, but she often wept for no obvious reason. Sometimes she said she felt ashamed to talk about the things the voices told her. Her mental illness had started fifteen years ago, and the symptoms fluctuated according to the psychiatric medication she was given each time. By the fiftieth day after starting homeopathic treatment, she had reduced the psychiatric medicines by 50 percent and said: "the tremendous depression I was feeling disappeared, I have no fear of going out of my house any more. I see the world differently now. I don't feel oppressed by fear. Those voices I was hearing have stopped." Three months after the onset of homeopathy, she stopped all psychiatric medication and commented: "I have become a completely different person, I feel free and reborn, I feel joy just by seeing the trees and the colors around me. I have gained self-confidence. My only problem is a physical weakness I feel." She looked much better and her relatives found her "absolutely normal." One year later, she married an architect and remains free from the mental illness to date, with no relapse and no need for further treatment.

A 38-year-old man came to the office in 1990 for a vision problem he had experienced for two years. During the investigation of his psychological condition, he described himself as "very authoritative and dictatorial with my children, very self-centered, tremendously egotistical, I feel I am the center of the universe, that no one around me is of as great a value as I am, I feel contempt for my wife, in any company I feel that all others are inferior. Insecure about my sexual ability (which is really poor). I deserve a better wife, and if I had no sexual problem I would divorce. I feel afraid to argue with others, and this is why I have never quarreled in my life. I am afraid in public places and have no self-confidence at all." He also suffered from anxiety about his health and fear of death.

It was clear that what we were dealing with here was mainly a personality disorder (what textbooks call narcissistic personality disorder) that touched, however, on the borderline of a delirious perception of reality, regardless of the fact that he came for the vision problem. All psychiatrists testify to the incurability of such cases, and of personality disorders in general.

The patient came back for a second visit after thirty-eight days of homeopathic treatment. He already looked much calmer and more relaxed. Strangely, he did not refer to his vision problem at all, but right from the beginning he expressed that "I gained an inner peace, self-confidence, joy for life, happiness. I had two professional failures this month that otherwise would have broken me to pieces, and they did not bother me. I feel very well. Less irritable. It is the first time in my life that I feel so happy. I live all the details of life. I see the same things as before but now they seem beautiful." His dictatorial behavior toward his children had diminished considerably, he didn't feel any contempt for his wife ("I have accepted her"), he felt no fear of death ("Now I go for walks around the cemetery"), he did not feel that he would divorce if he had no sexual problem. His sexual ability was slightly better, and for the first time he occasionally awoke in the morning with an erection. About his fear in public places, he commented that it was no longer so dramatic. His anxiety about health had decreased a lot. His vision problem improved during the third month of therapy.

☙

In the case of a 23-year-old woman with enuresis (bed-wetting) present from birth, we had to face the difficult task of finding the remedy her organism needed, and so our first eight different remedies failed to have any effect. Two months after the ninth — and indicated — remedy, her problem disappeared.

☙

In January 1990, a 17-year-old girl was brought to us by her mother for help with anorexia nervosa. In the last eighteen months she had lost more than 36 pounds and kept losing more. She weighed 107 pounds and her height was 5' 6". Her period had disappeared six months previously, her breasts had diminished in size, and she suffered from constipation. She used to hide food in closets and other places in the house, pretending that she had eaten it. "She is possessed by the persistent idea that if she eats even a small amount of food her body will become deformed," her mother said. Her mother described her as tremendously sensitive and very easily offended, while the girl described herself as "very closed and timid, not sociable at all, weepy, anxious about everything, so insecure that I rarely go out alone. I am afraid of others. I speak to no one at school." Having completed one month of homeopathic treatment, she commented that she felt no anxiety at all, she liked going out, had made some friends at school, slept more, and had no more constipation. She had wept only once, and had gained 2.2 pounds. One year after the first visit she said, "I have changed a lot in everything, I cannot believe the changes that are happening inside me." She had gained 10–12 pounds, but her menstrual period had not reappeared yet. Here we may note the priority that the organism gives to the restoration of the mental functions, leaving the physical problems for later. The reappearance of the period was delayed in this patient, because her organism could not endure the energy loss (blood loss) that this function implied. In the summer of 1991, she weighed 124 pounds she looked better than ever, and her mother stated that "psychologically she has improved in leaps and bounds. The difference is tremendous." The menstrual period reappeared two years after the onset of treatment, when she weighed 139 pounds (32 pounds gained). The total duration of homeopathic treatment during those two years was four months.

A 28-year-old man with a height of 5' 9" weighed 348 pounds. "As far as I can remember I have always been obese. I feel the need to eat often, otherwise I feel irritable and restless. When I sit down to eat, I feel as if it is the last time in my life, and I want large quantities of different foods." Three months after the first visit he had already lost 48 pounds, with no personal effort and no diet at all. His appetite had decreased. He felt much better psychologically. His vitality was improved. He did not feel irritable and restless when hungry, did not have the feeling of eating for the last time. He bit his fingernails much less than before, and almost stopped snoring at night. His sexual desire had diminished (it had been very frequent and he had been masturbating twice a day), and he was less anxious during work. Two years later he weighed 240 pounds. He never dieted. Psychologically he was much better.

A 37-year-old man complained of "restlessness felt inside my body, irritability, and difficulty in concentration. I drink alcohol that has a sedative effect on me, but afterwards I feel worse." He drank one liter of wine or three liters of beer every day, and had done so for the last five years. After one month of treatment, his consumption was reduced by 30 percent. Six months later he drank 70 percent less. Right from the first month after starting therapy he said he was "more optimistic, had better self-confidence, and was less timid," while during the fourth month a great improvement in vitality was added, plus an improvement in his sexual ability, concentration, and tendency to irritability. He looked much better. He never had a relapse.

A five-year-old girl was brought in by her parents for frequent colds and ear infections. During the psychological investigation of the child, her parents revealed that ever since she had started walking and going out, she stole things from any shop they visited. Her parents had to be very cautious about her, because of the subsequent problems, and were very hesitant to go shopping or even to visit friends with her. They described her as very lazy and jealous, weepy and obstinate. They said, "she is so difficult that very often we hit her." The second visit took place forty-five days later: the kleptomania had completely disappeared, she had become a child who was "much easier to handle, and we never needed to hit her again," her appetite and sleep had improved; and she wept much less. In later visits we were able to check that her tendency for frequent colds and ear infections had also disappeared.

Homeopathy can also be used to treat the following disorders: psychoses (popularly known as "insanity"), stuttering, elective mutism (often associated with excessive shyness, social isolation, withdrawal, clinging, school phobia or refusal, other phobias and enuresis (bed-wetting), creating a syndrome that is found in homeopathic textbooks to be cured very often with the remedy *Baryta carbonica)*, pica, sleep problems, attention deficit disorder with hyperactivity (also referred to as minimal brain dysfunction), and "psychosomatic" diseases (like asthma, ulcerative colitis, peptic ulcer, several skin diseases, and juvenile diabetes).

WHAT TO EXPECT

In order to find the correct remedy, we have to know how a particular patient functions physically, mentally, and sexually. We have to learn about their food desires and aversions (indicating the condition of his metabolism), sleep peculiarities, adjustment to all kinds of weather conditions, etc. All of these are investigated during the first interview, which takes at least one hour, in most cases. During the second interview, which for chronic patients usually takes place one month later, we try to find out the exact changes that the homeopathic remedy has brought about in each one of the patient's symptoms. The totality of the changes produced indicates the result of the remedy's action, and the need for possible continuation of the treatment, with the same or a different remedy.

There are no homeopathic psychotropic drugs or tranquilizers *per se*, because there is no direct correspondence between a given remedy and one specific "disease." Mental diseases disappear as the whole organism becomes healthier, and the improvement in mental health takes place at a faster rate than the improvement in physical health, since the body seems to tend to the most crucial functions first.

The percentage of cure and the number of diseases that will improve in a given period of time depend on the strength of the person and not on the name of the disease. Thus, five people with exactly the same psychiatric diagnosis will have different prognoses. This is also observed in conventional psychiatric treatment. If we succeed in finding the specific remedy needed by a particular patient, there will be an improvement in his or her mental illness no matter what diagnostic category this belongs to, from the very mild anxieties to serious organic mental disorders.

A precious gift found in homeopathic treatment is the restoration of health to a much better state than that existing before the onset of the disease, which means that given the same, or even worse, exciting causes, the disease will not reappear. The patient often expresses this new experience with phrases like "I have never felt better in my life," or "I feel a completely different person," or "my relatives are surprised by the changes."

Homeopathic remedies not only lack side effects or any undesirable interaction with any other therapy, they also bring about long-lasting results that may benefit the patient for the rest of his or her life. The therapeutic value of homeopathy is mainly tested by long-standing phobias that are persistent, heavy, and resistant to any other therapy, and by obsessive-compulsive disorder and suicidal depressions.

HOW TO CHOOSE A HOMEOPATH

Following are some criteria for assessing the quality and reliability of a homeopath:

1. A good homeopath prescribes one remedy at a time, to treat the whole organism, not just one symptom.

2. The first interview should not last less than one hour.

3. All the patient's symptoms at all levels (mental and physical) should be noted, otherwise it is impossible to recall them all from memory and evaluate them during the second, fifth or tenth reexamination.

4. The remedy should be prescribed to address the totality of the patient's problems, and not only the one that sent him or her to the homeopath in the first place. During homeopathic treatment, the organism begins with the most important matters and leaves the least important for the end. Only in acute conditions or acute exaggerations of chronic diseases are we justified in giving a local action remedy, based on the evaluation of the acute condition exclusively. This remedy will not improve total health (unless it happens to be the one the whole organism needed also), and the underlying long-standing illness will remain unchanged.

It is not advisable to use other alternative healing methods in combination with homeopathic treatment, as they may change the symptoms. This would

make it difficult for the homeopath to evaluate the true effect of a given remedy, and he or she would be prescribing based on false symptoms.

Following is information gathered by the editor of this book, Lynette
Bassman, on finding a homeopath in the United States.

For a national directory of homeopaths in the U.S., contact the National
Center for Homeopathy at:

NATIONAL CENTER FOR HOMEOPATHY
801 North Fairfax St., Suite 306
Alexandria, VA 22314
Tel: (703) 548-7790
or visit their web site at http://www.healthy.net/nch

The International Foundation for Homeopathy can provide referrals and
additional information about classical homeopathy. Write to them at:

THE INTERNATIONAL
FOUNDATION FOR HOMEOPATHY
P.O. Box 7
Edmonds, WA 98020
Tel: (206) 776-4147; Fax: (206) 776-1499

The National Council for Homeopathic Certification has established a
procedure for the certification of homeopaths. While their certification is not
mandatory, and is not a license, it is an important step in establishing the
national identity of the homeopathic profession, and assures certain standards
of training and competence. They can be contacted at:

THE NATIONAL COUNCIL FOR
HOMEOPATHIC CERTIFICATION
1709 Seabright Ave.
Santa Cruz, CA 95062
Tel: (408) 421-0565

Following is a list of homeopaths and homeopathic centers in Europe recommended by the authors:

THE FACULTY OF HOMEOPATHY   DR. BRIAN KAPLAN
OF THE ROYAL LONDON   136 Harlem St.
HOMEOPATHIC HOSPITAL   London WIN IAH, U.K.
Great Ormond St.   Tel: 00441-71-487-3416
London WC 1N 3HR
Tel: 00441-71-837-8833

CLINICAL TRAINING CENTER FOR
CLASSICAL HOMEOPATHY
12 Septemberstraat, 19
3940 Hechtel-Eskel Belgium
Tel: 0032-11-732355

CENTRO DI MEDICINA OMEOPATICA
Dr. Mangialavori M.
Via Rolda 91
41050 Modena Italy
Tel: 0039-597-48088

CENTRO DI MEDICINA OMEOPATICA
Dr. Stefano Barni
Via S. Vincenzo 59
36016 Thiene (VI) Italy
Tel: 0039-445-380348

GEORGE VITHOULKAS STIFTUNG FUR
KLASSISCHE HOMOOPATHIE
Heimstrasse 32B
D - 82131 Stockdorf Germany
Tel: 089-8561644

HOW TO LEARN MORE

Borland, D. M. *Children's Types*. London: The British Homeopathic Association.

Coulter, C. R. *Portraits of Homeopathic Medicines, Psychophysical Analyses of Selected Constitutional Types*. Berkeley, CA: North Atlantic Books, 1986.

Delinick, A., P. Bourkas, and K. Karagianopoulos. "Experimental Evaluation of the Potentization of Homeopathic Remedies." *European Journal of Drug Metabolism and Pharmakokinetics* 19, no. 2 (1994): 68.

Hahnemann, S. *The Organon of Medicine*. Calcutta: Roysinghand Co., 1962.

Herscu, P. *The Homeopathic Treatment of Children*. Berkeley, CA: North Atlantic Books, 1991.

Kent, J. T. *Lectures on Homeopathic Philosophy*. New Delhi: B. Jain Publishers, 1982.

Vithoulkas, G. *Materia Medica Viva, Volumes I, II and II*. London: Homeopathic Book Publishers, 1995.

Vithoulkas, G. *Homeopathy, Medicine of the New Man*. Second Edition. New York: Simon & Schuster, 1992.

Vithoulkas, G. *A New Model for Health and Disease*. Berkeley: North Atlantic Books, 1991.

Vithoulkas, G. *The Essence of Materia Medica*, New Delhi: B. Jain Publishers, 1990.

Vithoulkas, G. *The Science of Homeopathy*. New York: Grove Press, 1980.

ABOUT THE AUTHORS

George Vithoulkas was born in Athens in 1932. After studying civil engineering at the Polytechnicon in Athens in 1959, he worked as a civil engineer in South Africa. It was during this time that he first encountered homeopathy and dedicated himself entirely to studying it. He studied classical homeopathy in Noel Puddhephat's School in South Africa until 1962. He continued his homeopathic studies in India at the Bombay Homeopathic Medical College and after that at the Indian Institute of Homeopathy (Calcutta) until 1966. In 1967, he returned to Athens and began to teach classical homeopathic medicine which was almost unknown at that time in Greece. In 1970, Vithoulkas founded the Athenian School of Homeopathic Medicine. In 1971, he established the Greek Society of Homeopathic Medicine. In 1975, with a small team of doctors, he established the Centre of Homeopathic Medicine (K.O.I.) in Athens, which he still directs. The books of George Vithoulkas have been translated into seventeen different languages. He was recently awarded the Right Livelihood Award (the alternative Nobel prize).

Vangelis Zafiriou, M.D., psychiatrist, is 43 years old and was born in Greece. He graduated from high school in Minneapolis in 1969, and from Thessaloniki Medical School in 1977. He specialized in psychiatry in 1982 at the University Psychiatric Hospital in Athens, and is experienced in psychotherapy. Dr. Zafiriou studied homeopathy under the supervision of George Vithoulkas from 1979 to 1982 in the Athenian Center of Homeopathic Medicine, and has been practicing there since 1983. He teaches homeopathy at the Athenian Center, as well as at the Greek Homeopathic Association, and belongs to the educational committees of both. He has presented papers on ethnological, psychoanalytic, artistic, and philosophical issues related to homeopathy.

Alexander Neumeister, M.D.
Norman E. Rosenthal, M.D.

23 Light Therapies

WHAT IS LIGHT THERAPY?

Light therapy is a nondrug treatment used especially for depression, but it has shown promise for the treatment of other conditions as well (discussed below). Light therapy involves exposing a person to bright, artificial light, with an intensity of about 10,000 lux (the unit of measurement for light intensity), for about forty-five minutes in the morning and in the evening. The remarkable success of bright light therapy for seasonal affective disorder (SAD) makes it the treatment of choice for this condition (Rosenthal et al., 1984; Kasper et al., 1989; consensus report of the Society for Light Treatment and Biological Rhythms, 1990), but other treatments including antidepressants, stress management, exercise, and psychotherapy might be useful too.

SAD is a syndrome characterized by the annual appearance of depressive episodes during the fall and winter; these episodes go away during the spring and summer (Rosenthal et al., 1984). Symptoms of SAD include depressed mood, overeating with carbohydrate craving and weight gain, sleeping more than usual, fatigue, and social withdrawal. The depression can last for several months, depending on the person and the geographical location. The long duration of the symptoms distinguishes these depressive episodes from the so-called holiday blues, a psychological reaction to stress that typically occurs around the holiday season (Rosenthal, 1993). In most clinical samples of SAD, women outnumber men by about three to one, and studies have found that, in general, women report more of a seasonal pattern than men (Kasper et al., 1989; Rosen et al., 1990).

There are indications that light therapy can be useful for depression that does not follow a seasonal pattern; it can be used as an addition to medication therapy for people who have not had good results with medication alone. Further treatment indications for light therapy include the treatment of jet lag, shift-work, delayed-sleep-phase syndrome, and premenstrual syndrome. These problems all involve the capability of light to alter daily biological (circadian) rhythms in humans (for example, the sleep-wake cycle, temperature rhythm, and the cycles of hormonal rhythms).

HOW IT BEGAN

Although the beneficial effects of exposing people to artificial bright light have been well-known for some time, the "modern" era of light therapy began in the 1980s when a 63-year-old man came to the National Institute of Mental Health. He sought help with recurrent depressive episodes during the fall and winter months, which alternated with periods of stable or elevated moods during the spring and summer. This patient had reached the conclusion that the changes in length and intensity of environmental light might contribute to the cause of his depressive episodes. He was treated with light therapy (light intensity: 2,500 lux) for ten days; after four days of treatment he switched out of his depression (Rosenthal et al., 1983).

Since this initial case study, controlled trials have demonstrated the efficacy of bright light treatment for seasonal affective disorder. During recent years, physicians and patients have shown an increasing interest in the origins of SAD and the possibility of treating this disorder with light therapy. This interest is evident not only in the increasing number of scientific publications on the topic, but also by the appearance of books, newspaper articles, and radio and television programs on the topic. The Society for Light Treatment and Biological Rhythms (SLTBR) was formed in 1988 by the leading researchers and clinicians in this field, most of whom are still active in research and clinical work today. The society sponsors an annual conference on the latest research in this field.

HOW IT WORKS

Based on the knowledge that many animals exhibit seasonal changes in behavior and physiology (e.g., reproduction, migration, and hibernation), researchers explored the possibility that biological rhythms in humans might also be controlled by environmental light. It is widely acknowledged that biological rhythms in humans are controlled by an internal central pacemaker located in a region of the brain called the nucleus suprachiasmaticus (Duncan, 1996). From these findings a number of different hypotheses about the origins of SAD and the mechanism of action of light therapy have been investigated during recent years and are the focus of ongoing research.

WHAT THE RESEARCH SHOWS

Although no one knows exactly how light therapy works, there are some active areas of research that have shown promising results. Several researchers have explored the potential role of the brain chemical serotonin in depression (Asberg et al., 1976; Heninger et al., 1984), and how it relates to SAD and light therapy (Jacobsen et al., 1989; Kasper et al., 1996). Carlsson and colleagues found a seasonal rhythm in the amounts of serotonin present in the brains of people who had died during different seasons, with minimum levels during the winter months (Carlsson et al., 1980). Drugs that affect serotonin have been found to be effective in the treatment of SAD (O'Rourke et al., 1989; Lam et al., 1995; Blashko, 1995), and many of the symptoms of SAD, such as overeating, carbohydrate craving, and fatigue have been postulated to be closely related to problems in the functioning of serotonin in the brain (Fernstrom, 1988; Rosenthal et al., 1987; Rosenthal et al., 1989; Wehr et al., 1991). Possibly the strongest evidence that brain serotonin is involved in the mechanism of action of light therapy comes from two studies (Lam et al., 1996; Neumeister et al., 1997) showing that temporarily lowering brain serotonergic activity results in an increase in depressive symptoms in patients who were previously treated successfully with light. So far, we have no answer to the question of whether abnormalities in brain serotonergic functioning are confined to the depressive episode, or whether they are present even when the patients are free of symptoms.

Other theories of SAD involve abnormalities in hypothalamic-pituitary-adrenal (HPA)-axis functioning. This line of research (Rosenthal et al., 1997; Joseph-Vanderpool et al., 1991; Oren et al., 1996; Schwartz et al., 1997; Vanderpool et al., 1991) suggests that HPA-axis functioning may be underactive in SAD. This could be related to decreased brain serotonergic transmission.

Some researchers have suggested that the symptoms of SAD might be a result of abnormally delayed circadian rhythms, and that light therapy may work by shifting these rhythms to a normal pattern (Lewy et al., 1987). Yet other investigations support the hypothesis that abnormal nighttime secretion of the hormone melatonin might influence the development of symptoms in SAD (Rosenthal et al., 1986). Despite these promising leads, there is no consensus as to the cause of SAD or how light therapy works in the treatment of SAD (Rosenthal, 1996).

Use of Light Therapy on Nonseasonal Depression

There is an extensive literature on the use of light therapy for nonseasonal depression, but there are a number of unresolved methodological problems in these studies. Because of small sample sizes, short durations of treatment, and imperfect control of the placebo effect, we cannot say that light therapy is an effective treatment for this condition. Nevertheless, there are some studies that are designed well enough to give us the encouraging impression that light therapy may prove useful in this condition. For example, the group of Kripke and colleagues studied the effects of light therapy in nonseasonal depression most extensively and reported positive results (Kripke et al., 1992). They showed that bright light was significantly more effective than dim light in drug-free, nonseasonally depressed patients after only one week of treatment. This suggests an earlier onset of the antidepressant action than can be expected with antidepressant medications (Kripke et al., 1992). Schuchardt and Kasper (1993) studied nonseasonally depressed outpatients who had not gotten relief from antidepressant medication in a placebo-controlled trial. After four weeks of treatment, the group treated with bright light exhibited a 53 percent decrease of the depression scores, whereas there was just a 26 percent decrease in the dim light group. The results of this study suggest that bright light, but not dim light therapy, might be a valuable addition to drug treatment in patients resistant to medication alone. Another study (Neumeister et al., 1996) looked at light therapy in combination with a technique that has been useful in treating depression: partial sleep deprivation. Light therapy prolonged the antidepressant effects of partial sleep deprivation in the second half of the night for up to seven days after sleep deprivation. This finding is of clinical importance since there is often a relapse of depression following the post-sleep deprivation recovery night.

REAL PEOPLE AND LIGHT THERAPY

A 43-year-old schoolteacher was referred in November to the Seasonal Studies Program of the National Institute of Mental Health. She reported a history of fatigue and depressed mood, which has been recurring regularly during fall and winter for the past twenty years. As in all previous depressive episodes, she found it increasingly difficult to get up in the morning from the beginning of October. This year in particular she had difficulty concentrating on her teaching duties and had problems in organizing her family and herself. She had gained several pounds during the recent weeks before presenting to our outpatient clinic, and described increased appetite, especially for starches, chocolate, and noodles. During all her winter depressions, she felt rejected by her family, as well as her colleagues at school, and she felt like a failure. The patient grew up in the southern United States and reported no depressive episodes during her childhood and early adolescence. During her years at college, she lived farther north and started to develop symptoms of SAD as described above that led to regular difficulties at school during winter. During spring and summer, all her symptoms would resolve; she would once again succeed at school. During the winter, the patient withdrew from others, was irritable, tired, and unmotivated. She was too ashamed to discuss her problems with her family or her friends, believing that all people had difficulties during winter and that she had no right to complain about them. Consequently, she has never received a treatment for her depressive episodes. Family history revealed that her mother and her brother also suffered from regularly occurring depressive episodes that were not closely linked to any season. Since her symptoms were especially marked during this fall, the patient consulted her physician, who worked her up for several medical conditions, including mononucleosis and thyroid problems, but all laboratory findings were normal. Considering the regular occurrence of similar episodes during fall and winter, the physician referred the patient to the National Institute of Mental Health.

Routine physical examination, including laboratory work and

electrocardiogram, revealed that the patient was free of any medical difficulties. The patient was diagnosed as suffering from seasonal affective disorder (SAD), and light therapy was initiated. She was instructed to sit in
front of a standard 10,000-lux light box with a distance of 45 cm between
the screen and her eyes. She was asked to face the light box and glance at
it periodically but not to stare at it. Rather, she was encouraged to do
paperwork or to read during light treatment. Light therapy was prescribed
for forty-five minutes both in the morning and in the evening between
six and nine o'clock. She was encouraged to spend time outdoors during
her lunch break. Her condition began to improve after ten days of light
treatment. Within two weeks, she reported feeling almost completely better. She restarted her exercise program, which she usually undertook only
during spring and summer, and with continued light therapy the patient
remained well throughout the winter. She stopped light therapy in the
middle of March, and remained well, without treatment during summer.
In early September of the next year, the patient started light therapy as a
preventive measure before the development of her usual winter symptoms, and indeed, she succeeded in enjoying her first winter without
depression for years.

WHAT TO EXPECT

Currently, standard light therapy, as practiced at the National Institute of
Mental Health, involves exposing the patients with SAD to 10,000 lux light
intensity for forty-five minutes at a time, in the morning and in the evening,
although some controversy exists regarding the best timing for light treatments
(Lewy et al., 1987; Avery et al., 1990; Sack et al., 1990; Eastman et al., 1996;
Terman and Terman, 1996; Wirz-Justice et al., 1993). There is considerable
variation in the way light therapy is administered and the optimal duration of
daily treatment depends on the individual patient, the time of the year, and
the geographical location. Frequently, patients do best if light therapy is given
in divided doses through the day.

Usually, it takes about four to seven days until an antidepressant effect is felt.
In many cases where light therapy does not work within this time period, an

increase in the duration of daily treatment might optimize treatment response.

While there is general agreement that light treatment is often free of side effects (Gallin et al., 1995), the more common ones include headaches, eyestrain, increased irritability, and sleep disturbances, especially when the treatment is administered late at night. When side effects occur, they are usually mild and transient, and can be handled by decreasing the duration of treatments or increasing the distance between the light box and the eyes (Oren et al., 1991).

Although bright light therapy has been shown to be remarkably successful for treatment of SAD (Terman et al., 1989), not all patients show a favorable or completely successful outcome after light therapy, so treatment alternatives have to be found. As noted above, the first strategy for improving response is to increase the duration of treatment, but if light therapy is unsuccessful in alleviating the patient's depressive symptoms, it would be reasonable to try a psychopharmacological treatment, either in conjunction with, or instead of, light therapy. Antidepressants from the group called selective serotonin reuptake inhibitors (SSRI), e.g., fluoxetine (Lam et al., 1995) or sertraline (Blashko, 1995), are recommended as treatments of first choice. Light therapy and antidepressants can often be combined with good effect. SSRIs are associated with side effects such as sexual difficulties, changes in appetite, and weight loss or gain. The dosage of SSRIs and the level of side effects can be decreased by adding light therapy. Anecdotal evidence supports the value of stress management and exposure to outdoor light, and one controlled study of aerobic exercise has shown evidence for its efficacy. Patients should be informed about the different treatment options for SAD, and especially about the fact that bright light therapy is only effective when it is applied daily in a sufficient duration.

HOW TO FIND A PRACTITIONER

A list of names of practitioners who specialize in treatment of depression, and in particular SAD, can be obtained from the Society for Light Treatment and Biological Rhythms (SLTBR), listed in the next section. Although the incidence of side effects is low, we strongly recommend that patients see their physician on a regular basis to ensure an optimal treatment response. While patients with very mild cases of SAD (Kasper et al., 1985) may be able to treat themselves with enhanced environmental lighting, SAD, like all depressive disorders, can be a serious condition and should be treated with the help of a qualified professional.

RESOURCES

The SLTBR is a worldwide organization that includes scientists, students, and manufacturers of light boxes. There is an annual meeting where the latest research is discussed. Information about light boxes and light visors can be obtained from the SLTBR.

SOCIETY FOR LIGHT TREATMENT AND
BIOLOGICAL RHYTHMS (SLTBR), INC.
10200 West 44th Ave., Suite 304
Wheat Ridge, CO 80033-2840
Tel: (303) 424-3697; Fax: (303) 422-8894
Web site: http://www.webscience.org/sltbr
E-mail: sltbr@resourcenter

NOSAD was developed to support the interests of patients with SAD. Its membership is open to patients, relatives, friends, and interested professionals. NOSAD offers a newsletter, information about treatment options for SAD, and it organizes seminars for people interested in SAD.

NOSAD (NATIONAL ORGANIZATION
ON SEASONAL AFFECTIVE DISORDER)
P.O. Box 40190
Washington, DC 20016

The Internet has become a good source of information regarding SAD and light therapy, as well as alternative treatment options and other supporting groups and facilities. Following are some useful world wide web sites:

http://www.nimh.nih.gov/
http://www.mentalhealth.com/book/p40-sad.html#head_5
http://www.nyx.net/~lpuls/sadhome.html
http://avocado.pc.helsinki.fi/~janne/sad.html

Correspondence about this article can be addressed to Norman E. Rosenthal, M.D., at:

NATIONAL INSTITUTE OF MENTAL HEALTH,
CLINICAL PSYCHOBIOLOGY BRANCH
Building 10/Room 4S-239
Bethesda, MD 20892
Tel: (301) 496-2141; Fax: (301) 496-5439
E-mail: ner@box-n.nih.gov

HOW TO LEARN MORE

Asberg, M., P. Thoren, and L. Traskman. "Serotonin Depression: A Biochemical Subgroup Within the Affective Disorders?" *Science* 191 (1976): 478–480.

Avery, D. H.; A. Khan; S. R. Dager; G. B. Cox; and D. L. Dunner. "Bright Light Treatment of Winter Depression: Morning versus Evening Light." *Acta Psychiatr Scand* 82 (1990): 335–338.

Blashko, C. A. "A Double-blind, Placebo-controlled Study of Sertraline in the Treatment of Outpatients with Seasonal Affective Disorders." *European Neuropsychopharmacology* 5 (1995): 258.

Carlsson, A., L. Svennerholm, and B. Winblad. "Seasonal and Circadian Monoamine Variations in Human Brains Examined Post-mortem." *Acta Psychiat Scand* 61, no. 280 (1980): 75–83.

Eastman, C. et al., "Light Therapy for Winter Depression is More Than a Placebo." *SLTBR Abstracts* 8 (1996): 5.

Fernstrom, J. D. "Carbohydrate Ingestion and Brain Serotonin Synthesis: Relevance to a Putative Control Loop for Regulating Carbohydrate Ingestion, and Effects of Aspartame Consumption." *Appetite* 11, no. 1 (1988): 35–41.

Heninger, G. R., P. L. Delgado, and D. S. Charney. "The Revised Monoamine Theory of Depression: A Modulatory Role for Monoamines, Based on New Findings From Monoamine Depletion Experiments in Humans." *Pharmacopsychiat* 29 (1996): 2–11.

Jacobsen, F. M., D. L. Murphy, and N. E. Rosenthal. "The Role of Serotonin in Seasonal Affective Disorder and the Antidepressant Response to Phototherapy." In *Seasonal Affective Disorders & Phototherapy*, edited by N. E. Rosenthal and M. C. Blehar, NY: The Guilford Press, 1989.

Joseph-Vanderpool, J. R.; N. E. Rosenthal; G. P. Chrousos; T. A. Wehr; R. Skwerer; S. Kasper; and P. W. Gold. "Abnormal Pituitary-adrenal Responses to Corticotropin-releasing Hormone in Patients with Seasonal Affective Disorder: Clinical and Pathophysiological Implications." *J Clin Endocrinol and Metabol* 72 (1991): 1382–1387.

Kasper, S.; T. A. Wehr; J. J. Bartko; P. A. Garst; and N. E. Rosenthal. "Epidemiological Findings of Seasonal Changes in Mood and Behavior: A Telephone Survey of Montgomery County, Maryland." *Arch Gen Psychiatry* 46 (1989): 823–833.

Kasper, S.; S. B. Rogers; A. Yancey; P. M. Schulz; R. G. Skwerer; and N. E. Rosenthal. "Phototherapy in Individuals With and Without Subsyndromal Seasonal Affective Disorder." *Arch Gen Psychiatry* 46 (1989): 837–844.

Kasper, S., S. Ruhrmann, and H. M. Schuchardt. "The Effects of Light Therapy in Treatment Indications Other than Seasonal Affective Disorder (SAD)." In *Biologic Effects of Light 1993*, edited by E. G. Jung and M. F. Holick, Berlin: Walter de Gruyter, 1993.

Kasper, S.; A. Neumeister; N. Rieder; B. Hesselmann; and S. Ruhrmann. "Serotonergic Mechanisms in the Pathophysiology and Treatment of Seasonal Affective Disorder." In *Biologic Effects of Light 1995*, edited by M. F. Holick, Berlin: Walter de Gruyter, 1996.

Kripke, D. F.; D. J. Mullaney; M. R. Klauber; S. C. Risch; and J. C. Gillin. "Controlled Trial of Bright Light for Nonseasonal Major Affective Disorders." *Biol Psychiatry* 31 (1992): 119–134.

Lam, R. W.; C. P. Gorman; M. Michalon; M. Steiner; A. J. Levitt; M. R. Corral; G. D. Watson; R. L. Morehouse; W. Tam; and R. T. Joffe. "A Multi-centre, Placebo-controlled Study of Fluoxetine in Seasonal Affective Disorder." *Am J Psychiatry* 152 (1995): 1765–1770.

Lam, R. W.; A. P. Zis; A. Grewal; P. L. Delgado; D. S. Charney; and J. H. Krystal. "Effects of Acute Tryptophan Depletion in Patients with Seasonal Affective Disorder in Remission with Light Therapy." *Arch Gen Psychiatry* 53 (1996): 41–44.

Lewy, A. J.; R. L. Sack; L. S. Miller; and T. M. Hoban. "Antidepressant and Circadian Phase-shifting Effects of Light." *Science* 235 (1987): 352–354.

Neumeister, A.; R. Goessler; M. Lucht; T. Kapitany; C. Barnas; and S. Kasper. "Bright Light Therapy Stabilizes the Antidepressant Effect of Partial Sleep Deprivation." *Biol Psychiatry* 39 (1996): 16–21.

Neumeister, A.; N. Praschak-Rieder; B. Hesselmann; M. L. Rao; J. Glück; and S. Kasper. "Effects of Tryptophan Depletion on Drug-free Patients with Seasonal Affective Disorder During a Stable Response to Bright Light Therapy." *Arch Gen Psychiatry* 54 (1997): 133–138.

Oren, D. A.; A. A. Levendosky; S. Kasper; C. C. Duncan; and N. E. Rosentha. "Circadian Profiles of Cortisol, Prolactin, and Thyrotropin in Seasonal Affective Disorder." *Biol Psychiatry* 39 (1996): 157–170.

O' Rourke, D.; J. J. Wurtman; R. J. Wurtman; R. Chebli; and R. Gleason. "Treatment of Seasonal Affective Disorder with D-fenfluramine." *J Clin Psychiatry* 50 (1989): 343–347.

Rosen, L. N.; S. D. Targum; M. Terman; M. F. Bryant; H. Hoffman; S. Kasper; J. R. Hamovit; J. P. Docherty; B. Welch; and N. E. Rosenthal. "Prevalence of Seasonal Affective Disorder at Four Latitudes." *Psychiatry Res* 31 (1990): 131–144.

Rosenthal, N. E. *Winter Blues: Seasonal Affective Disorder: What It Is and How to Overcome It.* New York: Guilford, 1993.

Rosenthal, N. E.; A. J. Lewy; T. A. Wehr; H. E. Kern; and F. K. Goodwin. "Seasonal Cycling in a Bipolar Patient." *Psychiatry Res* 8 (1983): 25–31.

Rosenthal, N. E.; D. A. Sack; J. C. Gillin; A. J. Lewy; F. K. Goodwin; Y. Davenport; P. S. Mueller; D. A. Newsome; and T. A. Wehr. "Seasonal Affective Disorder: A Description of the Syndrome and Preliminary Findings with Light Therapy." *Arch Gen Psychiatry* 41 (1984): 72–80.

Rosenthal, N .E.; D. A. Sack; F. M. Jacobsen; S. P. James; B. L. Parry; J. Arendt; L. Tamarkin; and T. A. Wehr. "Melatonin in Seasonal Affective Disorder and Phototherapy." *J Neural Transmission* 21 (1986): 257–267.

Rosenthal, N. E.; M. Genhart; F. M. Jacobsen; R. G. Skwerer; and T. A. Wehr. "Disturbances of Appetite and Weight Regulation in Seasonal Affective Disorder." *Ann NY Acad Sci* 499 (1987): 216–230.

Rosenthal, N. E.; M. J. Genhart; B. Caballero; F. M. Jacobsen; R. G. Skwerer; R. D. Coursey; S. Rogers; and B. J. Spring. "Psychobiological Effects of Carbohydrate- and Protein-rich Meals in Patients with Seasonal Affective Disorder and Normal Controls." *Biol Psychiatry* 25 (1989): 1029–1040.

Rosenthal, N. E.; J. R. Joseph-Vanderpool; A. A. Levandowsky; S. H. Johnston; R. Allen; K. A. Kelly; E. Soutre; P. M. Schultz; and K. E. Starz. "Phase-shifting Effects of Bright Morning Light as Treatment for Delayed Sleep Phase Syndrome." *Sleep* 13 (1990): 354–361.

Rosenthal, N. E. "Diagnosis and Treatment of Seasonal Affective Disorder." *JAMA* 22 (1993): 2717–2720.

Rosenthal, N. E. "The Mechanism of Action of Light in the Treatment of Seasonal Affective Disorder." In *Biologic Effects of Light 1995*, edited by M. F. Holick, Berlin: Walter de Gruyter, 1996.

Sack, R. L.; A. J. Lewy; D. M. White; C. M. Singer; M. J. Fireman; and R. Vandiver. "Morning Vs. Evening Light Treatment for Winter Depression: Evidence That the Therapeutic Effects of Light are Mediated by Circadian Phase Shifts." *Arch Gen Psychiatry* 47 (1990): 343–351.

Schuchardt, H. M. and S. Kasper. "Lichttherapie in der Psychiatrischen Praxis." In *150 Jahre Deutsche Gesellschaft für Psychiatrie und Neurologie*, edited by U. H. Peters, Proceedings of Jubiläumskongreß in Cologne, Germany, September 26–30, 1992.

Schwartz, P. J.; D. L. Murphy; T. A. Wehr; D. Garcia-Borreguero; D. A. Oren; D. E. Moul; N. Ozaki; A. J. Snelbaker; and N. E. Rosenthal. "Effects of M-CPP Infusions in Patients with Seasonal Affective Disorder and Healthy Controls: Diurnal Responses and Nocturnal Regulatory Mechanisms." *Arch Gen Psychiatry* (in press).

Society of Light Treatment and Biological Rhythms. "Consensus Statement on the Efficacy of Light Treatment for SAD." *LTBR Bull* 3 (1990): 5–9.

Terman, M.; J. S. Terman; F. M. Quitkin; P. J. Mc Grath; J. W. Stewart; and B. Rafferty. "Light Therapy for Seasonal Affective Disorder. A Review of Efficacy." *Neuropsychopharmacology* 2 (1989): 1–22.

Terman, M., J. S. Terman, and B. Rafferty. "Experimental Designs and Measures of Success in the Treatment of Winter Depression by Bright Light." *Psychopharmacology Bull* 26, no. 4 (1990): 505–510.

Terman, M., and J. S. Terman. "A Multi-year Trial of Bright Light and Negative Ions." *SLTBR Abstracts* 8 (1996): 1.

van Cauter, E.; J. Sturis; M. M. Byrne; J. D. Blackman; R. Leproult; G. Ofek; M. L'Hermite-Baleriaux; S. Refetoff; F. W. Turek; and O. van Reeth. "Demonstration of Rapid Light-induced Advances and Delays of the Human Circadian Clock Using Hormonal Phase Markers." *Am J Physiol* 266 (1994): E953–E963.

Wehr, T. A.; H. A. Giesen; P. M. Schulz; J. L. Anderson; J. R. Joseph-Vanderpool; K. Kelly; S. Kasper; and N. E. Rosenthal. "Contrasts Between Symptoms of Summer Depression and Winter Depression." *J Affect Disord* 23 (1991): 173–183.

Wirz-Justice, A.; P. Graw; K. Kräuchi; B. M. Gisin; A. Jochum; J. Arendt; H. U. Fisch; C. Buddeberg; and W. Pöldinger. "Light Therapy in Seasonal Affective Disorder is Independent of Time of Day or Circadian Phase." *Arch Gen Psychiatry* 50 (1993): 929–937.

ABOUT THE AUTHORS

Alexander Neumeister, M.D., was born in Vienna, Austria. He did his medical training and received his M.D. from Vienna University in 1990. Immediately afterward, he began his residency in Psychiatry at the Department of General Psychiatry at Vienna University. He came to the Clinical Psychobiology Branch of the National Institute of Mental Health in September, 1996, supported by a fellowship from the Austrian Science Foundation. He has since returned to Austria and continues his work at Vienna University. During his residency, he started his scientific career and has focused on the biological basis of depression, in particular on seasonal affective disorder, and on nonpharmacologic treatment modalities for depression, such as light therapy and sleep deprivation. His work has been published in the leading scientific journals, including *The Archives of General Psychiatry*. Dr. Neumeister has received national and international awards for his scientific work, including the Raffaelson Fellowship Award in 1996.

Norman Rosenthal, M.D., was born in South Africa. He had his medical training and received his M.D. from the University of Witwatersrand in Johannesburg. He did his internship at the Johannesburg General Hospital, emigrated to the United States in 1976, and was resident and chief resident in psychiatry at the New York State Psychiatric Institute and the Columbia Presbyterian Medical Center. He came to NIMH in 1979 and has worked there since. He is currently chief of the section on Environmental Psychiatry.

Recognized as a worldwide authority on the effects of the seasons on mood and behavior, and on the antidepressant effects of light, Dr. Rosenthal has written a well-known book on the subject for the general public, *Winter Blues: Seasonal Affective Disorder — What It Is and How to Overcome It* (Guilford Publications, 1993). He has also written or co-authored over 175 articles and book chapters on the subject of mood disorders and biological rhythms.

He is past president of the Society for Light Therapy and Biological Rhythms, and has served as advisor on the DSM-III-R and DSM-IV task forces on mood disorders. Dr. Rosenthal has also been in part-time private practice for the past fifteen years. He has received a number of honors for his work, including the prestigious Anna Monika Foundation Prize in 1991.

David Briscoe

24 Macrobiotic Diet:
Whole Food for a Whole Mind

WHAT IS MACROBIOTICS?

Macrobiotics is an approach to living based on understanding the natural order of life. Natural order, according to the macrobiotic view, is the ever-changing interplay of complementary opposite energies within our environment, body, and mind. This interplay produces a dynamic balance and harmony in all aspects of life, including physical and mental health. When this balance is upset by extreme lifestyle habits and by consumption of poor quality food, physical illness and/or mental deterioration result. When we consciously align ourselves with the natural order by applying macrobiotic principles to our daily living and eating, we become the masters of our own destiny, steadily establishing true physical health and real mental vitality.

The first step in macrobiotics is changing to a diet based on whole grains and vegetables, in order to establish a healthy body and clear mind. With a healthy body and clear mind, we can go on to solve our difficulties, turning sickness into health, enemies into friends, sadness into happiness, and frustration into fulfillment.

In the macrobiotic view of mental health, psychological states are mainly a reflection of blood quality and internal physical condition. These things are primarily determined by the food we eat daily. Consequently, if you want to create and maintain true and lifelong mental health, you must select food each day with this in mind.

Food is an important aspect of macrobiotics, but there is more to it than that. Another part of macrobiotic practice is to make choices in all realms of living that are more natural and healthy for the individual and the earth. This includes choices about the kind of clothes one wears and the kind of personal health care products one uses. Living a personal life that uses the earth's resources wisely and without waste is a very important component of macrobiotic practice.

The macrobiotic way also encourages each person to take personal responsibility for his or her life. When we do this, we begin to live creatively and freely, without blaming other people, germs, bacteria, pollution, parents, or bad luck for our mistakes and misfortune. In the macrobiotic way, there are no excuses for illness and unhappiness; these are seen as the result of each person's own actions and choices. The heart of macrobiotic practice is accepting responsibility for one's own life without guilt or shame, and transforming it through personal effort and dedication. The macrobiotic road through difficulties, illnesses, and problems ends in happiness, health, and deep comprehension of life for anyone who cares to travel it all the way.

Until recently, the general macrobiotic view of psychotherapy was strongly influenced by its founding teachers, who came from a culture and generation that rarely used psychotherapy, nor had much understanding of its potential benefits to people of other cultures and generations. As a result, the traditional teachings of macrobiotics naturally didn't say much about seeking professional psychological help for mental and emotional problems. However, now that a new generation of Western-born macrobiotic teachers are stepping forward, more and more of them recognize the value of professional psychotherapy for those who need it. It is hoped that more psychiatrists, psychologists, and other mental health professionals will gain knowledge and understanding of macrobiotics. Psychotherapy combined with macrobiotic dietary practice can be a very effective partnership.

HOW IT BEGAN

The macrobiotic philosophy and dietary approach was introduced to the West in the 1940s by a Japanese man named George Ohsawa. Ohsawa developed macrobiotic philosophy out of traditional Eastern medical theory and cosmology. He became famous for its application not only to nutrition and healing, but to science, politics, sociology, psychology, and many other realms of life.

According to Ohsawa, the macrobiotic way of eating is based on the dietary tradition that all humanity practiced for thousands of years up until the last 200 to 400 years. Ohsawa taught that whole grains have always been the most important main food of all humanity, not only of Eastern people. He taught that if we go back to whole grains as our primary food, we will establish real health and well-being. He also taught that macrobiotic diet and lifestyle are the most economical, nourishing, and ecological ways of eating.

Today, the macrobiotic approach has grown into a worldwide movement with centers and communities all over the globe and hundreds of thousands of people living by its principles. Macrobiotics has been a major influence on the natural foods industry, the alternative medicine community, the organic agriculture movement, government food policies of the last two decades, and the new dietary views of major health organizations such as the American Cancer Society, the American Heart Association, and the American Dietetics Association.

HOW IT WORKS

In the macrobiotic view, our blood is the source of our health and well-being, so if we want to change anything about ourselves, we must consider changing our blood quality. From our blood come our body cells including nerve cells, body tissue, and internal organs. The health and proper function of our brain and nervous system determine our ability to judge, think, and express ourselves. Our emotions, behavior, attitude, and outlook are also affected by the function of our brain and nervous system. If our blood is of poor quality and contains chemicals and other substances that interfere with or weaken the function of the brain and nervous system, then all of our thoughts, dreams, decisions, expressions, and emotions will be effected adversely.

Where does blood come from? Food — plain and simple. Blood is a direct transformation of the food we eat. The quality of the food will determine the quality of the blood. So, to put it simply: food = blood = body cells = body tissue = body organs = physical condition, thoughts, emotions, actions, behavior, attitude, and so on. If we want to make a long-lasting beneficial change in any health condition of the blood, cells, tissue, organs, emotions, or behavior, we must go back to their primary source, daily food consumption. It is true that genetics, family circumstances, and upbringing do play a role in our physical and mental health, but according to the macrobiotic view, working on these areas alone as a means to mental health, without changing the daily diet, may provide little in the way of long-lasting results.

According to the macrobiotic approach, food provides two types of nourishment:

1. Basic nutrition. This is the kind of nutrition that many of us are familiar with already, and it includes the protein, fat, carbohydrate, vitamin, and mineral content of food. Consuming foods that are high in protein, fat, and refined carbohydrates leads to chronically elevated levels of acid in the blood. According to macrobiotic principles, over time this blood acidity causes chronic fatigue, mental sluggishness, moodiness, and weak function of all body organs, including the brain and nervous system. Numerous emotional and mental disturbances arise from this acidified blood and the weakened internal physical state that it causes.

    Also, foods and soft drinks that are loaded with simple sugars such as white sugar and honey are known to upset the body's glucose metabolism, which can lead to chronic blood sugar disturbance, causing mood swings. This has been widely reported in the news and in many scientific publications during the last twenty years.

2. Yin and yang nutrition. Each food has a unique quality that makes it different from any other. How a food is grown, where it is grown, the season it grows in, whether it grows slowly or quickly, whether it is of animal or vegetable origin, and what kind of sodium/potassium ratio it contains, will determine how a particular food affects the blood, body, and mental condition after it is consumed. In the macrobiotic view, all things, including food, can be divided into two opposite categories, called yin and yang. On the following page are examples of some of the foods in each of these categories.

Foods from the yang category, when consumed often, can lead to aggression, tension, violence, victimizing, and domineering behavior. Foods from the yin category can lead to spaced-out behavior, mental fatigue, lack of concentration, and other mental and emotional conditions characterized by loss of life direction and mental weakness. The foods in these two categories are considered to be very imbalanced in terms of yin/yang nutrition and are major contributors to mental illness and emotional imbalance. When a person eats foods from the yang category he or she will also crave foods from the yin category and vice versa. Opposites always attract.

Yang Foods	Yin Foods
Beef	Sugar (white, brown, fructose, "raw," etc.)
Eggs	
Chicken	Alcohol
Pork	Soft drinks
Hard cheese	Fruit and vegetable juices
Turkey	Soy milk
Heavily salted and dried food	Tropical fruits (pineapple, banana, oranges, grapefruit, mangoes, etc.)
All processed meat products such as lunch meat, hot dogs	Honey, maple syrup
Canned fish such as tuna, salmon	Artificial sweeteners
Crusty, crispy baked or deep-fried foods	Chocolate
	Spices
Overcooked foods	Marijuana and most drugs, prescription and over-the-counter medications
Grilled and broiled foods	

For foods that are more balanced, the macrobiotic approach recommends a daily diet consisting primarily of whole grains and vegetables. The following supplemental foods are also a very important part of the daily macrobiotic diet as they help to balance internal blood acidity by providing necessary alkaline-forming elements: Miso soup (miso is a delicious macrobiotic seasoning used in vegetable soups), sea vegetables, mineral-rich condiments such as gomasio ("sesame salt"), macrobiotic pickles, kukicha twig tea, sea salt for use in cooking, and natural high-quality soy sauce.

In addition, if the individual's health and condition permit, the following supplemental foods may also be taken, but usually less frequently: beans and bean products such as tofu and tempeh, fish, fruits, nuts, and seeds. There are other macrobiotic foods, too, including gourmet and international styles of macrobiotic cooking that are sometimes served at parties, holidays, and special dinners. However, the basic macrobiotic diet is recommended for daily use.

WHAT THE RESEARCH SHOWS

A study conducted in 1992 (Weidner, Connor, Hollis, and Connor) found that a low-fat, high-carbohydrate diet like the macrobiotic diet may lift depression and decrease aggressive hostility. According to researchers at the Massachusetts

Institute of Technology (MIT), whole grains and other foods high in complex carbohydrates have the ability to increase the brain's intake of tryptophan, an amino acid that aids in lifting depression and improving sleep (Kushi, 1987). According to Tom Monte, "It is becoming increasingly clear that brain chemistry and function can be influenced by a single meal" (Kushi, 1987).

One study found a seventy percent rate of chronic hypoglycemia in diagnosed schizophrenics, and another found an astonishing ninety percent hypoglycemia rate in a group of seven hundred neurotic patients (Goleman, 1988).

Dr. Stephen Harnish (1988), a New Hampshire psychiatrist, reported that macrobiotics had benefited many of his patients who were chronically and severely mentally ill. Dr. Stephen Shoenthaler (1982) reported positive changes in the behavior of juveniles in one detention home when the sugar content of their foods and beverages was covertly reduced.

Other research related to the role of the macrobiotic diet in reducing criminal behavior is too extensive to mention here. For a complete report of these projects, including one conducted with patients from the psychiatric ward of Shattuck Hospital of Boston, and for case histories of individuals whose behavior was changed by a macrobiotic diet, please read *Crime and Diet* by Michio Kushi et al. (1987).

REAL PEOPLE AND MACROBIOTICS

In 1967, at the age of seventeen, I was diagnosed by a team of psychiatrists and psychologists in Kansas City as paranoid schizophrenic. I spent the next five years on daily doses of Thorazine, Stelazine, and a parade of other medications whose names I have long since forgotten. I ran away to the then hippie paradise of Haight-Ashbury in San Francisco and I spent time locked up in psychiatric wards. My parents were told that they should prepare for a life of taking care of me well into their old age, and that, after they became too old to serve as my custodians, I would most likely end up in some sort of institution. I was extremely withdrawn and frightened. I didn't care about much of anything except hiding in my room and listening to my stereo for hours on end. I was unconsciously relieved to know that, with the doctors' diagnosis, I had a stamp of approval to go on living without responsibility or accountability for my life and actions. I was very lazy and let my parents take care of me. They felt sorry for me or guilty about me, so I could use my diagnosis as a rationale for my behavior and withdrawal. I withdrew more and more into my fears, anxieties, and bizarre inner world. I stayed in their home and attempted to function normally while under the steady doses of medication. Miracles do happen, though. In 1972, an acquaintance told me about the macrobiotic diet. I thought it was some kind of health cult and I didn't pay much attention to it. After all, I wasn't searching for a cure. I was strangely satisfied with my life of dependence on my parents, but somehow I became more and more interested in the macrobiotic diet, and I began cooking my own meals. Little by little, I began to notice subtle changes in my mind, and my thinking started to clear gradually. Within a year, I no longer needed to take the medications. Slowly but surely over the next few years, I became a healthier person. It was not at all easy and it was not immediate. There were still many ups and downs, but they didn't last as long as before. I slowly and painfully emerged from my shell and very gradually became a seasoned public speaker, something that still seems unbelievable considering my former state of withdrawal and fear. I went on to finish college and became a schoolteacher. I now have six children. I have already done all the things that my early doctors told my parents I would not be able to do. I know that changing my diet was the key to changing my life. The doctors and psychologists who say that diet can't make a difference in mental health should learn about macrobiotics. They would then understand how powerful real whole food can be. I am endlessly grateful to macrobiotics.

The following case study is excerpted from the *Vega News* (Miller, 1976): On the first day of tenth grade, James experienced an anxiety attack. Fits of vomiting accompanied the attack. This was the start of a seven year bout with mental illness. By the age of 16 he experienced numerous stomach troubles and developed an ulcer. He began medications for these and other physical problems and the doctor also prescribed Stelazine, an antipsychotic drug occasionally used for nonpsychotic anxiety. During the summer of his sophomore year, he experienced a nervous breakdown and kept himself sedated with the prescription medication while attending weekly sessions with a psychiatrist. During this time, Gregory also began a ten-year battle with a terrible case of acne. He loved sugar, soft drinks, and other junk food. None of the doctors or psychiatrists ever mentioned diet as a contributing factor in his physical and psychological problems. As he entered eleventh grade, his problems worsened and Gregory felt as though he was going to crack. The doctors prescribed Thorazine and then Elavil, and Gregory also began to experiment with drugs and alcohol. His condition deteriorated to the point of attempting suicide. He was now 20 years old. After getting out of the hospital, a friend gave him a copy of a macrobiotic book. He tried a simple macrobiotic diet for ten days and experienced incredible results. He began to live an increasingly more normal life. Within four years, Gregory was experiencing a better life than he ever thought possible.

WHAT TO EXPECT

When you begin using nutritionally complete and balanced foods, you can create very high blood quality, which will positively effect your physical and mental condition. You must be patient, though. The best changes are gradual ones and the internal condition doesn't change overnight. However, many people have reported feeling much better physically and mentally soon after changing to a wise and personally appropriate macrobiotic diet, as the blood quality has already been improved by the good food.

Changing lifelong dietary patterns and personal habits presents many challenges. Most of them can gradually be overcome when a person is patient and takes a gentle and thoughtful approach to making changes. If you rush too quickly into macrobiotics, or if you become fanatical and narrow-minded about it, the benefits of this kind of practice are reduced. Steadiness and continuity are essential, but if you backslide or get off track, don't despair. Just come back to your macrobiotic practice and continue on.

Macrobiotic counseling sessions can cost from $100 to $350 each, depending on the experience of the counselor. There is no predetermined number of sessions that are necessary. Most people have one or two sessions, while others may need regular follow-up sessions over a period of a year or two. This is determined by the client and the counselor.

I highly recommend attending macrobiotic cooking classes in order to learn from experienced and qualified instructors. Macrobiotics is primarily a do-it-yourself approach, but if you can receive good instruction in the beginning, you can establish a firm footing for your practice. Also, if you can connect with macrobiotic communities and individuals in your area, this will be very supportive of your own practice.

HOW TO FIND A MACROBIOTIC COUNSELOR

It is essential that people who have been taking medication or drugs receive guidance and support in their transition to macrobiotic practice from their personal doctor and a qualified macrobiotic counselor with experience in helping people who have been taking psychiatric medication or other long-term medication. Do not stop taking your medication to go directly into a macrobiotic practice. Take a wise and steady approach under the supervision of your doctor and a qualified macrobiotic counselor. Individuals who have been experiencing psychotic episodes, hallucinations, or extreme emotional states should wait until their state of mind is more stable before beginning a macrobiotic practice. Then, they should only proceed under the supervision of their doctor and a qualified macrobiotic counselor.

A qualified macrobiotic counselor is a person who has gained much experience and formal training in macrobiotic counseling at one of the country's major macrobiotic schools. Some also receive training through apprenticeship with senior macrobiotic counselors. If you are in doubt as to the qualifications of a particular counselor, you can call the macrobiotic centers listed below.

There are two major macrobiotic residential centers in the U.S. They are both long-established and offer a variety of classes, residential study programs, mail order service for foods, books, cooking supplies, and other macrobiotic services. Call them for information and for possible referrals to macrobiotic individuals in your local area:

THE VEGA MACROBIOTIC
STUDY CENTER
1511 Robinson St.
Oroville, CA 95965
Tel: (800) 818-8342 or
(916) 533-4777

THE KUSHI INSTITUTE
P. O. Box 7
Becket, MA 01223-0007
Tel: (800) 645-8744

As of this writing there are no macrobiotic mental health hospitals or clinics. However, I hope that in the future the mental health community will recognize the value of macrobiotic practice and begin to develop such facilities. Any mental health practitioners or organizations interested in incorporating macrobiotic principles into their program or who would like more information or are interested in sponsoring seminars can contact me at the Vega Study Center address above.

HOW TO LEARN MORE

Aihara, C. *The Calendar Cookbook.* Oroville, CA: George Ohsawa Macrobiotic Foundation, 1979.

Aihara, H. *Acid and Alkaline.* Oroville, CA: George Ohsawa Macrobiotic Foundation, 1986.

Aihara, H. and C. Aihara. *Natural Healing from Head to Toe.* Garden City Park, NY: Avery Publishing Group, Inc., 1994.

Briscoe, D. and C. Mahoney-Briscoe. *A Personal Peace: Macrobiotic Reflections on Mental and Emotional Recovery.* New York: Japan Publications, 1989.

Ferre, J. *Basic Macrobiotic Cooking.* Oroville, CA: George Ohsawa Macrobiotic Foundation, 1987.

Goleman, D. "Food and Brain: Psychiatrists Explore Use of Nutrients in Treating Disorders." *The New York Times,* March 1, 1988.

Harnish, S. "On My Awakening to the Macrobiotic Way." In *Doctors Look at Macrobiotics,* edited by Edward Esko, New York: Japan Publications, 1988.

Kushi, M. *Crime and Diet.* New York: Japan Publications, 1987.

Miller, G. "Whole Foods Saved My Life." *Vega News* 8 (1976): 2.

Weidner; G.; S. L. Connor; J. F. Hollis; and W. E. Connor. "Improvements in Hostility and Depression in Relation to Dietary Change and Cholesterol Lowering." The Family Heart Study. *Annals of Internal Medicine* 117, no. 10 (1992): 820–823.

ABOUT THE AUTHOR

David Briscoe became an internationally known macrobiotic teacher, counselor, and chef after recovering from schizophrenia through the application of
macrobiotic dietary principles. He is co-author of *A Personal Peace: Macrobiotic
Reflections on Mental and Emotional Recovery*. Before becoming a leading macrobiotic advocate, he was a teacher at the high school and college levels, as well
as an actor and director. He has appeared on numerous radio and television
shows and before medical audiences throughout the U.S. and abroad, sharing
the macrobiotic way with all who are interested. He is a consultant to psychologists and psychiatrists as well as other medical professionals. David is the general manager of the Vega Study Center in Oroville, CA, one of the world's
leading macrobiotic schools.

William J. Kaplanidis, M.A., C.R.C., L.Ac., M.T.O.M.

25 Martial Arts and Mental Wellness

WHAT ARE THE MARTIAL ARTS?

Martial arts is a broad term that incorporates many different fighting systems from various countries around the world. Perhaps the more well known or popular martial arts come from Asian countries; China, Japan, Korea, and the Philippines, but in today's world where global information exchange is much easier, martial arts from other areas such as Europe, Africa, South America, and the Middle and Near East are gaining recognition.

Martial arts training can include a combination of physical, mental, and spiritual exercises, and some incorporate various training methods like *Qigong* (pronounced *chi kung*), yoga, meditation, and acupressure.

The various training methods in the martial arts are not only helpful against physical attacks by others but can be applied to helping people face internal struggles as well. Studying the martial arts can be a process of self-exploration, self-expression, and self-cultivation. As training progresses you learn how to overcome obstacles in life through discipline and self confidence. The martial arts can help people cope with various emotional problems such as irritability, anger, anxiety, trauma, abuse, and depression. Martial arts strategies can be applied to breaking bad habits, dealing with feelings of frustration or helplessness, severe stress, and improving motivation, discipline, and self-esteem (Wing, 1988).

One also can use the martial arts as a way to honestly and creatively express oneself. Sometimes in the initial stages of training people get in touch with feelings of anger and aggression, which we tend to view as negative. Often, such feelings can be difficult to express. Martial arts can provide a forum for the expression, release, and transformation of these and other feelings. Through training, people can get in touch with feelings and emotions that can be further explored in individual psychotherapy. This can be very helpful in cases where a person feels a block or feels a need for extra support.

Many martial arts schools offer programs for children as young as six or seven years old. Martial arts training has many positive effects for self-esteem, concentration, and overall behavior through teaching discipline and respect.

HOW IT BEGAN

Historically, martial arts emphasized military and fighting aspects used in war or to protect one's self, family, country, etc. Over the centuries, the martial arts, particularly of China and Japan, incorporated religious, philosophical, and health-promoting components. Each martial art has its own unique historical and cultural roots. Many of the martial arts developed in China have Buddhist, Islamic, Confucian, and Taoist (pronounced: daoist) influences (Deng, 1990). In Japan we also see Shintoism or the Way of the Gods as a major influence (Random, 1977).

In both these cultures, martial arts became a way of life. The Scholar Warriors of China and the Samurais of Japan have left us with many methods of training and understanding that can be applied to our contemporary culture. For example, there are translations of Miyamoto Mushashi's *The Book of Five Rings* and Sun Tzu's *The Art of War* that describe how classic martial strategies and philosophies can be applied to success in business and in relationships in general.

After guns and other modern weaponry came into common use, the martial arts had to adapt to fit society, emphasizing their benefits in terms of health, discipline, self-cultivation, and almost any aspect of a person's life. Presently the martial arts continue to be practiced around the world. In China today there are organizations preserving the martial arts. In the late 1960s and early 1970s there was a surge of interest in the martial arts in the U.S. Today, we are seeing another period of increased interest.

HOW IT WORKS

Martial arts training can help one find balance between physical and mental, inner and outer, personal and social responsibilities (Deng, 1990). All martial arts have a component of self-defense that can help an individual physically and mentally defend against violent attacks. Some schools may emphasize training as a sport and as a method of physical fitness. However, a complete martial art should combine spiritual strength, mental power, technical proficiency, and physical strength to help people reach their greatest possible potential (Ochiai, 1991).

There are hundreds of martial art styles, each emphasizing various aspects of mind/body/spirit training. Chinese martial arts are often divided into two classifications: external and internal schools. External schools, the most famous being from the Shaolin Temple, emphasize a more physically demanding type of exercise; while internal schools such as *Xingyiquan* ("Hsing I Ch'uan"), *Pa Kua Chang* ("Baguazhang"), *T'ai Chi Ch'uan* ("Taijiquan"), and *Liuhebafa* emphasize the use of the mind and positioning over physical strength. Regardless of which style you choose, the training will usually lead to an understanding of both the external and internal. There is no true separation of mind and body.

I have made references to the martial arts as a way of self-cultivation, but I would like to clarify that Eastern approaches to self are different than our Western viewpoint. A basic teaching in Zen is that everything is constantly changing (Suzuki, 1983). Many of us in the West try to cling to a sense of self that is constant, because it gives us a sense of security. "There is no ego in the sense of an enduring, unchanging private soul or personality that temporarily inhabits the body" (Erlich, 1986). Our everyday self is seen in Buddhism as an illusion and to go beyond this state to a more un-self-conscious way of being can be a liberating experience. Part of applying these principles to martial arts training is learning how to go beyond one's ego and how to be fully present in the moment. It is a process of letting go and becoming at peace with one's mind, body, and the environment. Many masters describe themselves as "just doing" with no sense of self or ego. "The point is the doing of them rather than the accomplishments. There is no actor but the action; there is no experiencer but the experience" (Lee, 1975). Of course these higher levels come through discipline and perseverance. It is discipline that will liberate you (e.g., from bad habits) and make it possible for you to become whatever you want to be (Deng, 1990).

An important principle found in Taoism is the idea of yin and yang as pairs of opposing qualities. For example, yin can be seen as female, dark, and yielding, while yang can be seen as male, light, and active. Yin and yang are represented by the popular T'ai Chi symbol, which is shown in Figure 1.

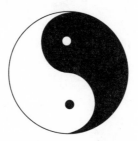

Figure 1. The T'ai Chi symbol representing yin and yang.

T'ai Chi Ch'uan as a martial art embodies the philosophy of yin and yang. For example, yin and yang can be applied to yielding and striking, and the harmony of body and mind training. In the West we tend to focus on one side of things while ignoring the other. An example is a man who sees only his male side while denying his female side. In general, in the West, the mind and body are seen as two separate parts of the self. Yin and yang are two equal powers that oppose and yet compliment each other (Liao, 1990). They represent the duality of our self-existence. Understanding and balancing yin and yang can help us go beyond our conditioned ego and reach a state of higher self or universal consciousness.

WHAT THE RESEARCH SHOWS

The physical and mental benefits of the martial arts are described in many books and research articles. Following is a sampling of the findings.

Weiser et al. (1995) mention that martial arts enhance self-esteem through the provision of physical activity and group experience, as well as the teaching of relaxation, concentration, assertiveness, directiveness, and honesty in communication. Martial arts are noted to be a form of therapy as well as a useful supplement to verbal psychotherapy.

Some of the research regarding the psychological aspects of martial arts training shows that longer training time is closely related to seeing positive change. For example, Kurian et al. (1993) note that groups of people who trained longer in *Taekwondo* scored significantly lower on anxiety and higher on independence questionnaires than those who had briefer training experiences. Daniels and Thornton (1992) suggest that participation in martial arts over time is associated with decreased hostility. Skelton et al. (1991) indicate a significant inverse relationship between children's Taekwondo rank and their aggression, implying a decrease in aggression with training time.

A pilot study by Gleser et al. (1992) found that a modified judo practice for seven blind, mentally retarded children with associated neuropsychiatric disturbances helped with improvements in physical health, as well as psychosocial attitude.

T'ai Chi may be the most well known martial art that benefits both physical and mental health. Although most of the literature about T'ai Chi training discusses cardiorespiratory, musculoskeletal, and other physical benefits, T'ai Chi is also known for its positive effects on mental health. Of course, as I mentioned earlier, the mind and body are not separated in ancient traditions and physical benefits can improve mental health and vice versa. One study by Wolf et al. (1996) investigated T'ai Chi and computerized balance training in reducing frailty and falls in older people. In addition to finding medical benefits of T'ai Chi, researchers noted psychosocial benefits such as a reduction in the fear of falling.

Edward C. Chang (1985) discusses the various healing aspects of T'ai Chi, including relieving neurosis and depression through calming the cerebral cortex, and effectively treating both anxiety and depression by producing a proper balance between sympathetic excitation and inhibition.

Although I feel it is difficult to analyze Eastern disciplines and healing systems from a Western perspective due to fundamental cultural and philosophical differences, I believe we will see more integrative studies as an increasing number of people see and experience the unlimited potential of combining the best of East and West.

REAL PEOPLE AND THE MARTIAL ARTS

Having been involved in T'ai Chi as a student and teacher, I have seen both subtle and radical changes in people's mental health. Over the years, I have noticed gradual changes in classmates who initially were perceived as having aggressive and ego-centered personalities. They gradually became more selfless, kind, and understanding individuals. People who suffer from chronic anxiety have reported to me a sense of being calmer and more in control of themselves. One of my former classmates, who studies both T'ai Chi and Aikido, related how some would-be muggers changed their minds about assaulting him after he met their threat with a calm and welcoming manner.

When I was a teenager, a number of sports injuries had left me unable to walk without some sort of external supports like braces and canes. I was told that I would never be able to participate in sports again, that I would walk with a cane the rest of my life, and be crippled with arthritis by the age of forty. Because I was an active child, and believed that my physical body was much of who I was, I was devastated by my inability to walk or to participate in the activities I loved most. As my mind became filled with rage, anger, sadness, and frustration, I realized I needed a way to express and heal myself that would incorporate my total being. T'ai Chi and meditation became a way for me to do just that. I felt that if I could regain the ability to do just some of the things that I had loved, I would choose the martial arts because I understood that they trained the body, mind, and spirit. This motivated me at a time when I felt hopeless, angry, and depressed. It was largely through T'ai Chi that I gathered the strength and balance I needed for healing myself physically, mentally, and spiritually.

Despite my physical limitations at that time, my teachers were very supportive and encouraging, giving me the guidance I needed. By practicing the slow moving T'ai Chi form, I began to feel calmer and more at peace, with a special connection to the world around me. Neighborhood cats and squirrels would often stop to watch me as I did my form. Learning how to apply the T'ai Chi philosophy to my life, and incorporating push-hands (a type of sparring done with a partner) and meditation as parts of my training, helped me transform many difficulties and obstacles into challenges that I could overcome, and from which I could learn some life lessons. Through these Eastern practices, I was able to prove the Western prognoses wrong, and to do things I was told I would never do again, such as walking, punching, and kicking.

Jerry, a 47-year-old male who became depressed after separating from his wife, decided to try T'ai Chi. He had heard it could help people find balance in their lives. At first, Jerry seemed enthusiastic and motivated to study T'ai Chi. But he soon began to experience performance anxiety and the fear that he would not be coordinated enough. These fears gained control over him and he began to make excuses for not participating in the class. He began to ask the teacher to make special arrangements for him, such as not having his classmates in the room when he was demonstrating his form. The teacher gave Jerry the space he needed but did not give in to all his demands. The teacher was nonjudgmental and encouraged Jerry to continue his practice and simply do his best. Jerry seemed to be a perfectionist and was very concerned about impressing the teacher. After about four months of practicing just part of the yang style T'ai Chi form, Jerry reported significant changes in his mood that were obvious to the teacher as well. Jerry seemed much brighter, more at ease, and more motivated as he began to study the movements in greater detail and found it easier to perform the set.

Jane, a 28-year-old single woman, sought help in resolving issues related to sexual abuse she suffered as a child. Her uncle was the perpetrator. The abuse began when she was five and continued for several years. Although Jane appeared to be doing well, working full-time, and leading a normal life, the aftermath of the abuse affected her intimate relationships as well as her menstrual cycle. Feelings of anger, rage, fear, guilt, anxiety, and hatred kept her from being free to love and express herself fully. Much progress was made through acupuncture, herbs, and hypnotherapy with this author, but it was through her involvement in a women's self-defense class known as "Model Mugging" that Jane further transformed herself. Some of the benefits of this physical, psychological, and martial arts training were that she felt stronger and more confident. She no longer expected others to protect her. Rage and anger were no longer paralyzing emotions. She learned how to accept these emotions and channel them constructively. There has been a significant improvement in her intimate relationships as well as her ability to maintain her personal boundaries. One can see a definite change in how she carries herself and how she faces life's changes. It has been a year since she took that class and she continues to be grateful for and aware of the many benefits.

Heather is a 40-year-old mother of two and a graduate student. She experiences stress from commuting over an hour each way to school five days a week, studying, working part-time, and raising a family. Worry, anxiety, overthinking, poor memory, and poor concentration have become part of her daily life. After eight weeks of *Qigong* classes, Heather noticed that on Mondays after her *Qigong* class, life seemed less stressful. Although Monday was just as hectic as any other day, she noticed that she got through the day with less anxiety and worry. She attributes this, along with improvements in her memory and concentration, to the *Qigong* and is inspired to exercise more regularly.

WHAT TO EXPECT

Studying a martial art requires a commitment of time and effort. Many of the positive physical, mental, emotional, and spiritual effects often come from years of training. The first things a person usually learns in martial arts training are various stretching and strengthening techniques to prepare the body. Various arts have different ranges of physical demands. Nevertheless, you can expect improvement in strength, flexibility, stamina, balance, coordination, reflexes, speed, etc.

In addition to learning basic methods of self-defense such as blocking, punching, kicking, throwing, grappling, etc., many martial arts include memorizing *katas* (also called forms or sets). Katas are sequences of prearranged defensive and offensive movements performed solo, in which one imagines she or he is fighting one or many opponents. Generally people learn shorter and easier sets first and progress to more complex and difficult ones. These sets are learned through modeling and repetition. Many people report that they develop better focus, concentration, and self-confidence from practicing these sets.

At its highest levels, kata becomes a kind of moving meditation (Ochiai, 1983). Katas can be performed at different speeds, emphasizing the integration of mind, movement, breath, and spirit. T'ai Chi is known for its slow movement sets. People turn their focus inward, concentrating fully on various aspects simultaneously, while moving the whole body as one unit. By continuing practice with a good teacher, one can discover hidden techniques and other subtleties through practicing katas.

Several martial arts focus part of their training on exercises that develop and help move energy or life's vital force, called *qi* in Chinese or *ki* in Japanese ("chee") throughout the body. Developing and circulating *qi* can create a balanced state of body and mind. *Qigong* or *qi* cultivation is the practice of doing therapeutic exercises that combine breath control, movement, concentration, and visualization. There are thousands of different forms of *Qigong*, some of which are more oriented toward fighting and others that focus more on promoting health. As with the martial arts, some *Qigong* sets are more meditative in nature, such as holding a standing, sitting, or lying posture while other sets may be more physically demanding. Similar types of exercises are also practiced in other traditions such as yoga and *pranayama* from India. Martial arts such as T'ai Chi and Aikido emphasize the power of the mind in the development of *qi/ki* and being calm and relaxed. Both these arts teach power and strength through relaxation and unification of mind and body.

Qigong, in addition to including meditation and other self-healing exercises, has a healing aspect. There are some *Qigong* masters who can direct their *qi*, as well as the *qi* around them, to help heal others. *Qigong* therapists may use a variety of touch and nontouch bodywork methods to help heal patients by moving, restoring, and balancing energy. Similar healing arts include reiki, therapeutic touch, acupressure, and Shiatsu therapy.

Breathing techniques are taught as part of many of the martial arts. Since breath and energy form a bridge between body and mind, breathing may be controlled either mentally or physically and is the only vital function that straddles the border of voluntary and involuntary control (Reid, 1989). Simple breathing exercises can have positive effects on health.

Another aspect of martial arts training is learning sets or katas that involve weapons. In the days before automatic machine guns, traditional weapons such as the staff or sword were part of a martial artists repertoire. Weapons training adds another dimension to personal development, beyond the self-defense function. People learn how to make the weapon an extension of their own *qi* and usually learn more advanced movements. Different weapons will have different unique health benefits on the body and mind (Deng, 1990).

In addition to solo exercises, martial arts often involve training with others. Besides working with a teacher, classmates might do exercises together. This may take the form of some sort of sparring. In T'ai Chi, a two person exercise called push-hands helps develop sensitivity to another person's energy and intention, which can be applied to self-defense. Various issues of boundaries and relating to others may be addressed through this type of exercise, as well as better self-understanding.

Meditation is often combined with the practice of various martial arts, and can be a way to counter and balance some of the aggression that may be associated with certain martial arts. Usually a good teacher and peer support can help, but some people might choose to seek psychotherapy in addition to their martial art training. In the self-defense course known as Model Mugging, women (and men) learn how to defend themselves against physical confrontations while their adrenaline is pumping. Often powerful emotions come up. The participants get a combination of individual and group support that helps them work through many emotional issues.

Many martial arts, particularly many styles of karate, have a colored belt system that is used as a way for the student and teacher to mark progress. As you progress in your studies, a different colored belt is awarded as you demonstrate proficiency in what you have learned. One of my teachers once said that historically there were only two belts, white and black. You began with a white belt, which, through years of practice, eventually turned to black, signifying the length of time you had studied.

Classes generally last from one to three hours and are offered once a week to every day. Usually people attend classes one to three times per week and are expected to practice at home what they learn. Some schools have specific uniforms that need to be worn while others recommend loose and comfortable clothing. You may be required to be barefoot, depending on the type of class. Some schools will incorporate the use of weapons and protective equipment such as padding, which are usually provided.

Whether the class is conducted in a more traditional, formal way, or a less formal way will depend partly on the type of martial art and partly on the instructor. For instance, the more traditional schools may require bowing to classmates and instructors and an understanding of a few traditional words in the native language of the art. In these schools, one would be required to show respect for classmates of higher rank and abide by certain rules of conduct. Less formal schools usually do not have the above expectations or they are less emphasized. The teacher may be seen more as a friend or peer rather than, or in addition to, being your master or coach. Sometimes the teacher takes on the role of parent to the student. It is important to be aware of your feelings, expectations, and your own responsibility and volition in the relationship with your teacher.

HOW TO FIND A PRACTITIONER

Choosing a martial art is a very individual decision based on numerous factors. One way to start is to explore what type of martial art schools and teachers are available in your area, or at least located close enough for regular training. If you do not have any leads, consulting your local phone book or looking in a karate or Kung Fu magazine may help you get started. Some martial arts are affiliated with professional organizations and have certain rank qualifications for teachers, while others do not. In addition to private schools, one may find instructors at community centers, colleges, and sports clubs. What to look for in a master or teacher is discussed at length by Deng Ming-Dao in his book *Scholar Warrior: An Introduction to the Tao in Everyday Life*. I like to encourage people to trust their feelings and intuition when choosing a teacher. People may need different teachers at different stages in their life and development. Your interest, motivation, and goals can help determine the type of martial arts teacher you choose. For instance, is your goal to learn practical self-defense techniques; are you looking for a teacher who will provide a rigorous workout and push you beyond your limits; or are you looking for more of a spiritual or lifestyle approach to the martial arts?

Once you find a school, inquire about the different aspects of training, such as the following:

- Are stretching and warming up part of the class time?
- Are any body-strengthening exercises taught?
- What if you cannot physically do some of the exercises?

- What is the focus of the training (e.g. for self-defense, competition, self-improvement)?
- Are there any lectures or meditation involved?

Ask if you can observe beginning and advanced classes. Look at and talk to senior students. See if you can get a sense of their physical, mental, and spiritual well-being. Observe the class and ask yourself if you feel comfortable with the teacher and classmates. Can you see yourself enjoying your training? Does the training and philosophy match with your needs and goals? Express your needs and you might get direction on where to go. Some schools may be more aggressive in the sense that getting hurt during training is part of the process. It is important to get a good idea of the training methods and what is expected of you at the various levels of training.

There is a wide range of costs for martial arts classes. Some schools require uniforms, start-up fees, etc., while others do not. Schools might offer a variety of payment plans. Of course individual instruction would cost more than group classes.

As I mentioned earlier, *Qigong*, which consists of self-exercises as well as therapy, can be explored in combination with another form of martial arts training, or by itself. If you are not very interested in the fighting aspects of these types of exercises, some T'ai Chi and many *Qigong* classes may be more suitable for you. James MacRitchie has put together an International Qigong Directory, available from:

THE BODY ENERGY CENTER
P.O. Box 19708
Boulder, CO 80301

Conversely for those of you, particularly women, who are interested in intensive self-defense training that incorporates the emotional and psychological aspects of being physically attacked, I highly recommend the Model Mugging program; for more information call (800) 443-KICK.

HOW TO LEARN MORE

"Bruce Lee: The Lost Interview Video." Calabasas, CA: Wolff Creative Group, 1994.

Chang, E. C. *Knocking at the Gate of Life and Other Healing Exercises from China.* Emmaus, PA: Rodale Press, 1985.

Cheng M. and R. Smith. *T'ai Chi.* Rutland, Vermont: Charles E. Tuttle Co., Inc., 1987.

Daniels, K. and E. Thornton. "Length of Training, Hostility and the Martial Arts: A Comparison with Other Sporting Groups." *British Journal of Sports Medicine* 26, no. 3 (1992): 118–120.

Deng M. *Scholar Warrior: An Introduction to The Tao of Everyday Life.* NY: Harper Collins Publishers, 1990.

Ehrlich, M. P. "Taoism and Psychotherapy." *Journal of Contemporary Psychotherapy* 16, no. 1 (1986): 23–38.

Gleser, J. M.; J. Y. Margulies; M. Nyska; S. Porat; H. Mendelberg; and E. Wertman. "Physical and Psychosocial Benefits of Modified Judo Practice for Blind, Mentally Retarded Children: A Pilot Study." *Perceptual and Motor Skills* 74, no. 3 (1974): 915–925.

Kurian M., L. C. Caterino, and R. W. Kulhavy. "Personality Characteristics and Duration of Ata Taekwondo Training." *Perceptual and Motor Skills* 76, no. 2 (1993): 363–366.

Lee, B. *The Tao of Jeet Kune Do.* Santa Clarita, CA: Ohara Publications, Inc., 1975.

Liao, W. *T'ai Chi Classics.* Boston: Shambala Publications, Inc., 1990.

Millman, D. *The Warrior Athlete: Body, Mind, and Spirit.* Walpole, NH: Stillpoint Publishing, 1979.

Musashi, M. *The Book of Five Rings.* New York: Bantam Books, Inc., 1982.

Ochiai, H. *Complete Book of Self-Defense.* Chicago: Contemporary Books, Inc., 1991.

Ochiai, H. "Kata." *Karate Illustrated* 14, no. 12 (1983): 38–41.

Random, M. *The Martial Arts.* London: Peerage Books, 1985.

Reed, W. *Ki: A Road that Anyone Can Walk.* Tokyo and New York: Japan Publications, Inc., 1992.

Reid, D. *The Tao of Health, Sex and Longevity.* NY: Simon and Schuster, Inc., 1989.

Skelton, D. L., M. A. Glynn, and S. M. Berta. "Aggressive Behavior as a Function of Taekwondo Ranking." *Perceptual and Motor Skills* 72, no. 1 (1991): 179–82.

Suzuki, S. *Zen Mind, Beginners Mind.* NY: Weatherhill, 1983.

Weiser, M.; I. Kutz; S. J. Kutz; and D. Weiser. "Psychotherapeutic Aspects of the Martial Arts." *American Journal of Psychotherapy* 49, no. 1 (1995): 118–127.

Wing, R. L *The Art of Strategy.* New York: Doubleday, 1988.

Wolf, S. L.; H. X. Barnhart; N. G. Kutner; E. McNeely; C. Coogler; and T. Xu "Reducing Frailty and Falls in Older Persons: An Investigation of Tai Chi and Computerized Balance Training." *Journal of American Geriatric Society* 44, no. 5 (1996): 489–97.

Wong D. and J. Hallander. *Shaolin Five Animals Kung Fu.* Burbank, CA: Unique Publications, 1988.

ABOUT THE AUTHOR

William J. Kaplanidis began his formal training in the martial arts at age nine. He has studied various styles of martial arts with T'ai Chi *(Taijiquan)* as his main focus since 1983. He teaches T'ai Chi and *Qigong* privately as well as at the Pacific Institute of Oriental Medicine in New York. He has over 10 years of experience working in the field of mental health including city and state psychiatric facilities as well as a private hypnotherapy/counseling practice. William is a licensed acupuncturist with a private practice in New York City. He combines his counseling training with acupuncture, herbs, T'ai Chi, *Qigong*, bodywork, and visualization, providing a holistic approach to healing. In addition, he currently teaches T'ai Chi and *Qigong* classes privately, at the Pacific Institute of Oriental Medicine and at New York sports clubs.

David DiDomenico, C.M.T.

26 Massage and Mental Health:
Touching the Mind

WHAT IS MASSAGE THERAPY?

Massage is a very general term that includes every form of "bodywork" therapy that exists. Many of these techniques do not use the word "massage" in their names, but all can be traced in some way back to our need as humans to touch and be touched. Massage, as we know it today, has grown out of our innate wisdom in caring for ourselves and others. The techniques of massage therapy have gone beyond what many people think of as massage. Rather than the "rub down" approach, which entails long soothing strokes, vigorous circular strokes, and friction strokes, there are additional techniques such as Japanese shiatsu, trigger point, and *jin shin* that place direct pressure on key points on the body. Passive stretching of the limbs and range of motion techniques might be used as well. This chapter will focus on those techniques practiced by body workers who refer to themselves as massage therapists.

HOW IT BEGAN

Massage has been around since the beginning of time, and not only for human beings. The licking of newborn puppies by their mother is one obvious example of massage in the animal world. The licking serves not only to cleanse the puppies of afterbirth but to stimulate the newly arrived organism into proper functioning. The muscular contractions of the human mother as her child is pushed through the birth canal serve to stimulate the newborn's organs, much like a massage. Examples of what can be considered massagelike stimulation are found everywhere in the animal kingdom

Human beings have an innate tendency to attend to sore areas with our hands. When we have a headache, for example, we will find ourselves rubbing our forehead or the base of the skull. Think for a moment about any area of your body where you experience sore, achy, or stiff sensations, and probably you will have a clear recollection of touching it in some way. We attend to these areas with touch because we can make a difference, however temporary, in how they feel. "Soothing" is a way we might define the sensation of touch in these instances.

In China, massage has been an integral part of the health care system for millennia. In Scandinavia, massage has been used for centuries as health care maintenance. Today in the United States, massage is beginning to be recognized as a valuable tool in the reduction of stress. It is also being used more widely as an adjunctive therapy for rehabilitation from trauma and in many soft tissue disorders. There are a multitude of massage techniques being taught and practiced in the United States, from ancient Chinese forms to forms developed this century.

HOW IT WORKS

Massage therapists generally believe that it is not possible to touch only the body or react only with the mind. When someone shakes your hand or pats you on the back, there is a response throughout the entire organism; you feel something. You may have a "gut" reaction or develop a "first impression" during a handshake by observing the firmness, dampness, and temperature of the other's hand. So when a massage therapist touches the client they do not just touch the body, they engage the entire person. The response or reaction to touch varies from person to person according to their prior experiences of physical contact, their perception of the therapist, their body image, their expectations, their physical condition, the pressure used by the therapist, and other factors. Following are some of the ways that massage can be used to foster mental health.

Shame

Frequently, issues of shame are raised and resolved through massage. One obvious example is the issue of nudity and having yourself exposed to another person. Even though the client is draped and never fully exposed, in massage it is common for clients to feel threatened by the fear of someone else seeing who they really are beneath the shelter of their clothing. In massage situations where clothing is not removed, these issues still arise from the intimacy of the therapist's touching. One of my clients said to me after a session, "I just realized I can't keep any secrets [about my body] from a massage therapist." This was a client who always remained fully-clothed during our sessions. Many people are ashamed of their bodies. How the client perceives her or his body and its functioning often is revealed in the initial meeting between massage therapist and client. Sometimes a client will apologize for being overweight, out of shape, scarred, excessively hairy, etc. A client once apologized to me for having dry skin and using up too much of my massage lotion.

It is important that the therapist respect these issues and work with the client to help them feel more comfortable with, and in, their body. Body image can be clarified and improved with the continuation of massage therapy. The client's awareness follows the hands of the therapist as they move over familiar and unfamiliar areas of the body such as the back, which is not easily accessed by one's vision or touch. This can help the client develop a greater awareness of her or his body which, in turn, provides a more complete picture of the self. Many times I have asked a client to touch him or herself to feel certain body parts such as bony structures or the texture of certain muscles. This can be an important step toward increasing self-acceptance.

A woman once came to me for help with her recovery from a shattered ankle. I felt it would facilitate her healing if she would massage her ankle herself at least once a day. When I suggested this, she cringed and said, "No way, I won't even look at it." After one of our sessions I asked if she would be willing to try touching her ankle. She agreed. I told her not to look at it but to begin to touch it, and then I would begin to guide her hands and show her some massage strokes she could do at home. We repeated this after each session until she reacquainted herself with her ankle. It is my contention that this helped her recover more quickly and completely.

Resistance and Defenses

The most important and well-known aspect of massage is that it is relaxing, yet massage clients commonly resist relaxing or "letting go." Feelings of vulnerability are a common response to a massage. This is a result of relaxing muscles that are chronically tensed in defensive patterns. A defensive pattern might, for instance, involve a collapsed chest and shoulders that are held rounded — a posture that might say "please don't hurt me." The individual displaying this type of muscular pattern probably had, or has, good reason for it. It is not uncommon for clients to recall, during massage, the incidents that caused them to create these defensive patterns. This awareness can occur when those muscles that are most involved are directly or indirectly manipulated or touched.

"Helping out" is a term used in massage to describe a situation in which the client uses her or his muscles to help the therapist to move them. For instance, when lifting the client's arm to massage it or do range of motion, ideally it is the therapist who lifts and supports the arm. Quite frequently the client "helps" — muscles tighten and the arm and shoulder become rigid. Sometimes a verbal cue is all that is necessary to help the client let go of the arm, but more often than not, the cue needs to be repeated throughout the work. Often the client believes they have let go, but when the massage therapist releases the arm, the client notices that the arm is actually still up in the air, and realizes his or her tension. This is a manifestation of resistance to relinquishing control. Control equals tension and can occur anywhere in the body. As clients begin to understand their impulse to help out (resist), they simultaneously learn how to let go. Many clients report that they caught themselves between sessions holding their shoulders up or tensing somewhere in their body and were able to release it. Clients in this process are developing a clearer communication with their muscles and gaining a higher form of control — the ability to let go. We all burden ourselves with enormous amounts of unnecessary muscle tension that only serves to eat up our much valued energy, causing fatigue, discomfort, and further distortion of our self-image.

People often have habitual patterns of resistance, patterns that may go as far back as infancy. An old injury, let's say the knee, may have caused an individual to adapt by decreasing the weight on the injured leg. If during a massage session the leg is moved in a direction that the client perceives as threatening to the knee, he or she automatically and unconsciously stops the movement, even if the knee has healed and the threat no longer exists. People who have been sexually abused sometimes make their body rigid or absolutely limp in an unconscious attempt not to experience their own sensations. They usually refer to this as "leaving the body." Since they were not physically capable of fending off the perpetrator, they did the next best thing to resist the threat to themselves. These defensive or resistive behaviors can become conscious through massage.

Trust issues also create resistance. A client will certainly not relinquish control over any body part if she or he thinks the therapist might drop it, nor will they deepen into a relaxed state with a person they don't trust. Some people's experiences have taught them that it is not safe to trust. This issue will often be raised in the massage therapy, which makes it more likely to be resolved.

A client who is a manic-depressive, and with whom I've worked with for many years, asked if I would work with her while she was hospitalized during a manic episode. I visited her several times in the hospital, where we talked and I did massage. I spoke with her after her release from the hospital and asked what she felt she gained from my visits. She said it was most important that I was someone she could trust from the "outside." She also said that it helped tremendously to "come back to my body" and feel more "grounded."

Allowing oneself to feel vulnerable is rarely easy. In many instances, just after receiving a massage, allowing the feelings of vulnerability is less of a struggle because of the safety of the massage office and trust in the therapist. It is when one tries to carry this out into the world that a conflict may arise. What is relinquished during a massage is a false sense of security created by excessive muscular tension, resulting in a potential experience of vulnerability. Excessive muscular tension heightens one's susceptibility to physical injury, as well as using up energy and contributing to many physical and emotional disorders. Rather than excessive muscular tension being a result of anxiety or neurosis, it is often the physical manifestation of what is taking place on a psychological level. When the muscular patterns of tension are released, neurosis can be more readily accessible to change.

Sexual abuse is trauma to the entire person and, as such, is displayed in all aspects of behavior. The feelings of vulnerability arising from massage can be terrifying to the sexually-abused individual. Those feelings can also open the door to healing. In cases of sexual abuse, it is not uncommon for the client spontaneously to recall traumatic events. Resistance to feeling pleasure from another's touch, or feeling out of control when relaxing, are two extremely important issues that often surface for the sexually abused individual during a massage.

In his book *Existential Psychotherapy*, Irvin D. Yalom writes: "During the course of therapy the patient opposes what he perceives to be the will of the therapist. Freud labeled this opposition 'resistance,' considered it an obstacle, and suggested various techniques to overcome it. To Otto Rank, this view of resistance was a serious error: he believed that the patient's protest was a valid and important manifestation of counter will and, as such, must not be eliminated but instead supported and transformed into creative will" (Yalom, 1980). This also applies to massage therapy, where, rather than a battle of wills (therapist vs. client), a client is often resisting movement, pressure, and/or relaxation because, either consciously or unconsciously, he or she is attempting to avoid unpleasurable sensations. Resistance then must not be considered an obstacle to be eliminated, but a manifestation of beliefs to be respected, explored, understood, and dissolved if the beliefs are no longer valid. The dissolution of resistance is accomplished by the client through his or her own creative forces, what Otto Rank called "creative will," while the massage therapist assists in the process.

WHAT THE RESEARCH SHOWS

There has been little research on the effectiveness of massage, and less yet in the area of massage and mental health. The Touch Research Institute at the University of Miami School of Medicine is conducting research on the effectiveness of massage with infants, children, adolescents, adults, and the elderly. Many of these studies are in progress or preparation, but preliminary results show reductions in stress and anxiety levels, as well as a decrease in depression. There is a study in progress on adolescents with eating disorders undergoing massage therapy.

REAL PEOPLE AND MASSAGE THERAPY

As I worked Mr. M.'s neck at the beginning of the session, I was aware of the small area I had to work with. His neck seemed much shorter than I would have expected from looking at it. When I picked up his head he instinctively shortened the muscles of the neck, shoulders, and upper back. I decided to begin working the shoulders one at a time, as he did not display the same reactive tendency there. I worked slowly and methodically to relax his shoulders, while simultaneously and surreptitiously introducing small rocking motions into his neck. Slowly, with some verbal cues to stop holding his head still, he began to allow the neck and upper back to relax. His head began to roll gently with my movements in a way that indicated he was not fighting gravity. Rather than going back to the neck immediately, I continued to work down his body, addressing his arms, chest, belly, and legs, introducing a gentle rhythmic rocking motion with each massage stroke. The intention of the gentle rocking was to continue the subtle rocking of the head that was established earlier.

I then returned to his head. I began by scooping my hands under his head very gently to avoid triggering the reactive shortening of his neck. There was a very low level of reactivity at first that passed quickly as I let his head rest quietly in my hands. I then began to make tiny movements with my hands, as if I was preparing to pull on his neck. This made him shorten his neck ever so slightly. After doing this a number of times his eyes popped open and he said, "I feel like a turtle wanting to pull its head in." Then continuing, as tears filled his eyes, he said, "I just remembered that my mother used to punish me, sometimes she just did it to be cruel, by hitting me on the head with something. I never knew when she was going to do it so I always had to protect myself."

We continued working for many sessions on overcoming his muscular reaction while he worked with his psychotherapist on related issues. We all tend to develop behaviors that our nervous systems believe to be protective. In the case of Mr. M., the protective or defensive behavior was causing pain, discomfort, and a limited range of motion. Mr. M. realized that this particular pattern was not only no longer necessary, but it was bad for his health. That recognition allowed him to free himself from the mental burdens stemming from an abusive parent. In this process, he risked being vulnerable to having his head bopped, even though intellectually he knew the chances were slim to none.

Ms. D., a woman in her mid thirties, came to see me to work with issues of sexual abuse. The psychotherapist that she was working with suggested that some massage might help her rediscover her body. She told me that she had some hip pain and that she always felt as if she were "holding back," but other than that there was nothing significant going on.

Lying on the table, she appeared very rigid, as if she were standing at attention. Her arms were tight to her sides and her legs were tight together. Her breathing was shallow and her eyes moved erratically beneath her closed eyelids. I proceeded very gently to massage her neck with long broad strokes, making sure not to make any sudden or startling movements. I continued with this approach over her entire body, taking extra care to help her feel safe. Ms. D. began to trust my work more and more as the weeks passed. This was evident in how quickly she responded to my touch when we began each session. Her breathing became deeper and more full, and her body began softening the moment I touched her. Eventually I began to introduce some gentle rhythmic rocking and, each time I did, she responded by tightening everything up. She pulled herself in toward her center. I immediately would stop the rocking motion and go over her body, suggesting with light massage and movement that she release those muscles she had just contracted. One session, after going through this process a few times, she began sobbing. She said she was feeling sad but didn't know why. I continued with a light nonintrusive massage and encouraged her to be in touch with the sadness.

During this session she had her first experience with feeling profoundly vulnerable. Rather than sending her out into the world with this new and frightening feeling, we sat and talked. After asking her how this vulnerable feeling affected her muscles, she came to realize that she tightened up. She agreed to experiment by noticing what muscles or areas of her body she felt like tightening, and then consciously tightened them and released them again. When asked what she felt after doing this exercise, she responded that she felt less vulnerable, but it didn't feel good to tighten back up. Her homework was to continue to explore this vulnerable/not vulnerable mechanism of tightening and relaxing muscles in the privacy of her home in front of a mirror or with a trusted friend. The tensing and relaxing that triggered the vulnerability or lack of it was so subtle that it was hard for a well-trained eye to tell she was doing anything. Yet she experienced it as gross movement. She realized that she could relax and not be "on guard" a great deal of time throughout each day.

Later in our work together, while Ms. D. was lying prone, I massaged her back and did a stroke that I had done many times before. The stroke involved pulling up with broad hands over her rib cage toward the spine. At one point in this stroke, my hands contacted the ribs under the arm and adjacent to the breast. When I performed that stroke on her right side, this time she tightened up. I stopped and asked if she was okay. Once again the tears came and she said she had just remembered her father touching her there and how she hated that he wanted to touch her breasts. After many massage sessions as an adjunct to her psychotherapy, Ms. D. is doing remarkably well.

WHAT TO EXPECT

In most professional massage sessions the client is first interviewed by the therapist. The interview can include completing intake questionnaires regarding health history and current problems one wishes to address with massage therapy, followed by a short talk about the same material. The health status of the client will determine the course of treatment, such as where on the body to begin, and what techniques will most likely be appropriate. A skilled massage therapist will continue to make adjustments to his or her work according to the changing needs of the client. Client feedback during and after each session is essential to the massage therapist's ability to facilitate healing. Massage, at its best, involves the massage therapist and the client working together to create change. The massage therapist is not there to fix you or heal you, but to help you discover and engage your own abilities to heal.

Most, but not all, massage therapies require that you be fully unclothed, or at least down to your underwear, though the use of sheets and towels ensure that your genital areas and breasts will not be exposed. This brings up the issue of whether you wish to use a male or female massage therapist. Some women, for example, feel too threatened by men to work with a male massage therapist. Some men feel threatened by the mere thought of being touched by another man, let alone enjoying it. I have worked with many sexually-abused women (abused by men) who specifically chose to work with me because I am a man, and they felt ready to deal with their issues. If you are currently working with a mental health professional and are considering massage as an adjunctive therapy, this is certainly a topic to discuss.

Some massage therapists may use oils or lotions for reducing friction or for their healing properties. This can be a consideration for some because of certain skin conditions. If you have to return to work after a massage, you might consider that your hair and makeup (if you wear it) will be a mess and, although you'll feel great, you might look like you just rolled out of bed. You can inquire about the availability of a shower.

Yet another consideration is your state of mind after a massage. Massage is usually very relaxing. This means that your muscles will be more supple, your mind more alert, and your breathing fuller, but you probably won't want to engage in vigorous activity, physical or mental, for a while. The state of relaxation achieved in massage can be profound. As mentioned above, many clients feel vulnerable immediately after a massage. With the muscles relaxed and reorganized, our everyday patterns of posturing are not active, or not as active. During the massage we may have relinquished the defensive patterns that seem to protect us against the world's dangers, such as an unconscious facial grimace that works well to keep people from engaging us in conversation. This can be refreshing or terrifying and, oddly enough, sometimes both at the same time.

Many people use massage therapy as part of their personal health maintenance program and receive massage on a weekly, bi-weekly, or monthly basis. Others use it as an adjunct to physical therapy or primarily for rehabilitation from injury. As described in this chapter, massage is very effective as an adjunct to psychotherapy. Treatment plans need to be developed through cooperation and communication between psychotherapist and massage therapist.

HOW TO FIND A MASSAGE THERAPIST

When selecting a massage therapist, most individuals want to have an idea of the number of sessions it will take to resolve the difficulties they are experiencing. Certain symptoms may go away during one session and may not return for hours or even days, but this does not mean the underlying cause has been resolved. The time it takes will obviously vary from client to client. I suggest that a client receive at least five sessions before determining whether or not they will benefit from massage. You must not, however, subject yourself to a massage therapist that you distrust or are not comfortable with. At all times while in session with the massage therapist, you are in charge. You can interview prospective therapists and get references to find one that fits your needs. Keep in mind that massage is inherently intimate. You will probably be touched and moved in ways that you are not at all used to.

Finding a massage therapist whom you feel comfortable working with may take some time. Many health clubs offer massage but these masseurs and masseuses generally do sports massage which, although excellent for health maintenance, is not appropriate (nor the setting) for someone seeking massage to include in their work with mental health issues. The American Massage Therapy Association (AMTA) is a professional organization serving massage therapists. They also accredit or approve massage schools. They publish a magazine called the *Massage Therapy Journal*, which is a good resource for names and locations of accredited massage schools that can usually provide the names and phone numbers of massage therapists in your area. References from trusted friends are worth following up, as well as those from mental health professionals who may already refer their clients to particular massage therapists.

RESOURCES

MASSAGE THERAPY JOURNAL
820 Davis St., Suite 100
Evanston, IL 60201-4444
Tel: (708) 864-0123

HOW TO LEARN MORE

Dychtwald, K. *Bodymind*. New York: Jove, 1977.

Feldenkrais, M. *Awareness Through Movement: Health Exercises for Personal Growth.* New York: Harper and Row, 1972.

Feldenkrais, M. *Body and Mature Behavior: A Study of Anxiety, Sex, Gravitation, and Learning.* New York: International Universities Press, 1950.

Hanna, T. *The Body of Life*. New York: Knopf, 1980.

Kurtz, R. and H. Prestera. *The Body Reveals*. New York: Bantam, 1977.

Masters, R. and J. Houston. *Listening to the Body.* New York: Delacorte Press, 1978.

Montagu, A. *Touching: The Human Significance of the Skin.* New York: Harper and Row, 1986.

Pelletier, K. *Mind as Healer, Mind as Slayer.* New York: Delta, 1977.

Todd, M. E. *The Thinking Body.* New York: Dance Horizons, Inc., 1979.

Yalom, I. *Existential Psychotherapy.* New York: Basic Books, 1980.

ABOUT THE AUTHOR

David DiDomenico, C.M.T. (Certified Massage Therapist), is also an authorized Feldenkrais practitioner. He is a graduate of the Boulder School of Massage Therapy and was a student of Moshe Feldenkrais. David is a former core faculty member of the Boulder School of Massage Therapy and has taught massage technique, movement, and stress management classes for numerous schools and organizations, in both the private and public sector. He currently resides in Boulder, CO, where he has a private practice in somatic education and massage, and continues to facilitate workshops and present keynotes in the field.

Barry Friedman, Ph.D., M.F.C.C.

27 Meditation and Prayer

WHAT ARE MEDITATION AND PRAYER?

Meditation and prayer are two distinct yet complementary spiritual practices that draw upon the deepest dimensions of human experience and reveal to us our hearts, psyches, and our relationship to the sacred. Meditation and prayer are gateways through which we can find inspiration, healing, and renewal for our spiritual journeys and for our mental, emotional, and physical needs.

From its Latin root *meditare*, meditation means to ponder, reflect, or contemplate; *meditare* itself may derive from the root *mete*, to measure. Thus, in its classical sense, meditation refers to a measuring of or reflecting upon an object of thought. In current usage, meditation is understood as a practice in which an individual gradually opens his or her mind to alternative states and levels of consciousness. These states are not apparent or present in everyday awareness, but they are understood to reside inherently and latently in the human psyche. These alternate levels of awareness are accessed through specific techniques of focusing attention.

Since World War II, there has been an influx of Eastern teachings and practices into the West. These have come together with indigenous Western meditation practices, and the result is that meditation has taken root in America in a myriad of forms, styles, and practices, each with its own teachings and philosophies. The uses and goals of meditation are also extremely varied, ranging from simple relaxation and calming, to healing physical, emotional, and spiritual "dis-ease," to the ultimate goal — variously described — of union with the Divine, Self/God realization, and complete enlightenment. The range of goals reflects the variety of traditions, Eastern and Western, that now flourish in the U.S. For the purposes of this book, meditation can be seen as a method for gradually and progressively enriching one's spiritual life, and for improving one's general mental health by bringing heightened, healing awareness to one's physical and emotional experience. Problems with depression, anxiety, confusion, addiction, anger, and fear, together with their physical manifestations such as low energy, high blood pressure, physical cravings, chronic pain, etc., may all be ameliorated or alleviated through ongoing meditation practice.

In this culture, prayer has come to mean communication with a "Higher Power." This communication begins in the heart; Larry Dossey describes prayer as "an attitude of the heart" (Dossey, 1996). While meditation may or may not involve a focus on a Divine Presence, prayer always seems to be an intentional act of "turning toward" a Divine Presence. This "turning of the heart" holds an intention of relationship with the Divine, and of communication in the form of dialogue, praise, thanksgiving, confession, petition, inquiry, and even for the purpose of struggling with the Divine.

As with meditation, prayer can significantly affect one's mental, physical, and spiritual health in a variety of beneficial ways. In fact, certain religious movements, such as Christian Science, consider faith and prayer to be the essential or only requirement for health and healing. Prayer can be a private, individual experience, or a communal one. Prayer takes an almost limitless variety of forms, based on the diverse spiritual traditions of the world's multicultural religious history. Each tradition has developed forms of prayer that are uniquely expressive and evocative for a variety of purposes and occasions. Please see the "How to Learn More" section later in this chapter for materials on prayer and meditation practice in Christianity, Judaism, Islam (Sufism), Hinduism, and Buddhism.

The principles that seem to link meditation and prayer together are inward/internalized attention, inquiry or searching, and attunement to a deeper — or higher — level of awareness or Presence. These actions facilitate the emergence of healing, vitalizing, transforming energies from the deeper mind and spirit that can, through practice, profoundly enhance an individual's life experience on various levels: physical, cognitive, emotional, and spiritual. In the deepest dimensions of the heart and mind, meditation and prayer can bring about an experience of wholeness and presence.

HOW IT BEGAN

Both meditation and prayer are practices rooted in the deepest emotional and spiritual yearnings of humanity from time immemorial. Throughout the world's cultural history, humanity has searched for — and taken part in — sacred and holy practices. Rudolf Otto, an early twentieth-century historian of religion, spoke of the sacred as a spiritual reality that bursts into the cultural matrix of every society, emanating majesty, mystery, and power, and inspiring the deepest awe, respect, and fear (Otto, 1976). Mircea Eliade, another eminent religious historian, traced the patterns and structures of religious experience throughout history, and suggested that humanity is engaged in the quest for a return to a sacred, transcendent, and eternal reality that holds our archetypal origins and that reveals itself symbolically in time and space. Through myth, ritual, and psychospiritual practices such as meditation and prayer, we attempt to attune ourselves to, and participate in, the sacred for the purpose of physical, emotional, and spiritual rebirth and renewal (Eliade, 1974). Meditation and prayer, then, are practices by which an individual or a community attempts to access the deepest dimensions of human experience, whether we call this experience God, Buddha, the Self, the Absolute, etc. However, I would like to add that these practices should not be viewed simply as attempts to "transcend" the human condition. In practice, meditation and prayer bring us to a very here and now experience of our humanness, as well as of our deepest nature and our relationship with the Absolute. Meditation and prayer often call into question distinctions between "sacred" and "profane," by inviting (or requiring) us to examine the totality of our lives with deeper, focused, and more encompassing awareness. Spirituality, after all, must be broad and deep enough to encompass all of who we are. As Jack Kornfield wisely attests, "The universal must be wedded to the personal to be fulfilled in our personal life" (Kornfield, 1993).

HOW IT WORKS

The variety of meditation techniques and modes of prayer seem limitless, given the range of cultures, religions, schools, and practices that have evolved in human history. For simplicity's sake, our discussion of meditation will refer to

Arthur Deikman's delineation of the subject into two principal categories —
concentration and mindfulness (Deikman, 1982). Concentrative meditation
involves a focusing of attention on a single object, e.g., a flame, a mantra (syl-
lable or series of syllables), the breath, a part of the body (the heart, the space
between the eyebrows), a feeling, an image, a holy person, or a representation
of the Divine. In this concentration, discursive thought, problem solving and
future-oriented goals are set aside so that the meditator's mind is in the immediacy of the present moment. In contrast, mindfulness meditation is not about
controlling one's attention at all. Rather, a steady, dispassionate, bare attention
is cultivated toward whatever sensations, thoughts, or emotions are arising
spontaneously in the moment. Though concentration and mindfulness techniques of meditation are distinct in practice, both promote the development of
an "observing self" (Deikman, 1982).

In the initial stages of meditation practice, the breath is often used as a
focus for the purpose of learning to relax. In fact, relaxation is, in my view, an
essential element of meditation on all levels of practice. With attention to the
breath, one gradually becomes calm and the body relaxes. Tension and pain in
various parts of the body often tend to dissolve as practice progresses. Along
the way, it may be necessary to "tune in" to the uncomfortable sensations and
let them "speak." Often, difficult physical sensations relate to unresolved events
and issues from the past that need to be remembered and cleared as one pro-
ceeds in the practice. Similarly, emotional impulses and feelings will arise as
one attempts to relax the mind; if these impulses and feelings (such as anxiety,
depression, anger) become unrelenting distractions, it may be necessary to
process (with a psychotherapist, for example) the feelings that are forcing themselves into our awareness. In truth, meditation tends to allow unresolved emotional conflict or trauma to surface so that we can bring healing awareness to
our past and present experience.

Initially, pleasant or unpleasant physical and emotional sensations and
impulses can seem like formidable obstacles to maintaining concentration or
prolonged attention. Gradually, however, the meditator learns to include these
"distractions" in moment-to-moment awareness. In fact, these distractions can
actually be viewed as opportunities to cultivate attention and mindfulness.
Distraction becomes an invitation to remember mindfulness in each emerging
moment. With continued practice of moment-to-moment mindfulness, the

need to "transcend" one's present state gives way to an experience of unfolding "immanence" and wholeness in each moment.

With continued practice, the meditator develops a familiarity with his or her psycho-physical organism. The observing self, or witnessing function of the mind, becomes increasingly attentive and tuned in to the subtle aspects of the body, mind, and spirit. Particularly in the traditions of Hindu and Buddhist meditation (*dhyana*), this observing self is seen as the vehicle by which an individual attains to progressively deeper (or higher) states of awareness and realization, culminating in complete spiritual enlightenment. In the Vedanta tradition of Hinduism, for example, concentrative meditation leads to the realization that the true self of the individual is identical with the ultimate, absolute Self (*Brahman*) of the universe. In Buddhism, the mindfulness meditations of the Zen, vipassana, and dzogchen traditions lead the practitioner to a gradual realization of "no-self," an awareness that our ultimate nature is beyond any conceptualization or conditioned feeling state, that our essence is the radiant, compassionate, wise, skylike emptiness of Buddha-mind.

As mentioned before, prayer is a heartfelt act of "turning toward" a Higher Power or Divine Presence that may be perceived as being inside or outside the self. The kind of communication and relationship we establish and cultivate depends to a great extent on what we seek from the relationship with the Higher Power, on our capacity for intimacy, and on our willingness to open ourselves, to "bare our souls" with honesty and integrity.

Prayer allows us to express the deepest yearnings of the heart for guidance, meaning, healing, and wholeness. Prayer is a resource for people who may be suffering from any type of physical, emotional, or spiritual "dis-ease." In prayer, one attunes him/herself to Divine Presence in order to establish and cultivate a relationship with the Divine. As this relationship evolves, personal problems can be held in a spiritual context of faith, love, compassion, and forgiveness. Dialogues with a Higher Power may not always be easy or joyful, but they can evoke tremendous insight, inspiration, courage, redemption, and resolution for the most difficult problems of body, mind, and spirit.

The practice of meditation and prayer deepens over time, and changes according to our needs and our capacity for intimate communication and connection with the Divine. I have found that with continued practice, the distinction between sacred and profane begins to dissolve.

WHAT THE RESEARCH SHOWS

As holistic approaches to the study of human experience, health, and healing have burgeoned in the last twenty years, meditation and prayer have become increasingly prevalent as modalities of prevention and therapy in the field of mental (and physical) health. Meditation and prayer have been shown to help with psychosomatic, mood (including anxiety, depression, and aggression) and other mental health disorders; facilitate recovery from drug and alcohol addiction; improve self-esteem and self-awareness; and stimulate cognitive abilities such as learning, memory, and concentration. Increasingly, studies are being undertaken to determine and verify the therapeutic effects of meditation and prayer. Authors such as Andrew Weil, Deepak Chopra, Herbert Benson, and Larry Dossey are not only documenting the benefits of meditation and prayer, but are also contextualizing these benefits in an integrated vision of body, mind, soul, and cosmos. A recent *Newsweek* (Woodward, 1997) article on the power of prayer underscores the growing interest in these alternative, spiritually oriented health practices for mainstream America.

REAL PEOPLE AND MEDITATION/PRAYER

Alice, a female in her early thirties, described herself as a successful physician who had achieved tremendous success in her professional life very shortly after becoming licensed. Not quite a workaholic, she nevertheless cultivated a very intense medical practice in which she became deeply involved in her patients' lives, hoping to promote their health and general well-being. Alice took great pride in her work and accomplishment, and was respected by colleagues and patients alike. Over the course of several years, however, gradually Alice began to notice that she was becoming increasingly anxious about the well-being of her patients. As her anxiety continued to grow, it began to interfere with the enjoyment of her free time and she developed insomnia. Over time, Alice's anxiety began to affect her physical health; she developed respiratory problems and, later, an inflammatory condition of the joints. Neither disorder had any apparent organic basis.

In our therapy sessions, Alice recognized the psychodynamic roots of her over-involvement with her patients; she was attempting to take too much responsibility for them. However, this recognition didn't fully relieve her anxiety or reduce her psychosomatic symptoms. I suggested a practice of mindfulness meditation in which, with eyes open but not focused on a point, Alice would allow her attention to be mirrored by the empty space in front of her. At first, distracting thoughts and feelings made it difficult for Alice to allow her mind to relax into emptiness. But with continued practice, she found that this mindfulness meditation became a deep experience of calm, peace, and self-awareness that greatly reduced her generalized anxiety. In addition, I suggested a prayer in which Alice would silently welcome her patients into the room with the intention of serving them well, and then silently bid them farewell as they left, praying for their healing and well-being, while recognizing their own responsibility and autonomy in the healing process. Within a few months, Alice's anxiety had greatly diminished, her psychosomatic symptoms mostly disappeared, and her enjoyment of her work returned.

∞

Jim, a gay African-American in his late thirties, came to therapy because, though he was extremely well-liked by the community at large, he had a very difficult time maintaining individual friendships. At a certain point in his relationships, he would inevitably feel slighted in some way and break off contact without explanation. While extremely intelligent and fairly well-educated, Jim lacked the self-awareness to understand how his own behavior perpetuated this pattern of failed friendships. His ego -strength and boundaries initially seemed inadequate to the task of containing his emotional pain about the loss of his friends. In therapy, I spent a great deal of time holding and containing Jim's emotional pain, and offering empathic reflection and insight, to the extent that he could receive them. Jim's ego-integrity, self-awareness, and capacity for intimacy began a steady development.

Then Jim received an AIDS diagnosis. With this diagnosis, Jim's sense of alienation from others returned and, in addition, he fell into a depression and despair which were at times overwhelming. He often wished to die. Fortunately, in the course of our work, I had discovered that Jim had access to a profound sense of spirituality within him. While supporting him emotionally in his struggle with a life-threatening illness, I also suggested that he might recognize his despair as a "dark night of the soul." Jim was questioning whether his life had any meaning. I gently encouraged him to pray for the guidance and understanding that he needed and sought. As Jim began to explore his connection to God and his Higher Self through prayer, he began to experience illuminating dreams and visions that allowed him to see himself more clearly and realistically, made his pain more intelligible, and offered him a sense of meaning and purpose in life. Before his death, Jim emerged from his "dark night" with a deep and grounded self-awareness and a profound spiritual presence.

WHAT TO EXPECT

Meditation and prayer can be practiced individually or in a group or community setting. There is a great deal of literature and taped material concerning both prayer and meditation that can assist you in beginning or cultivating these practices. With meditation, however, it would probably be best to begin studying with a competent and reputable teacher, either privately or in a group. Classes can usually be found in yoga schools, holistic health centers, or fitness clubs. Since there are many types of meditation practices, you might find that one fits your needs better than another. I recommend practicing a meditation technique for a month before deciding to try another, unless your mind and body give you very clear signals that a particular meditation is not for you. Whichever meditation you choose to practice, the time, energy, and commitment you give will determine the kind of results you achieve. In addition to a weekly session or class with your teacher, daily meditation is extremely useful. You might begin slowly by meditating once or twice a week for ten to fifteen minutes. Gradually build up to a daily routine of thirty minutes to one hour (depending on your time constraints). Meditation can be practiced sitting, lying down, standing, or walking. Usually, meditation is done in a sitting position, using a comfortable cushion to support the spine, which should be straight but relaxed. You may use a chair, if sitting on the floor is uncomfortable or inadvisable.

As a natural expression of the heart, prayer is a practice that you can begin and cultivate without the assistance of a teacher. However, many people find that some kind of "spiritual direction" or guidance is very useful in developing a prayer practice. Since you may be most comfortable with a specific religious tradition (either your family's or one that you have adopted), it might be very helpful to discuss your spiritual needs and intention for prayer with a spiritual director from that tradition, i.e., priest, rabbi, roshi, etc. As with meditation, prayer ripens with practice. A daily practice of prayer can engender an ever-deepening attunement with your Self and with God. Prayer is the cultivation of a very intimate relationship.

Meditation and prayer can be combined with other healing practices. Personally, I have found that psychotherapy is an excellent complement to the practice of meditation and prayer. Meditation and prayer often help us to "transcend" our ordinary consciousness or personality; psychotherapy helps us to "transform" those aspects of our consciousness or personality that impede our spiritual journey. Psycho-physical practices such as yoga and T'ai Chi are also excellent complements to meditation and prayer.

Whatever meditation or prayer you may choose to practice, the time, energy, commitment, and intention that you bring to your practice are the key elements that will condition your experience and the results you achieve. Also, remember that meditation and prayer tend to become part of a more inclusive way of life, which may call you to a gradual transformation and evolution in your life-path.

HOW TO FIND A MEDITATION TEACHER OR SPIRITUAL GUIDE

Meditation teachers are sometimes spiritual guides, and spiritual guides sometimes teach meditation, but this is not always the case. Meditation teachers and classes are often listed in the Yellow Pages under "Meditation Instruction" or "Yoga." Magazines such as the *Yoga Journal, Holistic Health Journal,* and *New Age Journal* list meditation teachers, schools, and classes, as well as offering useful articles on meditation and spirituality. You'll need to call and find out as much as you can about the particular meditation, tradition, and techniques being taught. Ask for literature. Find out about class schedules, length of classes and class size, the cost, the recommended dress, and if you need to provide your own cushion. You'll also want to tell a prospective teacher something about yourself, particularly your expectations for the class, and any relevant emotional and physical health concerns or constraints. Be sure to gauge how the teacher responds to you: Your initial feelings about the teacher can often be a useful guide to determine whether you want to study with him or her. Also ask about his or her credentials for teaching: training, certification, and teaching experience.

There is a common adage that searching for a guru or spiritual teacher is not useful — when the time is right, the teacher appears. This may or may not be true. However seeking spiritual advice or guidance in prayer can be very helpful. As mentioned, within your own religious tradition you might contact your local church, synagogue, mosque, Buddhist or Hindu temple, etc. to talk with a spiritual director. Again, some of the magazines cited earlier will list spiritual schools that you can contact to discuss your spiritual needs. And, simply, if you have thoughtful and compassionate friends or family who are interested in their own spirituality, you might talk with them about your interest in prayer. But be careful: Sometimes people who present themselves as spiritual teachers are unaware of their own ego or "shadow," and, in the guise of spiritual assistance they may try to subtly coerce you into accepting their beliefs and giving up your personal power to them. Always remember that you have free will and that what you are seeking is ultimately within yourself.

HOW TO LEARN MORE

There is an enormous body of literature on both meditation and prayer. The following list includes general reading on the role of meditation and prayer in mental and physical health, as well as secondary material on meditation and prayer from the five major religious traditions: Christianity, Judaism, Islam (Sufism), Buddhism, and Hinduism. For a deeper study, you may want to read the primary texts of some of the great mystics and masters of these traditions.

Benson, H. *Timeless Healing: The Power and Biology of Belief.* New York: Simon and Schuster, 1997.

Chopra, D. *Ageless Body, Timeless Mind.* New York: Crown Publishers, 1993.

Cooper, D. *Silence, Simplicity, and Solitude: A Guide For Spiritual Retreat.* New York: Crown Publishers, 1992.

Corless, R. *The Art of Christian Alchemy: Transfiguring the Ordinary Through Holistic Meditation.* Ramsey, NJ: Paulist Press, 1981.

Deikman, A. *The Observing Self: Mysticism and Psychotherapy.* Boston: Beacon Press Books, 1982.

Dossey, L. *Healing Words: The Power of Prayer and the Practice of Medicine.* San Francisco: HarperCollins, 1996.

Dossey, L. *Prayer is Good Medicine.* San Francisco: HarperCollins, 1996.

Easwaran, E. *Meditation.* Tomales, CA: Nilgiri Press, 1996.

Eliade, M. *The Myth of the Eternal Return.* Princeton: Princeton University Press, 1974.

Green, T. *When the Well Runs Dry: Prayer Beyond the Beginnings.* Notre Dame, IN: Ave Maria Press, 1979.

Goldstein, J. *The Experience of Insight: A Simple and Direct Guide to Buddhist Meditation.* Boston: Shambhala Publishing, Inc., 1987.

Helminski, E. *Living Presence: A Sufi Way to Mindfulness and the Essential Self.* New York: G.P. Putnam's Sons, 1992.

Kaplan, A. *Meditation and the Bible.* York Beach, ME: Samuel Weiser, 1988.

Kornfield, J. *A Path with Heart: A Guide Through the Perils and Promises of Spiritual Life.* New York: Bantam Books, 1993.

Otto, R. *The Idea of the Holy.* New York: Oxford University Press, 1976.

Schimmel, A. *Mystical Dimensions of Islam.* Chapel Hill: The University of North Carolina Press, 1978.

Suzuki, D. *An Introduction to Zen Buddhism.* New York: Grove Press, 1991.

Trungpa, C. *Training the Mind and Cultivating Loving-Kindness.* Boston: Shambhala Publishing, Inc., 1993.

Weil, A. *Spontaneous Healing.* New York: Ballantine Books, 1995.

Woodward, K. "Is God Listening?" *Newsweek*, March 31, 1997, 57–64.

ABOUT THE AUTHOR

Barry Friedman is a licensed marriage, family, and child counselor (MFCC) psychotherapist living in Oakland, CA, specializing in depth psychotherapy and spiritual inquiry. He received his M.A. in Divinity and Ph.D. in South Asian Languages and Civilizations from the University of Chicago, and an M.A. in Counseling Psychology from John F. Kennedy University. Barry has taught meditation, yoga, comparative mythology, and religion, and has been deeply involved in the field of death and dying. He is a student of Tibetan Buddhism and T'ai Chi Ch'uan.

J. Jamison Starbuck, J.D., N.D.

28 Naturopathy and Mental Health

WHAT IS NATUROPATHY?

Naturopathic medicine is a unique and distinct medical profession. Its practitioners are naturopathic physicians — primary care family physicians (and licensed as such in recognizing states) who are specialists in natural and holistic medicine. Naturopathic physicians treat a wide variety of physical, mental, and emotional illnesses, including depression, anxiety, addictions, eating disorders, trauma and abuse related illnesses, confusion and memory disorders, attention deficit disorder, obsessive/compulsive disorders, phobias, nightmares, insomnia, and issues related to self-esteem, self-actualization and personal growth.

Because of their role as primary care holistic doctors, naturopathic physicians are acutely aware of the interconnected nature of the mind and the body. In direct contrast to the mainstream medical model, in which a patient is "dissected" into many parts and directed to a different doctor for the separate treatment of each area of the body (a psychiatrist or psychologist for mental/ emotional complaints, an internist for fatigue, a dermatologist for skin rashes, and a gastroenterologist for stomach problems), the naturopathic medical model sees and treats a patient as one singular organism composed of many interrelated systems.

Naturopathic physicians routinely recognize the links between physical symptoms and mental and emotional complaints. In certain instances of mental or emotional illness, a physical imbalance underlies or causes the mental/

emotional disturbance. In other instances, the mental or emotional illness can create physical symptoms. In order to accomplish true healing, naturopathic physicians offer treatment for physical ailments in conjunction with treatment for mental or emotional complaints. This is done only when appropriate, based on each individual set of circumstances.

HOW IT BEGAN

The historical roots of naturopathic medicine lie in the nineteenth century eclectic, hygienic, and homeopathic schools of medical thought. In contrast to the "heroic" medical tradition of bloodletting, leeching, and purging with heavy metals such as mercury, the eclectic, hygienic, and homeopathic physicians employed gentler methods such as herbal formulas, specialized diets, exercise, lifestyle changes, and hydrotherapy.

The term "naturopathy," as a distinct medical profession, came into being in the United States between 1898 and 1902. In 1902, the first school of naturopathic medicine opened in New York City. At that time, the *Naturopath and Herald of Health* described naturopathic medicine as "standing for the reconciling, harmonizing and unifying of nature, humanity and God." Naturopathic medicine was "fundamentally therapeutic" because it offered "healing, education and empowerment . . . encompassing the realm of human progress and destiny" (Cody, 1996).

While today's language may be more down to earth than that of the lofty Victorian era, naturopathic medicine still offers healing, education, and empowerment. There are four recognized, accredited naturopathic medical schools in the United States, located in Portland, OR; Seattle, WA; Phoenix, AZ; and recently opened in Bridgeport, CT. Graduates of these schools take national licensing exams, and practice throughout the United States and other countries, as general naturopathic medical practitioners and family physicians.

HOW IT WORKS

Naturopathic medicine is based on several principles: *vis medicatrix naturae, tolle causum,* and *primum non nocere. Vis medicatrix naturae,* a term used by Hippocrates and dating to 400 B.C., means "the healing power of nature." This is the foundation of naturopathic medicine, the belief that the body and mind have innate healing mechanisms that can be enhanced and utilized in the treatment of disease. *Vis medicatrix naturae* also recognizes the healing properties of substances existing in nature: air, water, food, plants.

Tolle causum means "find the cause." This term encapsulates the naturo-pathic principle, which states that the most effective approach to disease involves not simply the treatment of symptoms, but the detection and treatment of the underlying cause of the illness.

Primum non nocere means "do no harm." Naturopathic physicians endeavor to use therapeutic modalities that are gentle, natural, and supportive to the body. Medicines that the body can utilize constructively, without difficult or dangerous side effects, are chosen to enhance the functioning of homeostasis.

Also worth discussing is the place of naturopathic medicine in the debate over vitalism vs. mechanism. The origins of these two medical philosophies can be traced again to Hippocrates and ancient Greece, while the history of their evolving schools of thought can be followed from ancient times into today. Mechanism essentially maintains that life is a series of complicated physical and chemical reactions; disease is a disruption of these reactions caused by some sort of external agent. Treatment therefore involves the swift eradication of the external agent, or the removal of its signs or symptoms. Examples of mechanistic philosophies at work in the orthodox medical community are: ear tubes in a child with chronic ear infections, anti-anxiety agents for a patient with panic disorder, Ritalin for a child with attention deficit disorder.

Vitalism, on the other hand, is based on the philosophy that each organism is unique and that life is more complex than simple chemistry. Vitalists acknowledge modern biological and medical science, and concurrently recognize the existence of something more — some special quality of homeostasis, of balance, of a vital force, that moves body and mind toward healing — that gives each individual his or her own uniqueness. Vitalism explains disease symptoms not as the action of the external agent, but as the body's *response* to the agent, and as the body's attempt to defend and heal itself. According to vitalism, individuality explains why not every person exposed to a flu virus will get flu symptoms, and why not every person exposed to the same event will display anxiety. Symptoms, according to vitalism, are relative to the vigor and uniqueness of the individual.

Naturopathic medicine is primarily a vitalistic system of medicine. Naturopathic therapies, such as botanical medicines, homeopathic medicines, nutrition, physical therapies, and counseling, largely work to strengthen the human organism and to enhance its capacity to fight disease. However, naturopathic physicians also agree that there are situations in which a mechanistic approach is necessary. Naturopathic physicians use their diagnostic and medical skills to make this determination, and, if mechanistic treatment is required, will use natural medicines whenever feasible and prescription medications if necessary. In many states, naturopathic licensing law allows naturopathic physicians to prescribe some pharmaceuticals that are natural in origin, such as penicillin, codeine, and thyroid medications.

Naturopathic physicians also recognize that there are individuals whose disease process requires mechanistic, medical intervention. Naturopathic medicine has a long history of cooperative interaction with orthodox practitioners and medical specialists. Naturopathic physicians will make referrals to medical specialists when necessary, and often work with patients who are concurrently seeing medical doctors and taking orthodox prescription medicine.

In the area of mental health care, naturopathic medicine works by gently strengthening and healing both the body and the mind. Areas of disease or illness are specifically treated while concurrently the whole organism is brought into balance.

WHAT THE RESEARCH SHOWS

Research on naturopathic medical modalities is increasing each year, with the most extensive research being conducted by the research departments at each of the four naturopathic medical colleges. Readers interested in ongoing or completed studies are urged to contact the research departments at National College of Naturopathic Medicine, Bastyr University of Natural Health Sciences, Southwest College of Naturopathic Medicine and Health Sciences, or University of Bridgeport College of Naturopathic Medicine (see addresses page 408). Numerous research studies on plant and homeopathic medicines have been, and continue to be, done in Europe. Interested readers can learn more about these studies through botanical and homeopathic journals.

REAL PEOPLE AND NATUROPATHY

T. L., an 11-year-old boy, was brought to the office for depression and attention deficit disorder. Among his symptoms were poor performance in school, suicidal thoughts and statements, many fears — of the dark, of the basement, of nighttime, of ghosts and monsters — and apathy alternating with quarrelsome behavior. This boy is also an artist, and at the time of his first visit, was making very dark drawings of people being killed with knives, of people hanging, and other scenes of torture and misery. At that time, T. L. was taking 50 mg of Zoloft daily. T. L. had taken a dislike to the Zoloft, and whenever possible, would hide the pill under his tongue and spit it out when his parents were not watching.

After a thorough case-taking involving a ninety-minute office visit, he was given one dose of a homeopathic remedy, stramonium 200C. During the first twenty-four hours, T. L.'s behavior worsened dramatically. He became very angry, volatile, and violent. His mother sent him outside to do laps around the yard in order to work off some of his frenzied energy.

By the next morning, T. L. had changed. He invited his mother into his room, usually a wild mess. His room was clean and tidy, organized for the first time. T. L. had arisen at 6 A.M. and spent over an hour straightening and cleaning his room. He was calm, able to be kind, and interact with family members.

Over the next two months, T. L. continued to improve. He lost his fear of the dark, began to do better in school, and no longer expressed any suicidal tendencies. His drawings changed to landscapes and scenes of boats, animals, and people enjoying themselves.

T. L. returned to the office several months later because of behavior that involved minor lying and stealing. His homeopathic case was taken again and at this visit he was given medorrhinum 200C. Again, T. L. had a significant reaction to the remedy, with lots of physical energy, anger, and mean behavior. Again, by the next morning he was calm. This time his mother found him sitting in bed, preparing his homework. Over the next few months, T. L. continued to improve in school and social settings.

T. L. was seen again for trouble at home involving power struggles and conflicts between him and his father. He had grown and changed, and the center of his disturbance was different than it had been several months previously. Lachesis 1M was prescribed. Again, T. L. had a similar disturbance, with angry words, hyperactivity, and meanness, this time for several days following the remedy. Again, he eventually settled down; he became happier and able to function well within his school and family system.

At the time of this writing, T. L. is doing well. He is happy, he is stable at home and at school, he is enrolled in a holistic tutoring program for certain subjects, and his grades have improved significantly. He has received no demerits in school this past term, and his creativity is showing itself in a positive fashion: T. L. is the only boy in his school to be selected for this year's all-city choir.

R. S., a 41-year-old female, suffered from anxiety, depression, and chronic fatigue. She had been born prematurely and grew up in an alcoholic family with significant physical and emotional abuse. She had been in therapy for several years. She liked therapy, though it drained her. Her therapist was urging her to take a prescription antidepressant medication.

On her first visit, R. S. refused any laboratory tests, claiming financial duress and an unwillingness to take any prescription medication. R. S. was asked to make dietary changes that included the elimination of caffeine, alcohol, and simple sugars. She was given a constitutional homeopathic remedy and a botanical formula including the herb St. John's wort.

At her two week follow-up, R. S. reported that she was feeling better; she was excited by the change and looked forward to what she called her "new life." R. S. did not return to the office for over two months, at which time she had had a 50 percent relapse in her symptoms, most significantly fatigue and a sense of black doom. Her homeopathic remedy was repeated, and she was also given a botanical formula to support her thyroid function. Again, R. S. felt better for a time, but was not able to completely sustain the improvement. Though she was attentive to her diet and self-care recommendations, R. S. was unable to work full-time without getting exhausted, unable to do the eight- and ten-mile hikes she used to enjoy on weekends, and she still suffered from a slight but ever-present sense of doom.

Finally, R. S. consented to laboratory tests, among them a thyroid profile test which revealed a hypothyroid state. R. S. agreed to try one grain daily of Armour thyroid (the most "natural" type of prescription thyroid hormone) in addition to her botanical formula. Within one week, her life had changed again. Within two months she had begun to work full-time and felt able to socialize, hike, and tackle projects long left untended.

Over the next six months, R. S. maintained her commitment to a healthy diet and was given another homeopathic remedy that helped her during a particularly difficult emotional period involving a job change. One year later, R. S. had begun a new romantic relationship, and was considering graduate school.

These two cases illustrate a broad application of naturopathic philosophy and treatments to several mental illnesses. In the first case, the treatment was vitalistic in nature, using homeopathic medicine to stimulate the vital force, and a minor amount of therapy to educate and balance the emotional functioning. In the second case, the vital force responded to natural medicines, but was unable to support and sustain the individual's vigor and verve for very long, due to a physiological deficit. When this was treated mechanistically with a small dose of prescription thyroid hormone, the homeopathic and botanical medicines were better able to support and strengthen R. S.

WHAT TO EXPECT

Typically, a patient schedules an office visit with a naturopathic physician. The first office visit ranges, depending on the practitioner, from thirty to ninety minutes. For a mental health patient, this first visit would involve a thorough history taking, a review of any records, and in-depth discussion of the problem at hand. Depending on the circumstances, a physical exam may be recommended or performed during the first visit, or may be scheduled for a subsequent visit. Because naturopathic medicine honors the individuality and uniqueness of each patient, issues of touch and of physical exams are managed in a sensitive manner. Patients are informed about the reasons for any physical exams or laboratory tests, and are empowered to make their own choices regarding their bodies.

In most instances, treatment protocols involve specific nutritional and lifestyle advice, one or more botanical prescriptions, homeopathic medicine, and recommendations regarding related therapies such as bodywork, hydrotherapy, exercise, and light therapy. Some naturopathic physicians have specific training in psychotherapy and thus offer counseling as a part of their treatment. Others are concurrently trained in acupuncture and Chinese herbology.

Naturopathic physicians take seriously the role of doctor as teacher; during the office visit, they educate patients about the disease and involve patients in the healing process. Patient participation may range from something very simple, such as taking a homeopathic remedy or brewing a medicinal tea, to more complex involvement such as keeping a diet diary, journaling, an exercise regimen, weekly counseling, or specific dietary changes.

The frequency of follow-up visits is also determined on an individual basis. Most patients working with mental health issues see their naturopathic physician once or twice a month. Others schedule visits as often as once or twice a week, depending on the treatment modalities utilized, the involvement of other practitioners, the extent of self-care, and issues related to geography, time, and finance. Typical costs for a first office visit range from $65 to $150; follow-up visits range in price from $35 to $75. Prices will vary depending upon time spent during the visit and upon local economic factors. Patients can also expect to spend additional money on medicines, such as herbal preparations, homeopathic remedies, and supplements, and on laboratory tests where indicated.

Symptom resolution is distinctly possible with naturopathic medicine. Because it is a broad spectrum, eclectic form of medicine, it offers a wide assortment of healing modalities, suitable for a variety of individuals. Most mental health patients notice a positive shift in symptoms within the first two weeks of treatment. Full resolution may come within several months. In some cases, continued maintenance is required over a period of years, and there are some cases where full resolution is not possible.

HOW TO FIND A NATUROPATH

It is essential for an interested patient to inquire about the training and licensing of a naturopathic physician. Patients should be certain that the naturopathic physician they are seeing is a graduate of an accredited naturopathic medical college, and is licensed as a physician by a state naturopathic medical licensing board. As mentioned, there are four accredited schools of naturopathic medicine in the United States: National College of Naturopathic Medicine, Bastyr

University of Natural Health Sciences, Southwest College of Naturopathic Medicine and Health Science, and University of Bridgeport College of Naturopathic Medicine. With few exceptions, graduation from one of these schools is required for licensing in the United States.

It is also a good idea to ask doctors, or their staff, if the doctor has had experience working with mental health issues. Patients should feel free to ask questions regarding training, licensing and practice specialties, practice style, and cost of treatment when making an initial inquiry and before scheduling an appointment.

The best source for locating a naturopathic physician is the American Association of Naturopathic Physicians (AANP), 2366 Eastlake Ave. East, Suite 322, Seattle, WA, 98102. The AANP has a referral line for patients seeking naturopathic physicians in their city or state: (206) 323-7610. There is a five dollar charge for an information packet. Interested persons can also contact one of the naturopathic medical schools:

NATIONAL COLLEGE OF
NATUROPATHIC MEDICINE
11231 SE Market St.
Portland, OR 97216
Tel: (503) 255-4860

BASTYR UNIVERSITY OF NATURAL
HEALTH SCIENCES
14500 Juanita Dr. NE
Bothell, WA 98011
Tel: (206) 823-1300

SOUTHWEST COLLEGE OF
NATUROPATHIC MEDICINE AND
HEALTH SCIENCES
6535 E. Osborn Rd., Suite 703
Scottsdale, AZ 85251
Tel: (602) 990-7424

UNIVERSITY OF BRIDGEPORT COLLEGE
OF NATUROPATHIC MEDICINE
221 University Ave.
Bridgeport, CT 06601
Tel: (203) 576-4109

Readers may also call or write their state naturopathic or medical licensing board for information about naturopathic medicine in individual states.

HOW TO LEARN MORE

Cody, G. W. "The History of Naturopathic Medicine." In *A Textbook of Natural Medicine*, edited by J. Pizzorno and M. Murray, Bothell, WA: Bastyr University Publications, 1996.

Pizzorno, J. and M. Murray eds. *The Encyclopedia of Natural Medicine*. Rocklin, CA: Prima, 1990.

Somerville, R. ed. *The Alternative Advisor*. Alexandria, VA: Time-Life, Inc., 1997.

ABOUT THE AUTHOR

J. Jamison Starbuck, J.D., N.D., has a practice in family medicine in Missoula, MT. At least 30 percent of her practice is devoted to the treatment of mental health issues, including A.D.D., depression, anxiety, and eating disorders. She also teaches homeopathy and botanical medicine, is a consulting editor for Time-Life Books, and writes and consults for various publications nationwide. She is a 1989 graduate of the National College of Naturopathic Medicine. She is also a graduate of Middlebury College and Willamette University College of Law, and is a member of the state bars of Montana and Oregon.

Donald M. Epstein, D.C.

29 Network Spinal Analysis:
A Chiropractor's Perspective on the Body/Mind Connection

WHAT IS NETWORK SPINAL ANALYSIS?

Network Spinal Analysis® is a leading-edge application of chiropractic methods available to anyone who wants a freer, more flexible, and more vibrant spine and nervous system. The shape, position, tone, and tension of the spine directly and indirectly affect our perception of life, the way we meet life, and the way we recover from life's circumstances. The ability of the spinal system to remain flexible, adaptable, and free from mechanical tension and interference is essential to the healing process.

The intent of Network Spinal Analysis is to locate and correct the subluxations (misalignments and resulting muscular tension) of the spine to empower the nervous system to express a fuller range of its healing potential. Network Spinal Analysis is not designed to remove uncomfortable situations from the patient's physiology or to help a person feel better (although this commonly happens). Network Spinal Analysis was not developed to cure any emotional or physical condition. The aim is to provide powerful assistance to the body's own self-regulatory and self-healing capacities through the spinal adjustment.

My colleagues and I have found that as a natural consequence of receiving Network Spinal Analysis, the nervous system often reexperiences the events that are the source of the suffering with new insight, as mechanical tension on the spinal system is released and the nervous system remembers the position the spine was in when traumas of the past initially occurred.

HOW IT BEGAN

My awareness of the relationship between the spinal structures and a patient's mental and emotional health began with the understanding that traumatic events could result in spinal distortion. At the beginning of my clinical practice, I had no idea that the significant correction of the spinal distortion could have a major impact on a patient's emotional and mental state, and experience of the world. In this chapter, I will describe some clinical situations that occurred in my practice, forever deepening my understanding of the spinal system as a modulator of consciousness, and of the dynamic relationship between traumatic events and the spine. These insights lead to the development of the work now called Network Spinal Analysis.

In my efforts to maximize the body's own self-corrective capacities in response to the force I applied to the spine in chiropractic technique, I discovered that not all subluxations of the spine were the same, and that the priority of addressing them needed to be explored. As I developed a sequencing of adjustments called a phasing system, and increased the precision of the timing, type, and location of force applied, emotional responses became more common. Later in the development of the technique, patients' spines began to undulate or wave. This was most often associated with altered states of consciousness, spontaneous emotional releases, and reduction of spinal tension. Further exploration of the significance of the body's self-generated wavelike motions and postures lead to the development of Network Spinal Analysis as it is presented in this chapter. There are two wave forms which may be generated during care, a respiratory and a somatopsychic (as compared to a psychosomatic) wave. Both are natural, spontaneous, and appear to be tools to dissipate energy and exchange information. Research has suggested that the appearance of these phenomena are positive influences for health and overall well-being (Epstein, 1996).

HOW IT WORKS

In my practice as a chiropractor, I have found that the shape, position, tone, and tension of the spinal system are directly related to the shape, position, tone, and tension in a person's life. It makes sense that when the spine loses its flexibility and natural contours, so does a person's life experience. A person with a spine that is less flexible and unable to recover from its experiences will most likely be stuck in one perspective.

When the spine cannot enjoy its natural, full range of motion, the body/mind is limited in the types of experience that it can have, as well as the ways it can express itself on physical, mental, emotional, and spiritual levels. At the same time, it will be predisposed to certain types of experience while being unable to respond to others. When your back and head are bent downwards, you may experience defeat or depression. When your spine is ramrod straight with the head pulled back, you will be more stoic and both emotionally and mentally rigid. When your head is tilted slightly upwards with full natural curves in your spine, you will be at peace, regardless of what is happening in your life. In this latter position it is actually difficult for you to experience anger or upset.

In addition, when a person has experienced a marked emotional, mental or physical trauma, certain parts of the spinal musculature will take on a characteristic tone. If someone experiences a significant loss (such as that of a loved one, a relationship, finances) their spinal musculature will tense. This is a natural process, but one that results in difficulty if the spinal system does not reset itself shortly after the experience. If the person's spine and nervous system do not recover from the event, then the musculature will take on a characteristic thickness associated with the length of time since the trauma occurred. This is not unlike observing the rings within a felled tree. We can determine how old the tree is by counting the number of rings. Someone who has had experience examining trees for their characteristic ring patterns can determine the types of traumatic events that the tree survived in its past, such as periods of drought, disease, or forest fire. Similarly, a skilled examiner can determine the nature of the trauma and the approximate period in a person's life when the situation occurred.

The body's movement and tension reveal its history to the trained observer or clinician. This occurs even if the person does not consciously remember the traumatic event that is expressed in the postural physiology. The nervous system will wall off the affected regions from the rest of the spine or body through restricted movement, tense musculature, restricted breath, and pain. It does this for as long as it needs to protect the rest of the nervous system, spine, and body from the traumatic history in that area. It may be years, if ever, before the nervous system can allow for a safe exchange of information, respiration, and movement between this particular region and the rest of the body-mind.

When the body is encouraged to reposition itself in the tension pattern that was originally associated with a traumatic experience, the body unwinds into and then out of the mechanical tension. With a movement of the body from high tension to low tension, an emotional release occurs. With this release, there is a return to a more peaceful and natural state of less tension, freer movement, and fuller respiration. Resolution of the tension may occur on many levels, including the mental and emotional realm, which is never separate from physical tensions.

I propose, based upon the model of Panjabi (1992), the following explanation for the process described above. The spine maintains integrity by the cooperation of its component systems. These systems are the passive system (the spinal bones), the active system (the spinal muscles), and the control system (the nervous system). When energy or information overwhelm the spine and nervous system, as in traumatic experiences, it may be stored as tension in at least one of these component systems. Muscle tension, altered spinal curves, and limited motion of the spine or extremities are examples of such adaptations.

An additional component is the emotional subsystem. The emotional subsystem is not located in any one place, as are the other systems. Instead it is a functional system derived from the tension and restricted motion of the body tissues. I theorize that this tension and restricted motion are processed through the nervous system, and experienced and understood as emotion or attitude.

The emotional subsystem shares information and energy with the other subsystems, and it must be able to dissipate its stored tension effectively for spinal stability to develop. The emotional subsystem may eliminate its tension through vocalization or through transferring the tension to the spinal muscles, which can release it through spinal motion, freeing the spinal bones to assume their natural range of motion. The less impaired the other spinal systems are, the more capable the emotional system will be to release its tension and share its information easily and safely. Network Spinal Analysis facilitates this process by removing impairments to the optimal functioning of the spinal bones and muscles.

WHAT THE RESEARCH SHOWS

A retrospective study was recently conducted at the Medical College of the University of California at Irvine. The study involved 2,818 patients in the U.S. and internationally. The results demonstrate that Network care is associated with statistically significant, profound, and consistent improvement in patients' self-reported health and wellness in many areas, ranging from general emotional well-being to improved work performance to making lifestyle changes and improving relationships.

Additional studies are in progress to assess Network patients longitudinally, and papers further detailing the results have been submitted to peer-reviewed journals for publication. For more information about this and other research projects involving Network Spinal Analysis, contact the Association for Network Chiropractic or Robert Blanks, Ph.D., at University of California at Irvine, Department of Anatomy and Neurobiology, Room 322 Med Surge II, Irvine, CA, 92697-1275, (714) 824-5984, E-mail: mdobson@uci.edu.

REAL PEOPLE AND NETWORK SPINAL ANALYSIS

The following clinical stories are taken from my book *The 12 Stages of Healing* (1994).

Arthur was brought into my office by his family. He was bent forward and to the side, using a stick to support himself, with one of his hands clenched in a fist, as if he was ready to punch someone. Arthur was experiencing extreme pain. He could not sit at all, because his pain was too severe.

He mentioned that he was bending over to make a repair when he felt a snap in his back. The pain that followed was excruciating. Nothing made it go away, not even the powerful medication and therapy given to him by his medical specialist. I consulted with him and his family about his past history, including his physical, emotional, mental, and chemical traumas and stresses.

On examining his spine, I discovered very tense, thick, and protective musculature, especially in his neck. Although his history did not reveal it, my physical findings suggested that a major trauma had occurred twenty years ago. When I questioned him about what might have taken place, his response was "Nothing." About two minutes later he recalled that his brother had died in Vietnam, "but that was twenty-three years ago." He got angry and was emphatic that there had been nothing wrong with him before he "snapped" his back.

I discovered a major region of mechanical tension in his upper spine, near where the skull meets the neck. I applied a force as light as you might comfortably place on a closed eyelid. Ten seconds after I removed my finger from his neck, Arthur's posture began to shift. He dropped his fists, brought his neck backwards, and tilted his head up. His spine began to straighten up, and he sighed deeply. He placed the tree branch he had used as a cane on the floor, and sat comfortably on the adjusting table.

Without my asking for any comments he offered, "You know, I almost cried today from the pain. I never cry. I never even cried when my brother died." He seemed surprised by the statement he heard himself make. It is common for a person to mention things about his or her past when spinal tension and interference are reduced with a specific spinal adjustment.

Arthur suddenly started to cry. His sobs resonated from deep inside his body. He spoke of God's participation in the world and of the beauty around him. This surprised him as it did his family. They had never seen him cry or talk about God in that way. He left the office at peace, with at least 75 percent improvement in movement, and periodic spontaneous deep sighs.

The very next time I adjusted this usually "self-controlled" man, a profound re-experiencing of a past event occurred. As I gently adjusted a different vertebra in his neck, he held his face, crying out, "Get away . . ." and some choice obscenities. He punched the air screaming, "Its broken! It's broken," holding onto his jaw and face. It seems that he was actually reliving an event that took place about three years after his brother died. This accounted for the twenty-year-old muscle tension I had discovered in his neck. The body never lies, and the body and mind are one.

He later related to me that he was re-experiencing his father's attempt to kill him, twenty years ago, by throwing a refrigerator on top of him. Within seconds of the spinal tension and interference being released, he actually re-experienced the sense that his teeth were knocked out, his nose broken, and that he was spitting blood. This was a holographic re-creation, as his nervous system was releasing the spinal holding patterns by which he had been limited all these years. This process continued for about an hour. Finally he stood straight and remarked that the pain was gone. Moments later, he began to shout obscenities at his father, and was once again immediately stooped over in pain.

His own body/mind connection was healing with the help of the tool called a chiropractic adjustment. He was learning from the inside that his body and mind are not separate. He recognized, without a word spoken from me, that he was responsible for what he had not been feeling all these years. Arthur told me that he was tired of not wanting to feel anything anymore. He now wanted not to *feel better*, but to *better feel.* His healing progressed rapidly. The release of spinal interference opened a new world to Arthur. This was the world of his own healing potential. He realized that there were things that he had placed in the "back of his mind." He also realized that his spine was indeed the "back of his mind."

Stories of healing such as Arthur's story occur commonly when patients receive Network Spinal Analysis care. It is important to understand that the use of Network Spinal Analysis by a chiropractor does not produce the emotional healing. The emotional healing spontaneously occurs as the spinal interference is reduced, allowing a greater degree of wholeness to spontaneously express itself. Life, or the power of self-healing, produces these changes. The chiropractic adjustment is the tool for the body to better express this power of life.

Ron had been a friend of my wife's family since high school. At thirty years of age, he was strong, well-built, and handsome. Ron was everyone's friend, and was always willing to do things for others. If your car broke down, he would stop what he was doing and fix it. If you needed money, he was glad to help out. Happily married to a fine woman, Ron had a twelve-year-old son who was the spitting image of him, as well as a nine-year-old daughter.

One afternoon, my wife received a phone call telling her that Ron had just returned from the hospital. He had been diagnosed with metastatic lung cancer that had spread to the bowel. He had undergone both surgery and radiation therapy. Ron's case was pronounced terminal, and he was sent home to spend his final days with his family. Ron's wife asked me to come over and attend to him as a chiropractor, not to treat his cancer, but in the hope that I could help free the spinal system of interference, knowing that this would empower his own self-organizing and self-healing system.

It was a shock to see him. Lying in a hospital bed that was set up in the den, Ron's head was bald, his body emaciated, and he had a sack to replace his intestines, which had been removed due to the bowel cancer. Ron's breathing was shallow and his eyes were glassy. He was not very responsive to conversation. Ron's legs had become paralyzed during his stay in the hospital, and they were propped up on pillows. Ron knew that his case was hopeless and that he was going to die.

Gathering my inner composure, I began by saying, "I cannot cure what is wrong with you, nor can I do anything for your distress." I told him that, as a chiropractor, I could only help free up that which was perfect within him, the coordinating intelligence of the body, by correcting spinal interferences (subluxations) in the central nervous system. I told him that I did not know if the cancer would go away, and that he would die eventually. However, I told him that I did not know *when* he would die, since none of our birth certificates have expiration dates. He looked up at me. With the assistance of his family, I performed a history of his physical, emotional, and mental traumas in addition to the conventional "medical" history. I then proceeded to examine his spine.

I stopped when I felt a band of thick muscles along his spine. It felt as though the associated trauma had occurred when Ron was about twelve years old. I asked what had happened in his life at that point in time. Ron's parents were in the room, and since he didn't respond, his mother said, "Well, he broke his hip that year." While that was indeed a physical trauma, the spinal posture indicated that an emotional trauma also occurred at that time. I asked if anything else had happened, and his mother replied that Ron had his appendix removed that same year.

Then his father mentioned that Ron almost lost both of his legs the following year, due to a bone infection. The situation was so serious that the doctors had considered amputation. Ron's history was becoming more clear to me: We had a boy who broke his hip in a bicycle accident, had an emergency appendectomy, and had nearly lost both legs at about the same time of his life. It appeared that there was a pattern involving the lower body reappearing at that point in his life. In clinical practice, I found that the body does not attract repeated physical crisis separate from emotional crisis or trauma. This is because the body and mind are not separate.

I then asked if there was an emotional loss that might have taken place. For the first time in his adult life, Ron began to cry, nodding in the affirmative. His mother said that at the age of twelve, Ron had witnessed the violent death of one of his closest friends. I continued to examine his spine, and located another major subluxation. I applied a gentle touch to a number of different vertebrae, and within minutes he raised himself up in his hospital bed and smiled. As his spine released its interference and holding patterns, his nervous system was slowly being freed from the perspective that it was in. His mood was changing.

When I saw him three days later, Ron's wife told me that he had revealed something that he never told anyone before. When he was twelve years of age, Ron challenged his best friend to catch a ride on the side of a moving bus. When his friend refused, Ron teased him and called him names until he agreed to do it. After barely grabbing onto the side of the bus, his friend lost his grip, fell under the bus, and was run over by the wheels. He was killed instantly. Ron watched in horror as his friend's legs and abdomen were crushed by the large vehicle. He never told anyone that he felt responsible for his friend's death.

After several days of adjustments Ron began to gain weight and to move around the house and yard. At the same time, he became more open with others, and he and his family began to have the most meaningful dialogues of their lives together. Music and laughter could be heard in the house once more. As Ron continued receiving regular spinal adjustments, I no longer saw a man who was dying, but someone who was reclaiming his life. Over the next few weeks, the quality of his life dramatically improved.

One night, an associate of mine visited Ron to adjust his spine, and Ron told him that he couldn't fight the cancer anymore and that he had decided to "move on." The following day Ron called his wife and children together and said that he was "going home." They held his hand and he described his ascension process as going through a door of light. Within a few minutes, he was gone.

Ron's childhood friend never made it to age thirteen. Ron was diagnosed as having cancer and passed on during his son's twelfth year of life. Ron's nervous system was stuck in a perspective: emotional, mental, and physical realities that paralleled each other.

Darlene came to my office for her first adjustment. After examining her spine, I asked her if a traumatic event had occurred in her life sixteen years earlier. She couldn't recall any such event, but I made a note of my findings in her clinical record.

After three or four spinal adjustments, she began to re-experience a situation sixteen years ago when her stepfather had raped her. As her spinal system was becoming freed of interference, it "remembered" the traumatic event, unwound itself past the experience, and Darlene actually re-created the experience from a place of greater flexibility. As a consequence of that merging, she experienced tremendous anger toward her stepfather that lasted for a couple of days. She chose to consult a personal abuse counselor. She soon totally forgave her stepfather. Please be aware of the fact that she did not "try" to forgive him. Instead, spontaneous forgiveness became a natural consequence of the healing she was experiencing, as her spinal system became more flexible, adaptable, and freed from its previous limited perspectives.

Darlene later related that her stepfather phoned her the same evening that she had forgiven him to say that he was sorry. This was the first time that they had spoken to each other since shortly after the rape. Darlene had not initiated direct contact with him. Her nervous system merged with whatever was behind her suffering, and as a result, she changed her perspective toward it from a higher state of consciousness. Her new perspective created a change in her life to which her stepfather somehow responded. I have found that it is not uncommon when an individual releases a major spinal source of tension and interference, for this to have an effect on others who were involved in the drama associated with the original spinal holding pattern.

Although I am not a psychologist and do not perform psychotherapy, I am aware of people's responses during the healing process. There is certainly a relationship between unacknowledged consciousness and the physical expression of disease. Somehow, in some way, the consciousness we are blocked from "being with" will often find a physical or emotional way to be with us. I have found, for example, that a high percentage of women who have had hysterectomies, or individuals who often complain of soft-tissue pain that does not respond to conventional treatment, often experienced some kind of marked physical or sexual abuse earlier in life.

I am not claiming that a particular disease is the result of a specific type of physical or emotional trauma. To make such claims would be a distraction from the message we are hoping to provide. What is important is to realize that being stuck in the perspective of a particular trauma can have physiological consequences and cumulative effects even years later. The spinal system appears to be a switchboard of consciousness and of a person's history. In Ron's case, the physical or emotional symptoms appeared to have been directly related to an earlier unresolved trauma. In other cases, they may appear to be totally unrelated to the original experience or event.

WHAT TO EXPECT

A thorough spinal examination will be performed on your first visit and periodically (often about every eight weeks) throughout treatment. Visual observation and palpation are essential tools, but practitioners may use additional forms of noninvasive evaluation. The patient will be asked about health-related life changes, and this information will be integrated with the findings of the chiropractor's spinal examination.

The treatment is built around a system of graduated "levels of care." There are two levels of corrective care and two levels of wellness care. Adjustments during the first level of care, which may in some cases last two months, are brief and involve gentle touch adjustments to the neck and lower spine, most often with the patient face down. Usually the sessions last no more than five minutes. The body's own self-corrective movements and respirations are seen as the body learns to dissipate energy from the spinal systems, releasing spinal tension and developing a long-term strategy for spinal stability. The second level of care may involve a more diverse range of adjusting techniques including, when necessary, gentle structural (moving the bone) types. This level of care is designed to correct the chronic subluxations and to engage the body's self-correcting and synergistic systems to a deeper level. Visits during this level of care may last fifteen minutes, though shorter or longer sessions are possible. Later levels of care involve positioning the patient in ways that allow for the body's own self-generated waves to correct the subluxations, and once again the visits are often less than five minutes each. All patients can progress through the four levels of care, but not all patients may choose to do so, depending on their needs and their goals for the treatment.

Patients are asked to wear loose-fitting clothes that are not bulky, so that the spine can be palpated through the garments. Periodic full examinations are most often performed with the patient in an examination gown, or dressed in a way that exposes the entire spine.

The fees vary from office to office with many offices offering substantial savings plans to accommodate frequent and family visits. Although the term Network Chiropractic was used to describe the earlier versions of what is now Network Spinal Analysis, the term Network Chiropractic is now used as a trade name by independent practitioners of Network Spinal Analysis.

HOW TO FIND A PRACTITIONER

Practitioners of Network Spinal Analysis are chiropractors, with all appropriate training and credentials required for their locations. In addition, they have taken basic or advanced, hands-on intensive seminars in the theory and practice of Network Spinal Analysis, offered through the postgraduate department of an accredited chiropractic college. Many have taken a series of certifying examinations covering that body of knowledge. A list of practitioners who have studied Network Spinal Analysis, support this conceptual model of body/mind integration, or have passed certification examinations can be obtained by contacting the Association for Network Chiropractic at 444 North Main St., Longmont, CO, 80501, (303) 678-810.

HOW TO LEARN MORE

Blanks, R. H.; W. R. Boone; D. Schmidt; and M. Dobson. "Network Care: A Retrospective Outcomes Assessment." (in preparation).

Craig, A., M. Dobson, and R. H. Blanks. "Changes in Lifestyle Practices Reported by Patients Undergoing Subluxation-based Chiropractic." (in preparation).

Epstein, D. M. "Network Spinal Analysis: A System of Health Care Delivery within the Subluxation Based Chiropractic Model." *Journal of Vertebral Subluxation Research* 1, no. 1 (1996): 51–59.

Epstein, D. M. *Theoretical Basis and Clinical Application of Network Spinal Analysis (NSA).* Longmont, CO: Innate Intelligence, Inc., 1996.

Epstein, D. and N. Altman. *The 12 Stages of Healing.* Novato, CA: New World Library/Amber Allen Publishing, 1994.

Dobson, M., W. R. Boone, and R. H. Blanks. "Women and Alternative Health Care: A Retrospective Study of Network Care Recipients." (Submitted for publication in 1996).

Panjabi, M. "The Stabilizing System of the Spine, Part I: Function, Dysfunction, Adaptation, and Enhancement." *Journal of Spinal Disorders* 5, no. 4 (1992): 384–389.

ABOUT THE AUTHOR

Donald Epstein graduated from New York Chiropractic College in 1977. The first articles about his networking of chiropractic methods and its impact on the healing response appeared in 1983. Dr. Epstein founded and developed the method of spinal evaluation and correction originally called Network Chiropractic, and more recently Network Spinal Analysis. He has taught thousands of chiropractors and chiropractic students his methods and theories. Over 15,000 people have attended his Transformational Gate™ weekend seminars. He is an international lecturer on chiropractic and healing. He is the author of *The 12 Stages of Healing,* published by New World Library/Amber Allen Publishing, and numerous professional publications. He serves on the Board of Regents of Sherman College of Straight Chiropractic, on the board of directors of EarthSave Foundation, and is president of the Association for Network Chiropractic.

Abram Hoffer, M.D., Ph.D., F.R.C.P. (C)

30 Orthomolecular Psychiatry

WHAT IS ORTHOMOLECULAR PSYCHIATRY?

Orthomolecular psychiatry is a branch of psychiatry, not yet recognized by the profession, that emphasizes the use of optimum amounts of essential nutrients to restore the health of psychiatric patients. Orthodox psychiatry depends entirely on the use of drugs such as tranquilizers, antidepressants, lithium, etc., and pays lip service to psychotherapy and counseling. It has been termed "toximolecular psychiatry" since it uses toxic drugs in sublethal doses. However, although tranquilizers initiate the process of recovery by helping reduce symptoms and making patients more comfortable, they also make healthy people sick. No person can be normal while taking the huge amounts of drugs that are prescribed for most patients. In other words, doctors who prescribe tranquilizers alone cause patients to develop a disease I call tranquilizer psychosis. This is characterized by physical and psychiatric problems including apathy, difficulty in thinking and concentration, retardation, tardive dyskinesia (a movement disorder associated with the long-term use of certain major tranquilizers), weight gain, and other side effects. This creates the tranquilizer dilemma. A doctor wants a patient to get well, and the drugs do initiate the process rather quickly. But as the patient starts to improve, their biochemistry becomes more normal, and the more normal they become, the more they react to the drugs as if they were normal — that is, they become sick. The patient

swings back and forth between the schizophrenic psychosis and the tranquilizer psychosis.

With orthomolecular therapy, the nutrients do not make people sick as
their mental health improves, although the initial results are much slower. So
in most cases it is possible to maintain the patient in a healthy state. The best
approach, then, is to use both: drugs for the rapidity of their effect, and nutrients because they will eventually allow the removal of the drugs. Patients will
remain well as long as they remain on the program.

Orthomolecular psychiatry has value in treating schizophrenia, mood disorders, children with learning and/or behavioral disorders, addictions (especially alcoholism), and a substantial proportion of the early senility and aging
changes.

HOW IT BEGAN

In 1951, Drs. H. Osmond, John Smythies, and myself hypothesized that there
might be a compound with the properties of mescaline present in the schizophrenic body, and that this compound might somehow be related to adrenaline. A few years later, we hypothesized that the compound might be
adrenochrome, a product of the oxidation of adrenaline. We tried using vitamin B_3 to inhibit the formation of adrenaline, and ascorbic acid to inhibit the
oxidation of adrenaline to adrenochrome. This was the world's first free radical
hypothesis, and the first suggestion of the usefulness of antioxidants.

The word orthomolecular was first used by Professor Linus Pauling in his
fundamental article in *Science* called "Orthomolecular Psychiatry" (Pauling,
1968). In 1966, he read our book *How to Live with Schizophrenia* (Hoffer and
Osmond, 1966). He was astonished by the fact that we were able safely to use
doses of nutrients up to 1,000 times the Recommended Daily Allowances
(RDA). He reconsidered the common belief that vitamins were needed only in
tiny doses, only for deficiency diseases, and developed a theoretical explanation
of why these high or optimum doses could be effective in many people who did
not have the classical deficiency diseases such as beri beri, pellagra, and scurvy.
Many other medical scientists had contributed toward the destruction of the
old ideas, but Dr. Pauling's contribution provided the impetus that forced the
scientific world to examine seriously the new ways of thinking about nutrients.

After several decades of resisting the idea that schizophrenia is a biochemical disease, the profession has now accepted this fact. However, most

psychiatrists are not interested in using nutritional methods for controlling the pathological process. They still reject it as alternative psychiatry when, in fact, it is more appropriately labeled complementary psychiatry and will one day be the mainstream of psychiatry.

Orthomolecular psychiatry, developed originally to treat the schizophrenias, has spread through the whole field of psychiatry and even more into medicine. Recently the International Society of Orthomolecular Medicine was established, with approximately 8,000 members worldwide. Over fourteen countries were represented at the first meeting of the society.

HOW IT WORKS

Most patients who consult orthomolecular psychiatrists have already been treated unsuccessfully by other psychiatrists, and they are well enough informed to seek other methods that they hope will be more effective.

I will outline the orthomolecular treatment process that I follow but this does not mean that every orthomolecular physician follows the identical program. Fortunately, orthomolecular psychiatry is still very fluid, allowing for innovation and the integration of new discoveries. We may differ in the details, but we all aim to use nutrition and supplements in the best way possible.

During the first interview, clinical material is obtained that includes the main symptoms and the development of the illness, as well as a history of other treatments and responses. Enough information should be obtained to make a provisional diagnosis. This might have to be modified when other information is obtained as the treatment is continued.

The diagnosis of schizophrenia is described in our book *How to Live with Schizophrenia* (Hoffer and Osmond, 1992). There are two main sets of symptoms essential to the diagnosis. These are perceptual changes (in the extreme degree, voices and visions, and to a milder degree, illusions) and thought disorder. These two sets of symptoms have been used over the past 100 years, and are still compatible with the recently changed criteria used by the American Psychiatric Association. In the large majority of cases my patients were diagnosed by previous psychiatrists before they came to see me.

Once the diagnosis has been established, treatment is recommended to the patient. Attention is given to the optimum nutrition for that patient, with recommended dietary changes, and explanations of the individual nutrients that will be used, their doses, and the reasons for their use. If the patients are already receiving medication, as most of them are by the time they arrive in the office, these are maintained in order to avoid relapse, since it may take the nutritional program several months to become fully established. But the aim is to discontinue medication as soon as possible, or to decrease the dose so that the drugs do not interfere with normal living. All of the patient's questions are answered.

Between visits, patients are advised to follow a program of fitness and to engage in as many social activities as they feel comfortable with. An estimate may be given of how long it might take the patient to recover. Usually acute illness responds more rapidly than chronic illness. Schizophrenics who have been sick many years may require up to ten years before they really recover. Chronic patients will also need rehabilitative help, including supportive psychotherapy (as opposed to psychoanalysis or the other probing therapies, which we do not find useful in the context of orthomolecular treatment), re-education, or education, and a lot of support.

The initial interview may last up to one hour. After that, patients are seen for follow-up therapy as often as indicated by the severity of the condition. Patients should expect to be treated as they would by their favorite internist or other specialists. Patients who are seriously ill should not try to treat themselves, but they are expected to be educated about nutritional medicine. This information is readily available from the more than 200 books available today that describe the various aspects of orthomolecular psychiatry and medicine.

WHAT THE RESEARCH SHOWS

Orthomolecular therapy is the first treatment modality that was introduced by double-blind methodology. It is also one of the very few therapeutic regimens that was not introduced by drug companies; the nutrients cannot be patented, and so are not of interest to these profit-driven organizations.

My initial work with Dr. Humphry Osmond and Dr. J. Smythies was published as the adrenochrome hypothesis of schizophrenia (Hoffer, Osmond, and Smythies, 1954), and included studies of the therapeutic value of two potential antidotes to adrenochrome: vitamin B_3 and vitamin C. We undertook the first double-blind controlled experiments to compare the value of both forms of vitamin B_3, niacin and niacinamide, against placebo. We doubled the two-year cure rate from 35 percent to 75 percent by adding these vitamins to the treatment used at that time. Large-scale clinical studies by the early pioneers in orthomolecular psychiatry confirmed these results (Hawkins and Pauling, 1973).

These experiments were terminated in the late 1960s. By that time, it had become too difficult to continue since tranquilizers had swept into psychiatry and psychiatrists would not allow their patients to be entered in these studies. But by that time we had amassed enough evidence to conclude that the addition of these two vitamins doubled the natural recovery rate by at least two years. At the same time, we continued to run clinical trials.

Other nutrients used in megadoses have not been examined as carefully with controlled comparison experiments. However, the mass of clinical evidence is so great that it is unlikely that controlled experiments will do more than confirm what is already known by orthomolecular physicians. For example, Dr. W. Shute and Dr. E. Shute of Ontario, Canada, proved that vitamin E was very therapeutic in preventing and treating heart disease. But when they published their findings they were considered quacks, and their work was totally discounted. The recent large scale studies at Harvard University have shown they were correct. Unfortunately, none of the Harvard scientists who reported these studies seem to be aware of the original Shute studies, and have not referred to them in their papers. Another example is the use of folic acid in preventing spina bifida. The first studies were clinical observational studies. They were severely criticized and laughed at until huge expensive studies showed that the original observation made fifteen years ago was correct. Now they are hastening to catch up and recommend the addition of folic acid to food to prevent this dreadful congenital complication. The cost of this fifteen-year delay is enormous.

I have personal experience with over 3,000 patients. Currently I have under my care about 500 chronic patients on Vancouver Island. They see me at intervals ranging from one month to several years. A survey of twenty-seven of these chronic patients who had been under care for at least ten years showed that more than half were normal, but that in some cases it had taken up to seven years for this recovery to occur.

Other corroboration comes from a large number of pioneer orthomolecular psychiatrists and many current ones. At a meeting many years ago we estimated that collectively we had treated about 100,000 patients in Canada and the United States. Every psychiatrist who has tried the orthomolecular approach has confirmed our results if they followed the procedure we had outlined. A few psychiatrists claimed they had not been able to reproduce our results. However, these researchers had modified the methods so much that it was no longer orthomolecular psychiatry, but simply their own idea of how it ought to be done. They used only chronic patients for short-term studies. This is like trying to treat chronic diabetics by giving them insulin for a month or two. If you bake a cake using a recipe that you do not follow, and the cake turns out badly, it is not the fault of the recipe.

Individual case histories are the stuff of medicine, and rightly so, since they are much more informative to clinicians. If all anecdotes were banished from medical schools, they would have to close down, yet often critics of orthomolecular psychiatry have dismissed the value of our work by saying that the results are purely anecdotal. I have read modern clinical papers in which no patients were mentioned. They presented a lot of statistics with probabilities but they didn't mention specific patients: what happened to them, how they liked it, and what the side effects were. I am proud of clinical medicine which, by the use of anecdotes only, has introduced some of the most effective treatment available today such as surgery, anesthesia, obstetrics, and the treatment of diabetes, pellagra, scurvy, beri beri, and other deficiency diseases.

REAL PEOPLE AND ORTHOMOLECULAR PSYCHIATRY

One young man I treated was advised by his psychiatrist that he would never recover from his schizophrenia, that he would never graduate from twelfth grade, and that he would never be off drugs. His father was devastated by this pronouncement, and he still became angry when he told me about it later on.

The family moved to Victoria, and the doctor they consulted referred him to me. He went on the total program of nutrition, with large doses of vitamin B_3, vitamin C, plus other nutrients and a small dose of a tranquilizer.

Four years later, I was invited to a graduation tea. My patient had been awarded his B.A. in Psychology from the University of Victoria. He had graduated with a high grade average and he planned to go on to postgraduate studies. His friends and family had gathered to help him celebrate. At the tea I met his cousin, who had been a successful psychologist and teacher, and had four years earlier been struck by schizophrenia. She was placed on tranquilizers and other drugs, and from then on went downhill. At the tea she was on lithium and several other drugs. She had gained about sixty pounds, and was puffy from ankles to her chest. She had severe tardive dyskinesia and needed someone to hold her cup so she could drink her tea. But she told me that at least she was no longer hearing voices. The contrast was obvious to the whole group of family and friends.

These two cases symbolize the two different approaches in treatment. With orthomolecular treatment a hopelessly ill young man began to improve, and four years later, he was normal. His cousin also became sick, but with standard treatment alone she had by now deteriorated to the point that she is hopelessly ill, and unless the treatment is changed, she will never again be a useful and productive member of our community.

In *How to Live with Schizophrenia* (Hoffer and Osmond, 1992) we briefly described the case of Mary, a chronic schizophrenic woman who had been resident in a mental hospital for fourteen years. She was admitted at age seventeen and was diagnosed as an imbecile (because her intelligence was tested and found to be under 25) and a chronic schizophrenic. I.Q. tests are totally invalid when given to very psychotic patients. She was one of their most difficult patients in the hospital. She had undergone every treatment known to psychiatry in an attempt to help her, including metrazole injections (the precursor to electroconvulsive therapy or ECT), insulin coma, and eventually repeated series of ECT every year or so whenever she became agitated and out of control. During her psychotic episodes she would go on a window-smashing rampage and break every window she could find. After a series of ECT, she was subdued and quiet. Tranquilizers had not yet been introduced.

We brought her into our home in Regina in 1953. The first month was very difficult for my wife, but our three young children took to her at once. She continued to hear voices. On one occasion during dinner she began to talk to her father. When I asked her what she was doing, she replied that her father was calling her from his grave and wanted her to join him. After a suicide attempt when she tried to strangle herself with an electric light cord, I started her on three grams of daily niacin. Slowly she began to improve. She learned how to use the telephone, how to read her bankbook, and other skills that she had never had or had forgotten. After two years with us, I got her a job on the cleaning staff at the general hospital in Regina. She moved into her own apartment. She continued to visit us, and whenever she had any difficulty, she would come to see me at the University Hospital. Mary remained well. Later she developed coronary insufficiency, but this was treated successfully.

In about 1980, Princess Margaret visited the hospital, presumably to officiate at the change of name from University Hospital to Royal University Hospital. Walking through the corridors, she saw Mary in her white uniform. Mary, unabashed, went up to her and said, "Dear, you look so nice." I imagine this is the first time a member of royalty was greeted by a chronic schizophrenic patient who had recovered on niacin therapy.

I spoke to Mary in August, 1996. She is retired, after working steadily for over thirty years, and she has been living happily with her boyfriend for the past eight years. A few dollars worth of vitamin B_3, and a couple of years of careful attention, support, and direction, has saved the province of Saskatchewan at least one million dollars. It is likely she would have died in the mental hospital or in some run down group home or nursing home if she had not come to work for us. But the minister of health of that province, several years ago, refused to consider this an appropriate treatment because he had been informed by the Saskatchewan Medical Association and by the Saskatchewan Psychiatric Association that this treatment was controversial. However, all new treatments are controversial when first introduced.

HOW TO FIND A PRACTITIONER

It can be extremely difficult to find an orthomolecular psychiatrist. There are no college or university courses available for the training of health professionals in these techniques. Most psychiatrists are either totally unfamiliar with the treatment or, if they have heard about it, they are hostile to it and believe that it can not possibly work. I suggest that the best approach is to read the literature, and to discuss this with your family doctor and try to persuade them to go along with the program. If your doctor will not, then seek another physician, and keep doing so until you find one willing to listen.

The International Society for Orthomolecular Medicine had its first organizational meeting in Vancouver, in the spring of 1996. This organization may be in a position in the future to have lists of physicians who are practicing this type of therapy, but no lists are available at this time. They may be contacted:

INTERNATIONAL SOCIETY FOR
ORTHOMOLECULAR MEDICINE
c/o Canadian Schizophrenia Foundation
16 Florence Ave.
Toronto, Ontario, M2N 1E9, CANADA
Tel: (416) 733-2117; Fax (416) 733-2352

HOW TO LEARN MORE

Hawkins, D. R. and L. Pauling, eds. *Orthomolecular Psychiatry*. San Francisco: W. H. Freeman and Co., 1973.

Hoffer, A. "Chronic Schizophrenic Patients Treated Ten Years or More." *Journal of Orthomolecular Medicine* 9 (1994): 7–37.

Hoffer, A. "Orthomolecular Medicine." In *Molecules in Natural Science and Medicine, An Encomium for Linus Pauling*, edited by Z. B. Maksic and M. Eckert-Maksic, Chichester, West Sussex, England: Ellis Horwood Ltd., 1991.

Hoffer, A. *Orthomolecular Medicine for Physicians*. New Canaan, CT: Keats Publishing, Inc., 1989.

Hoffer, A. "Nutrition and Behavior." In *Medical Applications of Clinical Nutrition*, edited by J. Bland, New Canaan, CT: Keats Publishing, Inc., 1983.

Hoffer, A. "Mechanism of Action of Nicotinic Acid and Nicotinamide in the Treatment of Schizophrenia." In *Orthomolecular Psychiatry*, edited by D.R. Hawkins and L. Pauling, San Francisco: W. H. Freeman and Co., 1973.

Hoffer, A. "Megavitamin B-3 Therapy for Schizophrenia." *Canadian Psychiatric Association Journal* 16 (1971): 499–504.

Hoffer, A. "Treatment of Schizophrenia with a Therapeutic Program Based Upon Nicotinic Acid as the Main Variable." In *Molecular Basis of Some Aspects of Mental Activity, Vol II*, edited by O. Walaas, New York: Academic Press, 1967.

Hoffer, A. *Hoffer's Law of Natural Nutrition*. Kingston, Ontario: Quarry Press, 1966.

Hoffer, A. and H. Osmond. "Treatment of Schizophrenia with Nicotinic Acid - A Ten Year Follow-up." *Acta Psychiatrica Scandinavia* 40 (1964): 71–189.

Hoffer, A. and H. Osmond. *How to Live with Schizophrenia.* Revised Edition. New York: Citadel Press, 1992.

Hoffer, A. and H. Osmond. *How to Live with Schizophrenia.* New York: University Books, 1966.

Hoffer, A. and H. Osmond. "In Reply to The American Psychiatric Association Task Force Report on Megavitamin and Orthomolecular Therapy in Psychiatry." Regina, Saskatoon: Canadian Schizophrenia Foundation (Now at 16 Florence Ave., Toronto, ON, Canada M2N 1E9) August, 1976.

Hoffer, A.; H. Osmond; M. J. Callbeck; and I. Kahan. "Treatment of Schizophrenia with Nicotinic Acid and Nicotinamide." *Journal of Clinical Experimental Psychopathology* 18 (1957): 131–158.

Hoffer, A., H. Osmond, and J. Smythies. "Schizophrenia: A New Approach II. Results of a Year's Research." *Journal of Mental Science* 100 (1954): 29–45.

Hoffer, A. and M. Walker. *Putting It All Together: The New Orthomolecular Nutrition.* New Canaan, CT: Keats Publishing, Inc., 1996.

Hoffer, A. and M. Walker. *Smart Nutrients - A Guide to Nutrients That Can Prevent and Reverse Senility.* Garden City Park, NY: Avery Publishing Group, 1994.

Pauling, L. "Orthomolecular Psychiatry." *Science* 160 (1968): 265–271.

See also the *Journal of Orthomolecular Medicine* published by the Canadian Schizophrenic Foundation.

ABOUT THE AUTHOR

After being awarded his Ph.D. in biochemistry, Abram Hoffer enrolled in medicine at the University of Saskatchewan and completed his education at the University of Toronto in 1949. He interned for one year and then joined the Department of Public Health, Psychiatric Services Branch, Saskatchewan, to head a psychiatric research division. He was Associate Professor of Psychiatry and director of research until 1967. In 1967, he entered private practice, moving to Victoria in 1976. He has been actively involved in searching for the causes of schizophrenia and in developing a treatment called orthomolecular psychiatry. He is president of the Canadian Schizophrenia Foundation and editor of the Journal of Orthomolecular Medicine. Readers may visit his home page at: http://www.healthy.net/bios/hoffer/advisory.htm

Roger Woolger, Ph.D.

31 Past Life Therapy

WHAT IS PAST LIFE THERAPY?

Past life therapy (also called past life regression therapy) is the process of accessing information or images from possible former lifetimes, usually through hypnotic regression or some form of altered state of consciousness, for therapeutic purposes. Accessing emotionally or physically traumatic life memories can be helpful for promoting cathartic release, reframing attitudes, changing old habits or behavior problems, and gaining conscious insight into the lessons of that life or memory. The information can be used to resolve deeply buried attitudes, beliefs, or experiences that effect current life problems. This is different from the practice sometimes referred to as past life regression, where the unconscious mind is probed to retrieve historical memories or information with no expectation of follow-up counseling to help understand or deal with the information. Past life therapy is a truly transpersonal psychology that assumes a spiritual dimension to human experience and addresses the deeper question of meaning.

As a therapeutic technique, past life therapy superficially resembles hypnotic age regression, where a client is encouraged, in trance, to re-experience a childhood trauma as if he or she were a child of four, for example. The difference with past life therapy is that the imagination is given a much wider range of possibilities, as in the work of Jung or the psychodrama of J. L. Moreno and its derivative, Gestalt therapy. Much like hypnotic regression, the client is guided back to, and encouraged to relive, scenes from the past that have been lost to consciousness. But instead of being regressed to the patient's current childhood, a strong suggestion is given that he or she go back to a "previous life" where the trauma originated.

What is remarkable about this technique is that the client need not believe in reincarnation for it to be effective. He or she simply relives a distressing scene from some other historical time frame or culture as if it were real. During the re-enactment, the client may temporarily identify strongly with a quite different character and a different body image, but always with the conscious awareness that "this is only a regression." The therapeutic effectiveness of reliving the "past life" trauma — accident, abandonment, violent death, rape, betrayal, etc. — is similar to the therapeutic effect of recalling traumas in the current life. The past life trauma will usually mirror the present situation quite precisely, but will allow it to be experienced far more intensely and fully. For example, a fear of suffocation may be replayed as originating in a "past life" all the way through an imagined death, which brings release and a sense of detachment. Such reliving is like a fictional psychodrama that leads to a complete cathartic discharge of blocked feelings, such as rage, fear, grief, guilt, or shame. This method allows an irrational symptom — say, a baseless fear of knives — to be taken seriously and played out through these images, rather than being interpreted as a metaphor or a psychological defense mechanism.

Past life therapy is a short-term, intensive therapy that is often reserved for patients who have already made considerable headway in conventional psychotherapy. It is particularly helpful for those who are blocked in particular areas of conventional therapy; it supplies a new modality for those "stuck in a groove" to finish unresolved stories. The following kinds of problems often respond particularly well to past life therapy: difficulties in relationships, abandonment and separation issues, power and money issues, chronic guilt, phobias, compulsions, some depressions, anxieties, and various physical complaints, such as back pain and asthma. It has also been extremely effective in releasing dissociative reactions such as severe shock and emotional shutdown arising from physical and sexual abuse. Birthing and fertility problems have responded to this approach and it has brought much relief to sufferers from sado-masochistic compulsions.

HOW IT BEGAN

Past life therapy developed from a growing awareness of ancient spiritual traditions and experimental psychologies. The concept of past lives or reincarnation has been around since the beginning of human culture, recorded in pictures, words, and cryptic symbols by cultures ranging from the Egyptians and Tibetans to Christian Gnostics and Native Americans. Reincarnation is the belief in the survival of the soul beyond the life of the body. The Egyptians mummified bodies and buried servants with their rulers so their afterlives would be as rich as their earthbound lives. The Hindus believe we live cycles of birth and death, progressing up an evolutionary path, including lives as animals before birth as humans.

The early pioneers in past life therapy came from several different fields and philosophical roots. Colonel Albert De Roches, who claimed to have regressed patients back beyond childhood to *in utero* and previous life memories, was a turn-of-the-century French psychoanalyst and hypnotherapist. Edgar Cayce, the American clairvoyant venerated as "the sleeping prophet" because he gave medical readings and other advice while in a trance, was a simple country man. His channeling often connected past lives to present health problems, though his limited education and strict religious upbringing caused him to reject many of the concepts he communicated while channeling.

In the 1950s, the public was entertained by regression stories, such as the case of Bridey Murphy (Bernstein, 1965), and a debate on proof of reincarnation, while past life therapy was quietly taking shape. An English psychiatrist, Dr. Denys Kelsey, began exploring reincarnation as an explanation for behavior problems when more conventional therapeutic approaches had failed. A member of the Royal College of Physicians, Kelsey was one of the first to go public with his use of prenatal and past life regressions.

Morris Netherton, whom many consider one of the founders of past life therapy, documented past life traumas affecting current life health conditions. His 1978 book, *Past Life Therapy*, related case studies of chronic illnesses such as migraines, ulcers, and epilepsy.

In the 1970s, the American public really took note of the philosophical underpinnings of past lives with Dr. Raymond Moody's ground-breaking study of near death experiences (NDEs) in *Life After Life*. While several other explanations for NDEs are proposed and may be possible, Moody's work, and further research by Kenneth Ring, Ph.D., have further opened the window to belief in survival of the soul.

Meanwhile, the field of psychotherapy was beginning to shift from the cognitive and interpretive "talk therapy" to more experiential forms. These theoretical developments validated what past life therapists were seeing in their work with clients. Hypnotherapists, for example, had discovered the use of spontaneous images of other lives to release emotional and physical traumas to help clients overcome mental and physical health problems.

Hazel Dening, Ph.D., one of the founders of the Association for Past Life Research and Therapy (APRT), is a quintessential example of the kind of regression therapist coming to the fore. Her first regression into a past life was an accident. A client's hypnotic regression to childhood overshot and spontaneously landed in a life during the Civil War. Like most hypnotherapists who have experienced a similar surprise, Denning used the imagery therapeutically with her client, achieving positive results. She did not talk about it for a long time, but she did use the technique with success on other clients.

The APRT was established in 1980 for past life therapists to come together and share experiences, research, and expertise. The APRT holds annual conferences, publishes the *Journal of Regression Therapy*, and trains clinicians interested in incorporating past life therapeutic techniques into their practices.

HOW IT WORKS

Past life therapy builds upon the common experience that the psyche imagines itself to have lived many times, a fantasy that has been rationalized variously as the doctrine of reincarnation or metempsychosis, the transmigration of souls. One could say that past life "stories" are the spontaneous products of right brain consciousness — much like dreams or memory images — while "reincarnation" or "metaphor" are theories constructed by the left brain to explain and organize the experience logically. One does not, therefore, need to believe in the philosophy to benefit from regression material. But for those who do believe in reincarnation, the work they do on themselves in this life is part of moving further along their particular evolutionary or spiritual path. Psychological healing is part of spiritual growth.

Stanislav Grof, a leading researcher in experiential psychology, is particularly known for his theoretical work on the influence of the birth experience on personality and health. He has found that we humans carry major unconscious imprints of physical accidents and emotional traumas, including the birth experience. Grof called such an imprint a "system of condensed experience" or a COEX; Jung used the term complex, now widely used to describe the same phenomenon. The new psychologies recognize that we "embody" our complexes — express them through many parts of ourselves. Every complex has six aspects to it, which are all available to consciousness, as illustrated in Figure 1.

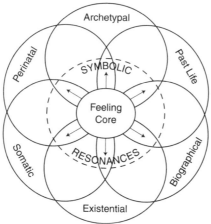

Figure 1

Traumatic influences can show up as a physical symptom, a neurotic complaint or behavior, a dream, or even a secondary personality. Past life therapy extends these concepts to past lives. Past life therapy thus treats "past life complexes" as well as current life ones.

There are three levels of processing the material in past life therapy. The first level involves reliving the story, and asking and answering questions "as if" it were a "real" lifetime and not a free-floating fantasy. In order to clear negative past life patterning, the client must fully experience the body sensations as well as the emotions until they are completely released. This might involve actual pain as the events from the past are actually experienced. Next, the symbolic or metaphorical content is explored. For example, pains in the neck that were first experienced as beheading may indicate a feeling of being cut off from life. Feeling crippled and being starved for love in a past life may now be seen to be metaphors for our current life patterns. Full mental understanding of the karmic or symbolic meaning of the patterns must occur or else the symptoms will simply recur in physical and/or emotional form. The client begins to see that he or she no longer needs to live life "as a constant sacrifice" (past life of martyrdom), or crippled by a fear of public humiliation (past life of persecution), or that he or she has to live in terror, "without any guts" (past life of disemboweling). Then, finally, the insights are applied to daily living, in the interest of creative productivity and service. Transformed rage at injustice may now be channeled into starting a new political organization; chronic performance anxiety, when reversed, may produce a fine teacher; grief at devastating loss may lead to work as counselor with the bereaved.

WHAT THE RESEARCH SHOWS

The most thorough research on past lives as memories has been conducted by Dr. Ian Stevenson (1987, 1974). For over thirty years from many parts of the world, he collected the spontaneous past life memories of children, details of which were meticulously followed up and examined. Research on past life regression as therapy, however, remains scant, largely due to the difficulty of getting scientific funding and backing. In Holland, a recent study took two groups of clients with similar symptoms and randomly selected half of the group for past life therapy and the remainder for conventional therapy. Measured by standard tests, those undergoing past life therapy recovered at about twice the speed as the control group. In the U.S., the American Psychological Association has not yet formally recognized parapsychology and transpersonal psychology as genuine disciplines. This is a major impediment to serious research on these topics.

REAL PEOPLE AND PAST LIFE THERAPY

A woman of thirty-four, a professional painter, sought therapy for a number of problems related to her marriage and her overly involved relationship with her mother. During the relaxation part of the induction procedure, she had great difficulty letting go. Her shoulders and neck were very tense. As we worked to relax them, she spontaneously began to tell the story of a life as an impoverished male Dutch painter during the seventeenth century. The painter had a wife and a very young baby, whom he could barely support. In his obsession with finishing a certain painting, he severely neglected both wife and baby, even when the baby became sick. To his horror, the baby grew worse and died, and his embittered wife deserted him. The key scene in our work was as follows:

THERAPIST: Where are you now?

CLIENT: I'm wandering along the canals. I can't find my wife. She's left me for good.

THERAPIST: Where do you go now?

CLIENT: I think, back to the house. Oh, no! I don't want to go back there. (Her shoulders begin to tense up very noticeably.)

THERAPIST: Breathe deeply and go back to the house and see what happens. (At this point, the young woman shot up from lying on the couch to a sitting position, grabbed her neck, and began to scream).

THERAPIST: What has happened?

CLIENT: Oh God! I hanged myself (sobs deeply).

For a short while we worked on letting go of the death experience and the emotions connected with the loss of wife and child. Then, when asked to move forward in time, she spontaneously found herself re-experiencing her birth in this life — with the umbilical cord wrapped around her neck! Full understanding came moments later when, as a baby, she looked up at her mother, having survived this second trauma.

CLIENT: I know why I'm here.

THERAPIST: Why are you here?

CLIENT: To be close to my mother (sobs). I know who she is now. She is the baby who died. I see that I've been trying to make it up to her all these years.

In subsequent sessions, she was able to release the guilt that had become locked in her neck and shoulders. She also felt that the pressure had been taken off her marriage.

Melinda had consulted several therapists about her failure to form close relationships with men and her near frigidity when it came to sexual contact. For a period she had been in a lesbian relationship, which helped her somewhat, because her lover wanted companionship more than physical contact. Yet the root issue remained untouched. She reported a clear memory of sexual molestation at 11 years of age. A 12-year-old boy from the neighborhood had enticed her into an unused garage and had fondled her genitals, though he had not attempted penetration. Her retelling of the story was cold and detached; she seemed to hold herself clenched as she told it. Apparently she had talked about this event many times with her previous therapists and, though she had also beaten out her rage on pillows and mattresses, part of her was still holding unfinished anger.

When I invited her to lie down on a mattress to recall the event in more detail, her clenching became even more pronounced:

"I don't want to do this," she said, with markedly more anger in her voice.

"Lie down anyway and keep repeating that phrase to whoever it applies to," I urged gently.

With her eyes closed, the following monologue emerged with very little prompting from me other than to direct her to repeat certain phrases and to exaggerate her bodily posture:

"I don't want to do this. I don't want to do this. Don't make me. DON'T MAKE ME. NO! NO! NO! You're hurting me. Get away."

She started to kick, shake her head, and writhe. "Get away. Get away. No. Don't make me." For a while she continued this way, her body becoming more and more tense, her outrage more pronounced. I imagined that she must be re-experiencing the incident from her childhood. Then suddenly, her words indicated that we had slipped into another lifetime:

"They're raping me. They're raping me. Help! Help! HELP! There are six or seven of them. They're soldiers. I'm in a barn. My arms are tied. It's Russia somewhere. I'm a peasant girl about eleven or twelve. God, it's awful. They don't stop . . . I don't want to do this. I don't want to be here. LEAVE ME ALONE. I'm not going to feel this. I won't feel this. I won't show them anything."

Her pelvic area was stiff, her legs taut, her head turned from side to side. I urged her to let those parts of the body speak and express what was going on with them.

"I'm not going to feel this, I'll never show you I like it" (pelvis and genitals).

"Don't touch me! Get away! I'll kill you. I hate you . I hate you. I'll kick you" (legs).

"I'm not going to see this. It's not happening" (head).

For a while, we worked through this awful scene, and I encouraged her to let her legs kick, to let her genitals record exactly what they felt, and to allow her head to see and understand all of it. There was kicking and weeping and rage and terrible confusion as, for a while, her genitals registered both pleasure and pain. Gradually, as these sensations and movements surged through her body, she seemed to experience a huge releasing and letting go of the earlier clenching, all of which culminated in a bout of intense sobbing and convulsive movements in her pelvis.

Suddenly she was no longer with the soldiers:

"I'm in that garage. I don't want him to touch me. I don't want to do this. Don't make me. I just freeze up, but he doesn't hurt me. He's quite gentle, but my thighs just go rigid and I'm not really there."

I urged her to breathe deeply and see the similarity to the earlier rape scene.

"Oh, yes!" she says. "My body was remembering something else. It was like a flashback, a nightmare, but I didn't want to see it."

As Melinda surveyed the two stories and gave herself permission to see them, she had all kinds of spontaneous recognitions: how just being touched always leads to a kind of freezing, how she is always somehow not present in sex, how she has always had fantasies of wanting to kick men, and so on. In a later session she reclaimed more of the Russian girl's story: how she had become pregnant, raised the child — a boy — alone, and had bitterly avoided contact with men from then onward, dying quite young from a wasting disease. The crucial events, however, were clearly locked into the rape scene at 11 or 12. Her unconscious compulsion laid down in the previous life had led her — unconsciously of course — to repeat a similar but far less violent sexual trauma in this life. The contemporary trauma served to reawaken the latent past life level of the complex, fraught as it was with terror, humiliation, and rage.

WHAT TO EXPECT

Past life therapy work generally consists of a series of two-hour sessions. Most patients complete their work in about five to ten of these intensive experiences. The therapist will usually start with a detailed personal history from birth through the present time, noting illnesses, accidents, or impairments such as deafness, the need for glasses, high blood pressure, etc., and any emotional upheaval that occurred shortly before or around the same period of life.

Actual regression starts with induction into an altered state. This can be either a light state, such as when doing visual imagery, or a deeper state, often identified with hypnosis. You may be asked to lie down. The therapist will use a current issue and its emotional charge to act as a bridge to imagery that will lead you to a past life that directly mirrors and amplifies your issue. For example, if you suffer from a fear of crowds, you may be asked to repeat the phrase, "I've got to get out of here," until images surface of crowds and panic and possibly violent death in a past life scenario. When you have arrived at a time and place, the therapist will probably ask you to describe what you see, your surroundings and other people, your own body, and what you are feeling. This helps anchor the images or impressions and bring them into focus. You may see images, hear sounds or voices, smell odors, or simply get thoughts; each of us has our own way of seeing and knowing. You should keep up communication with the therapist so she can guide you and help you if the experience is confusing or frightening. You do not necessarily have to dramatize or act out what you are experiencing, but letting out the tears, laughter, or anger may be very therapeutic. The therapist may ask you to look at the times just before and during the moment of death, in an effort to determine what you might learn by the experiences. This might help you capture the meaning of that life and death, seeing that emotional decisions, judgments made, and strong negative feelings and assumptions were locked in at the moment of death.

Bear in mind that the therapist is there to watch over you and your experience, creating a safe environment for you to explore deep images and emotions. You can come out of the altered state whenever you choose to.

The following kinds of clients are not well suited to past life therapy: people with schizophrenic tendencies, people with strict religious upbringings for whom the idea of reincarnation is offensive, people who are vulnerable to intense or overwhelming feelings, and overly intellectual people. All people should be aware that this kind of work can bring up painful feelings about the darker sides of ourselves, and there is a natural tendency to get caught up in dramatic fantasies of past lives in an effort to avoid the real therapeutic work of knowing yourself.

HOW TO FIND A PRACTITIONER

The following organizations can make referrals to psychotherapists who have had training in past life therapy. It is best to work with a past life therapist with extensive psychotherapy training in addition to in-depth study of past life therapy. He or she should be licensed or certified as a psychologist, psychiatrist, counselor or social worker.

ASSOCIATION FOR PAST-LIFE RESEARCH
AND THERAPIES, INC. (APRT)
P.O. Box 20151
Riverside, CA 92516
Tel: (714) 784-1570

WOOLGER TRAINING SEMINARS
126 Boggs Hill
Woodstock, NY 12498
Tel: (914) 679-7823
Fax: (914) 679-6491

HOW TO LEARN MORE

Bernstein, M. *The Search for Bridey Murphy*. New York: Doubleday, 1965.

Cranston, S. and C. Williams. *Reincarnation: A New Horizon in Science, Religion and Society*. New York: Julian Press, 1984.

Fiore, E. *You Have Been Here Before*. New York: Ballantine, 1979.

Hall, J. *Past Life Therapy*. London: Element, 1996.

Moody, R. *Life After Life*. New York: Bantam, 1981.

Netherton, M. and N. Shiffrin. *Past Lives Therapy*. New York: William Morrow, 1978.

Stevenson, I. *Children Who Remember Past Lives*. Charlottesville: University Press of Virginia, 1987.

Stevenson, I. *Twenty Cases Suggestive of Reincarnation*. Charlottesville: University Press of Virginia, 1980.

Weiss, B. *Many Lives, Many Masters*. New York: Simon and Shuster, 1988.

Woolger, R. *Other Lives, Other Selves: A Jungian Psychotherapist Discovers Past Lives*. New York: Doubleday, 1987.

ABOUT THE AUTHOR

Roger Woolger, Ph.D., is a British-born Jungian analyst trained at the C. G. Jung Institute in Zurich, with degrees in psychology, religion, and philosophy from Oxford and London Universities. He leads workshops at the New York Open Center and Esalen Institute, has taught at Vassar College, the University of Vermont, and Concordia University, Montreal. He is a member of the Association for Transpersonal Psychology, the Scientific and Medical Network (U.K.), and the British Society for Psychical Research. His book, *Other Lives, Other Selves* (Doubleday, 1987), a definitive work on past life therapy, has been translated into six languages. He is also the author with Jennifer Barker of *The Goddess Within* (Ballantine, 1989), and articles on dream work, meditation, and mysticism. He runs professional trainings in soul drama and regression therapy in Europe and North America and currently lives near Woodstock, NY.

John Beaulieu, N.D., Ph.D.

32 Polarity Therapy and Mental Health

WHAT IS POLARITY THERAPY?

Polarity therapy is a holistic healing art based on balancing life energy. At the heart of polarity therapy is the view that each individual is animated by a universal life energy. Imbalances in the circulation of life energy lead to mental and emotional distress and physical illness. When our life energy is balanced, the result is a healthy body and clarity of thought and emotion. A polarity therapist is trained in different methods of finding and correcting life energy imbalance, which include hands-on bodywork, counseling on diet and nutrition, guidance in a series of exercises called polarity yoga, and counseling that emphasizes the importance of positive thinking.

Polarity teaches us that distress and pain are signals for us to learn, change, and realign our lives. Dr. Randolph Stone, the founder of polarity therapy, quoted the old saying: "Obstacles are God's design to make man or woman with a spine." Through understanding, meeting, and resolving life's obstacles and challenges, we evolve and grow stronger. Polarity is a comprehensive clinical system for understanding the energy dynamics of a challenge, as well as methods for cultivating and expressing the energy necessary to meet challenges.

Webster defines mental health as "psychological well-being and satisfactory adjustment to society and to the ordinary demands of life." Polarity therapy expands this definition. We say that mental health is the ability of an individual to maintain an ongoing harmonious interrelationship of body, mind, and emotions in resonance with the requirements and challenges of daily life, thereby creating an internal state of mental, emotional, and physical well-being.

Polarity therapy is a great integrator of different therapeutic modalities. Within the mental health field, polarity therapy works very well with mild to severe depression, especially when combined with cognitive and Gestalt therapy. Polarity is exceptionally effective in resolving traumas from accidents and helping with unexpressed emotions. The deep relaxation of a polarity session works very well with guided visualization and shamanic journeying. Polarity therapy enhances all twelve step and recovery programs. Polarity therapy combined with cranial therapy works well with learning disorders and autism. In general, polarity supports and adds an extra dimension to the many already existing psychotherapeutic processes. It is important to keep in mind that polarity therapy is not a panacea. Severe depression usually requires a multidisciplinary approach.

HOW IT BEGAN

Polarity therapy was founded by Dr. Randolph Stone, D.O., D.C., N.D., (1890–1981) who traveled around the world studying and integrating many healing arts including chiropractic, osteopathy, naturopathy, homeopathy, ayurveda, and Chinese medicine. Dr. Stone believed that life was much more than chemistry and that healing was greater than freedom from symptoms. He saw life as a spiritual journey based on life energy principles and he saw healing as our total alignment to that journey.

In 1972, Dr. Robert Hall discovered Dr. Stone and Polarity Therapy while visiting an ashram in India. He watched Dr. Stone treat many people at the ashram clinic, including his wife, who was very sick. Dr. Hall was so impressed with Dr. Stone and polarity therapy that he organized polarity therapy seminars in the San Francisco area. From these humble beginnings, polarity therapy has grown into a profession under the guidance of the American Polarity Therapy Association (APTA). Today there are over 600 registered polarity practitioners in the United States and many more throughout Canada, Mexico, Europe, Australia, and Asia.

HOW IT WORKS

Polarity practitioners work from the premise that people are fields of pulsating life energy made up of specific qualities known as the five elements: ether, air, fire, water, and earth. When our thoughts, emotions, and physical body are aligned with the elemental energy necessary to meet a life challenge, health and well-being result. When we are out of alignment, energy imbalances result that appear as mental and emotional distress and physical symptoms. Polarity teaches us that mental, emotional, and physical distress are signals for us to learn, change, and realign our lives.

To begin to understand the polarity model of holistic health, imagine a pyramid inside a circle.

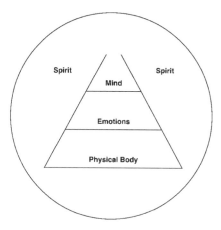

Figure 1
(Illustration by John Beaulieu)

The circle represents all-encompassing Universal Energy. This energy is the source of life and healing. Our individual life energy can be visualized as a drop of water in an ocean of Universal Energy. Dr. Stone created the term ultrasonic core to describe our own unique and individual animating life energy. He believed that all true healing must resonate with the fundamental qualities of our ultrasonic core.

Our mind is located at the top of the pyramid. Dr. Stone believed that "right thinking" was the highest aspect of polarity. Right thinking is the art of aligning our thoughts and actions with Universal Energy. It has nothing to do with the right or wrong judgments of daily life. When our thoughts and actions are out of alignment with our energy source, we experience mental, emotional, and physical dissonance.

Our physical body is located at the bottom of the pyramid. The physical body is our vehicle for expressing life energy. One can imagine Universal Energy as a laser light that shines through a prism (our mind) creating a three-dimensional holographic form we call our physical body. For a polarity practitioner, touching and aligning the physical body is a method of communicating with our emotions and thoughts to help an individual receive and express life energy.

Emotions are located between the mind and physical body. When our thoughts and physical body are aligned, emotions serve as a force that fills us with universal spirit. These are called our higher emotions or passions. When our thoughts and physical body are not aligned, our emotions become sandwiched between the mind and body and they build up pressure. For example, it is a well-known fact that laughter is an excellent release for emotions and has a tremendous healing ability. This is because the act of laughing distracts us from negative thinking, allowing our physical body to loosen and release emotional energy.

The following story illustrates the polarity relationship between mind, emotions, and body. A man came to his therapist's office believing that it rains every Tuesday although he lives in an arid climate. Every Tuesday he puts on his raincoat and adjusts his physical posture, emotions, and thoughts for a rainy day. Because all his friends began making fun of him, creating dissonance in his life, he decided to seek a therapist. On Wednesday, he saw a brilliant therapist and he discovered that it, in fact, does not rain every Tuesday. From Wednesday through Monday, he is ecstatic and tells everyone not to expect rain. When Tuesday arrives, his body automatically adopts the posture of a rainy day and he finds himself having thoughts of rain and walking around in his rain coat.

Polarity therapists say that when Tuesday came, the physical body was not in balance with the mind. The result was a state of disharmony between mind and body, creating emotional pressure. In this case, a dysfunctional sense of relief came when he chose to go back to an old pattern and walk around in his raincoat. Even though he had mental insight, he lacked the physical repatterning and emotional flexibility to holistically "embody" his new thought.

A polarity practitioner would help this person by evaluating his posture in relationship to thought and, through gentle touching, repattern the body to accept the new thought. A polarity practitioner accomplishes this through a knowledge of body structure and a highly refined sense of touch related to life energy. When the mind and body align, there is a sense of resonant tone in the tissues and symmetry of hips, shoulders, and neck. One can literally see a change in how the person stands and walks.

WHAT THE RESEARCH SHOWS

Research studies on polarity therapy are in progress. The American Polarity Therapy Association is sponsoring and promoting new research. Large scale polarity therapy studies have begun in America and England. Results are not yet available. Until these studies and others are published, we have to rely on the many testimonials of satisfied clients.

REAL PEOPLE AND POLARITY THERAPY

Susan came to her polarity session wanting help with recurring back pain. During the history taking, she talked about the specifics of her pain and said her life was otherwise fine. During the evaluation process, the tissues around her joints were found to be contracted and shaking, and her back muscles were tense and hard. I gently placed a hand on her lower back and slightly decompressed her hips, allowing the tissues of the lower back to relax and unwind. As the tissues softened, Susan began to cry and she talked about losing her father to cancer over a year ago. As she talked, a wave of grief moved effortlessly through her body, causing her tissues to elongate and than relax.

When Susan got up from the treatment table she looked like a different person. Her face was relaxed and her eyes glowed. Her shoulders were lowered down and her breathing was full and natural. Susan said she thought she had worked through her father's death and was surprised at her own response. I told her that she had worked through a lot and her body just needed to let go. During the week Susan reported that her back pain disappeared. During follow-up sessions, I continued to work with Susan's spine and she talked about how her father had supported her and how much she missed him. Susan then talked about new ways she could take responsibility for her life and support herself.

Mike came to his session feeling depressed and confused. He said he was a recovering alcoholic and he often went through "feeling down." As he sat in the chair, his body appeared pulled in and compressed. During the evaluation, the tissues of his cranium were tense and his neck, shoulders, and hips were contracted. I slowly began to loosen his lower back, followed by his shoulders and neck. I finished the session gently holding his head, allowing the cranium to unwind. Mike got up from the table and said he felt very relaxed. The next day Mike called me to let me know that he could think clearly for the first time in weeks. He wasn't sure what had happened, but he was happy with the results.

In the twelve step addiction recovery program the second step states: "We came to believe that a Power greater than ourselves could restore us to sanity." When I aligned Mike's body and his tissues relaxed, the Universal Energy began moving through him. The Universal Energy is a power greater than any addictive pattern. Mike opened himself to the energy and was willing to express it in his life, although he did not understand how polarity worked.

WHAT TO EXPECT

Polarity practitioners work from the premise that healing comes from within. The practitioner and client work together to allow the client's own inner healing response to emerge. By developing an understanding and sensitivity to life energy, a polarity practitioner can systematically evaluate its movement. During the process of a polarity bodywork session, clients may spontaneously experience emotions and/or feel the need to talk about their life. This often happens when tense and/or compressed tissues begin to relax and unwind. The polarity practitioner then reflects back a client's thoughts and emotions while continuing to facilitate the unwinding process. At any time the client may stop talking and the session then moves naturally back to silent bodywork.

Polarity bodywork is very gentle and painless, and polarity verbal communication is non-directive, with the intention of helping a client become aware of his or her process. A polarity practitioner may also recommend simple nutritional changes and/or exercises to support the energy balancing. Polarity session times vary from thirty minutes to one hour, based on the issue being addressed. Clients are asked to wear loose-fitting cotton clothing. The number of sessions a client receives is based on individual needs and progress. Most polarity clients have sessions every week or every other week. However, different clients require different interventions.

A polarity practitioner's office normally contains two chairs and a treatment table. Usually the practitioner begins by asking the client's reason for coming. This is followed by taking a history, which may take ten to thirty minutes. The client is then asked to lie on the table and the practitioner does an energy and structural evaluation. The evaluation touch is gentle and soothing and the client may become very relaxed during the process. Based on a client's reasons for coming and the overall evaluation, the polarity practitioner may begin bodywork, make nutritional recommendations, give exercises, and/or enter into verbal counseling. During subsequent sessions the practitioner focuses on continuing energy evaluation to monitor progress.

HOW TO FIND A PRACTITIONER

Polarity Therapy is under the guidance of the American Polarity Therapy Association which oversees educational standards, professional registration and ethics, national and international networking, and conferences. Two levels of training are accredited by APTA: Associate Polarity Practitioner, which requires 60 hours of training; and Registered Polarity Practitioner, which requires 615 hours. Accredited trainings are based on the APTA Standards For Practice and include studies in Polarity theory, evaluation, bodywork, nutrition, exercise, and communication.

When seeking a Polarity practitioner for mental health reasons, one should first make sure the practitioner is APTA Registered (RPP). RPP-trained practitioners are trained to be verbally supportive. However they are not trained in psychotherapeutic or counseling methods. RPPs can work very well in conjunction with a psychiatrist, psychologist, counselor, or social worker. However many RPPs are also psychotherapists with degrees in psychiatry, psychology, social work, or counseling. You should always ask prospective Polarity practitioners about their training in the mental health field. Many Polarity practitioners work with a supporting therapist who can focus on the verbal aspect of therapy while the Polarity work focuses on the bodywork. It might be wise to inquire about how a given Polarity practitioner handles this.

You can contact the American Polarity Therapy Association for a list of Registered Polarity Practitioners at the following address:

AMERICAN POLARITY THERAPY ASSOCIATION
2888 Bluff St., Suite 149
Boulder, CO 803301
Tel: (303) 545-2080; Fax: (303) 545-2161

HOW TO LEARN MORE

Beaulieu, J. *Music and Sound in the Healing Arts: An Energy Approach.* Barrytown, NY:
Station Hill Press, 1987.

Beaulieu, J. *Polarity Therapy Workbook.* New York: BioSonic Enterprises, Ltd., 1994.

Sills, F. *The Polarity Process: Energy as a Healing Art.* Longmead, England: Element
Books, 1989.

Stone R. *Health Building: The Conscious Art of Living Well.* Reno, NV: CRCS
Publications, 1987.

Stone R. *Polarity Therapy: The Complete Works. Vol. 1.* Reno, NV: CRCS Publications,
1987.

Stone R. *Polarity Therapy: The Complete Works. Vol. 2.* Reno, NV: CRCS Publications,
1987.

ABOUT THE AUTHOR

John Beaulieu, N.D., Ph.D., is a registered polarity practitioner who has been
practicing and teaching polarity for twenty years. He is a graduate of Purdue
University, Indiana University, Westbrook University, and the International
College of Naturopathic Medicine. John has served as a supervising therapist
and research coordinator at Bellevue Psychiatric Hospital and worked as a pro-
fessor at City University of New York and Fairleigh-Dickenson University.
Currently he maintains a private polarity practice in New York City and directs
the International Polarity Wellness Network. John is a member of the American
Polarity Therapy Association and the American Naturopathic Medical
Association and is the author of the *Polarity Therapy Workbook* and *Music and
Sound in the Healing Arts: An Energy Approach.*

Jeffrey Maitland, Ph.D.

33 Rolfing:
The Whole Body Approach to Well-Being

WHAT IS ROLFING?

Rolfing® is one of the twentieth century's most influential and most often imitated forms of soft tissue manipulation. As a direct result of its ability to dramatically alter posture and structure, Rolfing can create greater ease of movement and enhance the overall functioning of the whole body. If you can imagine how it feels to live in a fluid, light, balanced body, free of pain, stiffness, and chronic stress, at ease with itself in the gravitational field, then you will understand the purpose of Rolfing. Professional athletes from NBA superstars to Olympic champions, movie stars, dancers, students of yoga and meditation, business people, musicians, and people from all walks of life and of all ages have sought the benefits of Rolfing. Not only do people seek Rolfing as a way to ease pain and chronic stress, but also as a way to improve performance in their profession and daily activities. Rolfing is useful in overcoming a variety of emotional problems because as the overall structure of the body is improved, old patterns of emotional distress that have been held in the body are released. This enables people to move beyond their habitual patterns of painful emotions and maladaptive functioning.

Rolfing was named structural integration by its founder and creator, Dr. Ida P. Rolf. But Rolfing is the nickname that many clients spontaneously gave this pioneering system of soft tissue manipulation, and it is the name that stuck.

HOW IT BEGAN

Ida Pauline Rolf was born in 1896 in New York. She earned her Ph.D. in Biological Chemistry in 1920 from Columbia University. Later she became an associate in the Rockefeller Institute's Department of Organic Chemistry, where she did research and published many articles for well over a decade. For most of her life, she was fascinated with and studied many forms of alternative healing, including homeopathy, osteopathy, and yoga. Of all the systems of manipulation she studied, Dr. Rolf was most influenced by osteopathy. She experienced the power of osteopathic manipulation when she was cured of pneumonia by one its practitioners. From that time on, she remained convinced of one the first principles of osteopathy, that structure determines function. For almost fifty years of her professional life, she studied and worked with osteopaths and chiropractors.

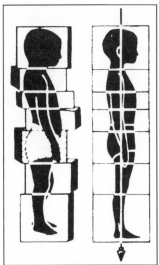

Figure 1
(The Little Boy Logo® is a registered trademark of the Rolf Institute of Structural Integration.)

Dr. Rolf had an uncanny ability to see whole body alignment and misalignment as they were displayed in the soft tissues of the body. Driven to find a solution to her own problems, as well as those of her two young sons, she spent years exploring and experimenting with different systems of healing and manipulation. When she combined her discoveries with her remarkable powers of observation, Rolfing was born.

Her original vision was broad and deep. She saw the need to explore her work from the points of view of philosophy, medical science, and psychology. Her life's work was devoted to the philosophical and scientific investigation into the conditions that must be fulfilled in order for the person as a whole to function optimally. Recognized around the world as the leader and pioneer in whole body alignment through soft tissue manipulation, she died in 1979 at the age of 83. Since Dr. Rolf's death, the philosophy, science, and art of Rolfing have continued to evolve significantly and profoundly.

In 1972, Dr. Rolf founded the International Rolf Institute in Boulder, CO. The Rolf Institute is the education and research center and professional association for Certified Rolfers® worldwide.

Figure 1, traced from an actual photograph of a little boy who underwent ten sessions of Rolfing, has become the official logo of the Rolf Institute. The logo is an excellent representation of the remarkable postural and structural changes for which Rolfing is known.

HOW IT WORKS

Science has known for years that proper body alignment, physiological function, and anatomical structure are related. Other systems of manipulation, such as osteopathy and chiropractic, were created and based on this insight. But Dr. Rolf pioneered the discovery that a long-lasting improvement in alignment and overall sense of well-being required a deeper understanding of the impact of gravity on our bodies. The key to this deeper understanding is the myofascial system. The myofascial system is composed of muscle tissue and a form of connective tissue called fascia. Fascia surrounds and penetrates the muscles and all other structures of the body. In conjunction with the bones and muscles, it is largely responsible for the unique form that each of our bodies displays. Everyone who has either skinned an animal or cut a piece of meat has seen fascia. It is the white, filmy substance that compartmentalizes and binds everything together in the body. Although a practical impossibility, if everything but the fascia could be removed from the body, what would be left over would be a perfect three-dimensional blueprint of the entire body — in essence, an intricate web of connective tissue in the form of a fascial body. It would look something like a huge loofah sponge in the shape of our body. In it, we could see where every single bone, nerve, blood vessel, organ, and so forth belongs.

At every level, our health and well-being are very much a function of the architectural integrity of our body, of the span and balance of the myofascial system within gravity. Distortions and patterns of strain within the fascial network can be the expression of injury, illness, stress, and long-standing psychological and emotional conflicts. Just as a tent will be dragged down by gravity if the guy wires and the fabric lose their appropriate stretch and span, our body will lose its architectural integrity as some muscles and fascia become too tight and others too flaccid.

Since the entire body is connected through its fascial network, lines of stress and strain within any section of fascia can be immediately transmitted throughout the entire fascial network much in the same way snagging part of a sweater can distort the shape of the entire sweater. These patterns of strain in the fascial network contribute to the unique form that each of our bodies displays, as well as to our unique ways of standing, sitting, and moving. Like a pair of well-worn shoes, these patterns of fascial strain display our unique struggles with gravity.

Fascia is made up of a colloidal ground substance and collagen fibers that give it strength. Fascia is a highly adaptive tissue that shortens and thickens in response to injury, sustained or traumatic emotional conflict, imbalance, and diseases. In this process of shortening and thickening, the ground substance of fascia loses its elasticity and fluidity. Dr. Rolf discovered that the ground substance of fascia could be softened and lengthened by the intelligent and appropriate application of pressure through her hands. To most people, Rolfing sessions look like a form of body sculpting. Using their fingers, knuckles, and elbows to ease and lengthen fascial strain patterns, Rolfers reshape and reorder the whole body from head to toe. Through a careful and systematic application of pressure coupled with keen observational powers, Rolfers bring the human body to a higher level of flexibility, balance, organization in gravity, and economy of function. As clients approach an easy upright posture, they report shedding their aches and pains, performing better in their daily activities, and attaining a much higher state of well-being. Some even experience life-transforming changes as they release deeply repressed patterns of trauma and emotional conflict.

Metaphorically, Rolfing attempts to transform the sky, not push the stars. Any manipulative system that symptomatically adjusts bones back into place in order to release local joint fixations, or manipulates local areas of tight fascia or muscle, is a star model of manipulation. Star models of therapy and myofascial release often provide people with effective and beneficial help. But Rolfing is a sky model of manipulation and somatic education. As such it is a holistic system that has the potential to not only release the body from its local aches and pains, but to transform the whole person. The sky that Rolfing works with is the myofascial system of the body in its relationship to gravity. By transforming the fascial sky and organizing the whole body in gravity, the various stars of the body not only find their appropriate place, but they also function better. Rolfers understand that symptomatically releasing local areas of dysfunction rarely creates integration and lasting change — if the whole body is not properly prepared to receive the effects of local manipulations, either the change will not be maintained or strain will show up in other areas. By transforming the sky, Rolfing can and does release the body from its aches and pains and restrictions. Symptoms tend to disappear, not because the body has been manipulated symptomatically and piecemeal, but because the whole person has been engaged and educated to find optimal balance in the gravitational field.

Rolfing has continued to evolve in rather significant ways. Rolfing began as a rather painful style of manipulation and over the years sustained this reputation in the mind of the public. Fortunately, however, through the creative efforts of some of the Rolf Institute's teachers, the techniques of Rolfing have broadened to include a softer and more discriminating sense of touch. The new Rolfing is both less invasive and more precise in its ability to release and organize the body at every level. Many clients who have felt this gentler approach are often surprised to discover that their experiences of massage are actually more uncomfortable than Rolfing.

The advanced Rolfing faculty have also evolved new techniques that can easily release joint fixations in the spine and other bones of the body with as much precision as any other system of manipulation. But unlike other systems of manipulation, Rolfing can accomplish these results without resorting to thrusting techniques which typically "pop" bones into place by forcefully releasing joint fixations. As the strain patterns in the fascia and ligaments that are responsible for the joint fixations are gently and systematically eased under the intelligent pressure applied by the Rolfer, bones and the other structures of the body quietly shift back to where they belong as motion restrictions at many levels of the body dissolve.

Some of the advanced Rolfing teachers also pioneered a way of teaching and performing the work of Rolfing. Dr. Rolf had developed a ten session protocol she called "the recipe," her notion of ideal body alignment. Today's advanced teachers have replaced the recipe with an approach that is tailored to the unique differences among people. As a result, Rolfing has become more a process of discovery in which Rolfer and client explore the most effective ways to enhance the inherent being of the whole person.

The new Rolfing program of instruction has been broadened and expanded in many ways. Along with the principle-centered decision-making process, the new understanding of how to release joint fixations, and the introduction of gentler techniques, it now includes, for example, a rich and diversified training in how to enhance our inherent potentials for free, fluid movement. These and other advances in Rolfing are continually being refined as new insights and discoveries are integrated into the work. There is a growing body of research that supports many of the claims of Rolfing.

WHAT THE RESEARCH SHOWS

Research conducted at UCLA (Hunt and Massey, 1977) showed that Rolfing creates a more efficient use of the muscles, allows the body to conserve energy, and creates more economical and refined patterns of movement. More recent research conducted at the University of Maryland (Cottingham, Porges, and Richmond, 1988) demonstrates that Rolfing significantly reduces chronic stress and changes body structure for the better. In these studies, Rolfing significantly reduced the spinal curvature of subjects with lordosis (sway back). The research also indicates that Rolfing enhances neurological functioning. Surprisingly, these changes in structure and function are long lasting and rarely require further maintenance sessions.

REAL PEOPLE AND ROLFING

Like many people who seek the benefits of Rolfing, Marcie's body was collapsed, round shouldered, and much too soft. Her psychotherapist suggested she try Rolfing as a way both to improve her posture and deepen her therapy. Marcie complained that she was much too sensitive, often to the point of being overwhelmed by the negative aspects of her world. Her comportment gave the appearance of a fearful person. Until she began Rolfing, however, she rarely experienced her fear directly. She said she felt insecure, needy, ineffectual and, at times, experienced a kind of inner vacancy. Because she did not like her posture and believed herself to be too soft and skinny, she tried weight lifting and rigorous exercise programs as counter measures. She was frustrated by how ineffective these programs were for her.

After a number of Rolfing sessions, Marcie's body began to lengthen and lift out of her collapse. But she still carried her head and neck too forward of the rest of her body. Her shoulders were still pulled up and in as if she were frozen in fright. During a session devoted to balancing and organizing her shoulders, neck, and head, Marcie began to shiver uncontrollably on the table as if she were suddenly freezing cold. From embarrassment she tried to control herself. Soon she realized this strategy only made her feel worse. On the advice of her Rolfer, she let herself go into the shaking. Almost immediately, she complained of a constriction in her throat. Her jaw began to quiver and she trembled even more intensely. These actions were followed by whimpering and then what sounded like a series of muffled screams.

After the trembling and whimpering subsided, Marcie reported that she had relived the fear she felt as a toddler when her mother went into a rage and yanked her around the room by her hair. The constriction she felt in her throat was both the repression of her screams and the expression of being invaded by undeserved and powerful forces that threatened the integrity of her developing self. Reliving these experiences on the Rolfing table proved to be a significant turning point for Marcie. In therapy, she finally was able to explore these traumas and begin the lengthy process of overcoming and resolving her repressed fear.

By the end of her Rolfing series, Marcie's posture and gait changed dramatically. She stood taller and moved with a sense of grace that caught the attention of all who knew her. As her legs came directly under her, she experienced her feet more squarely on the ground. As a result, she felt more secure and her upper body lifted elegantly upward. She looked and felt much less fearful. Marcie continued to integrate the changes in her body as her life began to change. She found a better job, which brought in more money, required regular hours, and demanded more interpersonal skills. She took up karate and finally began to firm up her body to her satisfaction. Karate also allowed Marcie to explore and enhance her newly discovered sense of power and bodily integration. And she began cleaning up her personal life which had been a mess for years.

∞

Trudy came to Rolfing after a number of years of psychotherapy. She and her therapist felt that Rolfing could help speed up her therapy which had begun to bog down. Her body was dense and tight, and she had a mild scoliosis. She gave the appearance of great sadness and her eyes expressed confusion. She blinked a lot, and had trouble looking at her Rolfer when they talked. She reported that, as a child, she felt invisible to her parents, as if they hardly even knew or cared whether she was there. In addition to making her feel invisible, her parents never protected her from the relentless beatings she received from her brothers. She said that she did not trust men and often felt anxious. She also felt she had never been seen for herself and often experienced a desperate need to be.

Before beginning Rolfing, Trudy effectively blocked awareness of her sadness by making her musculature dense and tight. Unfortunately, the act of suppressing her sadness had the unwanted consequence of suppressing her joy, her exuberance over simply being present. Trudy's density was the armor she needed to protect herself from her brothers, from her anxiety, and to block awareness of her sadness.

Her dense musculature also served another important and vital function in her life. She said that when she experienced anxiety, it felt as though she were losing herself — as if she were vanishing into nothingness. In response to this ever-present threat to her being, she tensed the musculature of her body as a desperate way of forcing herself to be present. Since her parents were never there for her, Trudy had to develop her sense of self in a vacuum of neglect filled with her brother's unpredictable beatings. Lacking a healthy parental mirror of love in which to see herself, Trudy was forced to develop her own sense of self and grew up sad and alone. Thus, she worked hard at being present by tensing her musculature in a desperate attempt to force herself to be here. Her body said, "Look at me, I am not invisible. I am here!"

During her early sessions, she often tensed her body in response to the manipulations of Rolfing. Soon it became clear that tensing was part of her desperate need to be. Not surprisingly, she said she was afraid to give in to the profound relaxation that Rolfing produced, for fear that she would become a "blob." She said that this strategy of tensing her whole body for the purpose of being seen felt like she was taking amphetamines, and that she had trouble coming down at night. No wonder she resisted the pressure of Rolfing — the feeling of "coming down" or "becoming a blob" brought her too close to her anxiety, making her feel as if her presence were vanishing into nothingness.

Trudy continued to work on her anxiety with her therapist, and finally after a series of Rolfing sessions, her dense musculature began to ease. Her eyes became bright and clear and lost much of their confusion. Her body looked longer and she moved with a more graceful ease. She said she was finally hired to do the job she had trained for in college and loved her work. Because she was able to trust her male Rolfer, she was more trusting of men and now, a couple of years after a difficult marriage and painful divorce, she was looking forward to a relationship with a man. She also said she used to hate being alone, but now she really appreciated and enjoyed the time she could spend by herself. Being alone no longer meant being lonely to her. And best of all, she said she was beginning to know happiness. Her sadness and the loss of presence she had been defending against all her life were dissolving. In its place she was just beginning to experience the joy of life — her own sense of exuberance over just being present.

WHAT TO EXPECT

Rolfing is designed not just to restore function and help you with your aches and pains, but to systematically align and organize your body in gravity in order to enhance how you function at many levels. Some Rolfers still work within the ten session protocol, while others work in a more individualized way. The client is usually clothed in underwear, shorts, or a bathing suit. In order to create an effective strategy for organizing the client's body, the Rolfer usually begins the session by observing and evaluating the client standing and walking. The client then lies on a specially designed padded table and the work begins. A typical Rolfing session takes between an hour to an hour and a half, and includes hands-on manipulation coupled with movement analysis and corrective suggestions. Prices for a Rolfing session vary around the world. One session can cost anywhere from $80 to $130.

HOW TO FIND A ROLFER

Only practitioners certified through the Rolf Institute can call themselves Rolfers and perform Rolfing. A candidate desiring to train as a Rolfer must have a college degree. Upon acceptance into the Institute's training program, the student must first complete the basic program of instruction. Within four to seven years of graduating from the basic level, every certified Rolfer must complete the advanced level of instruction. To find a qualified Rolfer or make sure that a practitioner is a certified Rolfer, contact:

THE ROLF INSTITUTE
INTERNATIONAL HEADQUARTERS
205 Canyon Blvd.
Boulder, CO 80302
Tel: (800) 530-8875; Fax: (303) 449-5978

HOW TO LEARN MORE

Cottingham, J., S. Porges, and K. Richmond. "Shifts in Pelvic Inclination Angle and Parasympathetic Tone Produced by Rolfing Soft Tissue Manipulation." *Physical Therapy* 68 (1988): 1364–1370.

Cottingham, J. *Healing Through Touch: A History and Review of the Physiological Evidence.* Boulder, CO: Rolf Institute, 1985.

Hunt, V. and W. Massey. *A Study of Structural Integration from a Neuromuscular Energy Field, and Emotional Approaches.* Boulder, CO: Rolf Institute, 1977.

Maitland, J. *Spacious Body: Explorations in Somatic Ontology.* Berkeley, CA: North Atlantic Books, 1995.

Oschman, J. L. *The Connective Tissue and Myofascial Systems.* Berkeley, CA: Aspen Research Institute, 1981.*

Rolf, I. *Rolfing: The Integration of Human Structures.* Boulder, CO: The Rolf Institute, 1977.*

Rolf, I. *Ida Rolf Talks About Rolfing and Physical Reality.* Edited by Rosemary Feitis. New York: Harper and Row, 1978.*

* These titles are available through The Rolf Institute.

ABOUT THE AUTHOR

Jeffrey Maitland, Ph.D., Certified Advanced Rolfer and Advanced Instructor, is one of four advanced Rolfing instructors worldwide. He is faculty chairman and Director of Academic Affairs for the International Rolf Institute. Dr. Maitland is also a Board Certified Diplomate in the American Academy of Pain Management. He was a member of the Council of the National Certification Program, which helped to establish standards in somatic education and massage therapy by creating a national certification exam. Prior to becoming a Rolfer, Dr. Maitland was a professor of philosophy at Purdue University for thirteen years. After experiencing the dramatic results of being Rolfed for a debilitating back problem, he gave up his tenured position to pursue a career in Rolfing. He has published and presented many papers on Rolfing, on the theory of somatic manual therapy, and on philosophy. He is the author of *Spacious Body: Explorations in Somatic Ontology* (1995, North Atlantic Books).

Rolfing® is a service mark of the Rolf Institute of Structural Integration.

The case studies used in this chapter were abbreviated and excerpted from Jeffrey Maitland's book, *Spacious Body*.

Ilana Rubenfeld

34 The Rubenfeld Synergy Method

WHAT IS THE RUBENFELD SYNERGY METHOD?

The Rubenfeld Synergy® Method is a contemporary form of body-centered psychotherapy and education that integrates the body, mind, emotions, and spirit. Its goal is to teach people how to recognize, understand, and deal with their physical, emotional, and mental problems. This dynamic system uses gentle, noninvasive and nonsexual touch, talk, and movement simultaneously.

The Rubenfeld Synergy Method has a beneficial impact on people's self-image, health, spirit, and personal and family relationships. Among the people who can benefit from it are:

- people who are anxious, depressed, phobic, or who suffer panic attacks
- survivors of war, displacement, sudden loss, violence (including those diagnosed with post-traumatic stress syndrome)
- those with addictive behaviors such as eating disorders and substance abuse
- people in high-stress occupations, such as performing arts, business, government, and education
- people dealing with debilitating health problems
- couples and families suffering from dysfunctional patterns

There are no known contraindications for the Rubenfeld Synergy Method. Its practitioners — called Rubenfeld Synergists — are trained to recognize when they need to refer clients to other professionals.

The Rubenfeld Synergy Method is unique in its ability to address physical and emotional issues in an integrated way. The original creators of Rolfing, Alexander, Trager, Feldenkrais, and Swedish massage focused on clients' physical conditions and intentionally did not include verbal processing of emotional experiences that arose during the body work. The Rubenfeld Synergy Method is a useful adjunct to other approaches. Many psychiatrists and talk therapists refer clients for Rubenfeld Synergy. Body therapists who are not trained to deal with emotional material also refer clients for Rubenfeld Synergy.

Clients remain fully clothed at all times in a Rubenfeld Synergy session. The Rubenfeld Synergy Method does not include massage techniques, such as deep tissue manipulation, the use of oils and lotions, hydrotherapy, or adjustments of spine and joints.

HOW IT BEGAN

In the 1950s, I was a conducting student at the Juilliard School of Music when a debilitating back spasm changed my life. Seeking help, I found Judith Leibowitz, a teacher of the F. M. Alexander Technique, who taught me how to use my body efficiently and avoid re-injury. During my Alexander lessons, I sometimes expressed intense emotions. Untrained in processing emotions, Leibowitz suggested that I see a psychoanalyst. I took her advice but by the time I saw him, the intense feelings were gone. For the next few years, I saw Leibowitz, who touched but wouldn't talk, and the analyst, who talked but wouldn't touch. I realized that it was her touch that accessed my memories and his verbal processing that helped me understand them. I wanted someone to do both — talk and touch.

This yearning marked the conception of the Rubenfeld Synergy Method. Its gestation took many years of research, study, and experimentation. I became a master teacher of the Alexander Technique and trained extensively with Moshe Feldenkrais in the Feldenkrais Method®. For years, I taught both of these body-mind methods, but found that they missed what for me was the most vital element — processing the emotional material that emerged during lessons. I longed to know the emotional history, stresses, and life problems that created physical dysfunctions in the first place. This curiosity led me to train and collaborate with Dr. Peter Hogan (an Adlerian psychiatrist) and Fritz and Laura Perls (co-founders of Gestalt therapy), and to further refine the integration of these somatic methods and psychotherapy. These theoretical and practical elements formed the harmonics in my orchestration of a new therapeutic and educational paradigm.

Buckminster Fuller, the creator of the geodesic dome, suggested the word "synergy" at a conference after watching me demonstrate my work, which was still nameless at that time. He said "integration" did not accurately express what I was doing and explained that "synergy" would be a more appropriate name. (With synergy, the results are greater than — and different from — the sum of the results of the component parts.) At last I had found a word that expressed the dynamics of my method. The Rubenfeld Synergy Method was born.

In 1975, bodywork practitioners and psychotherapists approached me to train them in the Rubenfeld Synergy Method. How would I teach them the individual elements while also teaching them how to integrate them all into an organic whole? This was the challenging puzzle I had to solve. My training as a music conductor rescued me. Keeping track of twenty or more simultaneous activities, while retaining the entire gestalt of a composition, is part of every conductor's education and daily practice. I accepted the first group of trainees in 1977 and designed the program to be highly experiential, with discussions, individualized supervision, body-mind exercises, demonstrations, and lectures. Trainees learn to practice self-care and maintain high standards of integrity, competence, and ethics (the Synergists' code of ethics deals with respect and confidentiality, avoiding personal relationships, maintaining clear boundaries, and more. Copies of the code are available — see Resources.).

Since that first professional certification training program, my faculty and I have certified over 350 Rubenfeld Synergists. After certification, they have additional opportunities to continue their education, training, therapy, and supervision.

HOW IT WORKS

Rubenfeld Synergy works by addressing the client's current complaints or problems, such as anxiety, inability to concentrate, or aches and pains. During sessions, clients may become more self-aware and discover for themselves the source of the complaints. What is the body doing that contributes to the tension, anxiety, or pain?

The Synergist-client relationship is one of partnership in the unfolding of the body's wisdom and self-healing. Safety and trust between client and

Synergist are key to the development of a successful healing partnership. If an emotional issue emerges during a session, the Synergist is qualified and trained to deal with this material, as well as the physical.

The following principles, philosophies and theoretical foundations (Rubenfeld, 1996) guide Rubenfeld Synergy sessions:

1. *Each individual is unique:* Rubenfeld Synergy respects the uniqueness of each individual. Synergists approach each session with no pre-determined agenda, choosing instead from options of touch, verbal interaction, imagination, and movement ways to support the client's unique path to growth and change.

2. *The body, mind, emotions, and spirit are part of a dynamically-interrelated system:* Each time a change is introduced at one level of a person's being, it has a ripple effect throughout the entire system, changing the equilibrium of the whole person. For example, changes in the posture and breathing affect the person's mood and spirit, and vice versa.

3. *Awareness is the first key to change:* Each of us has physical and emotional habit patterns. We may not be aware of them and how they affect our life because we learned them unconsciously. To change these habit patterns, we need to become aware of them. Through the Synergist's use of movement, touch, verbal intervention, and creative experimentation, clients become aware of their habit patterns and can begin to make different life choices.

4. *Change occurs in the present moment:* Clients may experience their memories of the past and fantasize about the future, but change itself can occur only in the present. When memories of painful past experiences emerge in a Rubenfeld Synergy session, clients have the opportunity to relive and review the experience in the present moment through active imagination and visualization. They can re-script the remembered events and look at them from another vantage point. They can also resolve unfinished business and integrate their new insights.

5. *The ultimate responsibility for change rests with the client:* There is no way a therapist can force an individual to change. Sometimes the very resistance to change is what keeps the client together, even though it may be dysfunctional. The Synergist can help clients recognize the dysfunction,

emotionally and physically, and slowly guide them to try a new behavior. Eventually this newly learned behavior can replace the old habits of the past.

6. *People have a natural capacity for self-healing and self-regulation*: The client's innate healing ability already exists, waiting to be actualized. The Synergist doesn't "correct" it but facilitates its development.

7. *The body's life force and energy field can be sensed*: There are many ancient energy systems, in use for millennia, that have become known in the West. The body's energy has many names. *Chakra* is a Sanskrit word that describes swirling circles of energy (prana) at various locations in and around the body, from the base of the spine to the top of the head. The Japanese *qi* and Chinese *chi* refer to the life force that circulates along meridians in the body. "Orgone" was Wilhelm Reich's term for the life force. Synergists often sense a marked change in the quality of energy, its pulsations and movement, when tense holding patterns in the body-mind are released.

8. *Touch is a viable, accurate system of communication*: Since touch is a powerful language that communicates, Synergists develop "listening hands." They can hear the story of the body and convey trust and safety back to the client. This specific touch opens new gateways to clients' mental and emotional awareness and creates dialogues with the unconscious mind.

9. *The body is a metaphor*: Our postures and other physical manifestations may mirror mental and emotional problems. Complaints of "She's a pain in the neck," or "He makes me sick to my stomach," or "I can't shoulder the burden anymore" are often body metaphors for real life issues.

10. *The body tells the truth*: When people communicate verbally, their bodies may tell another story. The body's story usually reflects their unconscious and authentic state. The Synergist's listening hands are able to detect this incongruence and use it as a guide for questions and other explorations. The goal, in this situation, is for the body and mind to "talk to each other."

11. *The body is the sanctuary of the soul*: All beings — from the smallest creature to the most complex systems of the universe — embody spirit. Rubenfeld Synergy sessions may progress toward a spiritual dimension

when clients deal with their "soul" issues — questioning their life values in relationships, families, communities, and the world.

12. *Pleasure needs to be supported to balance pain:* Grief, anger, pain, joy, and laughter are all housed in the body. Some people have become addicted to repeating their most painful stories and thereby ignore opportunities to experience joy and pleasure in the present. Pain-addicted clients can grow to recontact their long-forgotten strengths and joyous playfulness lost since childhood, and learn to use them to create a more well-balanced life.

13. *Humor can heal and lighten:* When clients get stuck somatically or emotionally in a painful and repetitive loop, using appropriate humor — not sarcasm — interrupts their habitual pattern. Laughter can dissolve fear and make it possible for clients to deal with past emotional wounding that is otherwise too painful to bear. Laughter can free tight holding patterns, invite deeper breathing, enhance creativity.

14. *Reflecting clients' verbal expressions validates their experience:* Hearing their stories retold by the Synergist confirms that they are being heard and understood. Clients often use this opportunity to reflect on their initial statements and take them to a deeper level.

15. *Confusion facilitates change:* Confusion interrupts dysfunctional habit patterns. During this window of opportunity, the Synergist invites the client to experiment with nonhabitual behavior, which then needs to be integrated emotionally and somatically.

16. *Altered states of consciousness can enhance healing:* During altered states of consciousness, the client's attention may focus acutely on certain sensory modalities and internal states of being. Altered states can facilitate the client's ability to contact old physical and emotional memories that are still present in the body and can expand the Synergist's ability to dialogue with the unconscious body/mind.

17. *Integration is necessary for lasting results:* Many physical habit patterns can be changed and integrated only when their associated emotional material is processed. Unless clients incorporate their new insights and behaviors into their daily lives, they are likely to revert to old, habitual patterns. Integration within a session can take place on many levels: The client

integrates words and movements, sensation and emotion, memories and images. The "re-entry" phases of a session allow the client to integrate the new awarenesses physically, mentally, and emotionally.

18. *Self-care is the first step to client care.* Synergists are trained to protect themselves from "burnout." They learn to maintain personal boundaries. If they identify with clients, they do so without merging with them. This clarity keeps Synergists from transmitting their problems and tensions to the client through their hands and also from taking on the client's somatic aches and pains.

WHAT THE RESEARCH SHOWS

Much research has documented the therapeutic effects of touch in general on self-healing (for example, Pert, 1985; Field, 1986; Weil, 1995). One Ph.D. dissertation (Junglas, 1994) documents the experiences with Rubenfield Synergy of eleven adults, and elucidates eight themes common to all.

Although no other studies about Rubenfeld Synergy have been published, many unpublished pilot studies have been conducted by Rubenfeld Synergists. These include studies of the effects of Rubenfeld Synergy on self-esteem, body image, eating disorders, alcohol and drug abuse, anxiety, panic attacks, depression in cancer patients and their caregivers, migraine and chronic headaches, fibromyalgia, diabetes, multiple sclerosis, fibrocitis, stuttering, creativity, and self-expression. More information about these studies may be obtained from the Rubenfeld Center.

REAL PEOPLE AND THE RUBENFELD SYNERGY METHOD

Susan came to me because of unremitting anxiety. By the end of a session, Susan successfully released her bound-up shoulders and allowed them to drop down, but the following week, she again sat in the chair with her shoulders hunched up toward her ears. In one session, she began to sob in a very high-pitched voice. Recognizing the significance of that moment, I quietly asked her how old she felt just then.

"Two years old," she replied, crying. With my hands touching her upper back and right shoulder, I asked her to close her eyes and go back to that time. There was a sudden shudder as she squirmed in the chair and pulled her knees up to her chest so tightly that she resembled a small ball. She opened her eyes briefly to check that I was still there. A distant memory surfaced — of her hands being tied with brightly colored ribbons to the bars of her crib. Slowly her story unfolded: her mother wanted to keep baby Susan from touching her genitals. This position was frozen in her body even while the memory had been repressed for so many years.

In successive sessions she continued to release her shoulders further. Now her arms moved more freely, allowing her hands to be closer to her genitals. This new position scared her, and her shoulders often returned to their old position. After months of working through this emotional trauma and its somatic implications, she was able to express anger, resentment, and pain about her mother's behavior. Later, Susan was able to reclaim her sexual feelings in a healthy way and forgive her mother. She had integrated her relaxed shoulders and open chest into her present life and relationships.

∞

John, a depressed and sad young man, lay motionless on the table. I tried gently to move his head. It was stuck. When I slipped my hands under his back it felt like a sheet of steel. He explained that his fiancée had left him suddenly and he was confused. I asked him to imagine his fiancée and speak to her. In a soft, placating voice he said, "Joan, I forgive you . . ." As he spoke, his back tightened even more, as if it were saying, "You must be kidding! I'm furious!"

His back clearly contradicted what he was saying. "If your back had a voice, what would it say?" I asked. He began to pound the table, yelling, "I'm so angry at what you've done!" Even though he thought he should forgive her, his body was expressing his inner emotions. After several sessions, he was able to contact and express his grief and sadness. Then, looking and feeling more relieved, he was genuinely ready to forgive her. His body, mind, and emotions were now congruent.

∞

WHAT TO EXPECT

Sessions usually begin with verbal conversation about issues the clients present and may move to the past and future depending on clients' needs. No diagnoses are made nor cures promised.

Clients are invited to lie down fully clothed on a padded table. Sessions may also take place with the client sitting, standing, and moving. The Synergist honors and responds to their pace and focus. A gentle touch, with healing intention, is introduced when they are ready. Clients are reassured that they can stop the session at any time, for any reason.

Once clients are aware of how their dysfunctional habit patterns have contributed to their issues, the Synergist may invite them to experiment with some nonhabitual behaviors. As each session comes to a close, clients usually integrate some insights and learning from the session and prepare to re-enter the outside world.

Single sessions, usually forty-five minutes long, are most often scheduled once or twice weekly. When long distance travel is required, double sessions (ninety minutes long) may be appropriate. Although Rubenfeld Synergy may bring life-changing insights in a short time, weekly sessions for at least several months, and perhaps for several years, are advised to allow for fully integrated and lasting benefits.

When appropriate, the Synergist may teach Rubenfeld Bodymind Exercises, which develop strength, ease specific tensions, foster mental and physical flexibility, and teach "inner listening." These simple exercises can be practiced between sessions anywhere. Practicing them helps to replace old habit patterns — which may contribute to the presenting problem — with new, more life-enhancing ways to move.

HOW TO FIND A PRACTITIONER

In the U.S., the Rubenfeld Center can provide referrals to a Certified Rubenfeld Synergist in your in area. In Canada, you can call or write to the Canadian Association of Rubenfeld Synergists.

The Rubenfeld Synergy Training Program is currently a 1600-hour program. It is the only source of training and certification of Rubenfeld Synergists.

Take your time to interview and consult with several Synergists. They will probably see you one to three times before agreeing to an ongoing weekly process. If you do not continue together, the Synergist may refer you elsewhere.

RESOURCES

The Rubenfeld Center can provide more information about the Rubenfeld Synergy Method and the Rubenfeld Synergy Training Program, audiotapes and videotapes, reprints of articles, and a current schedule of workshops and conferences. You can contact the Center at:

THE RUBENFELD CENTER
115 Waverly Place
New York, NY 10011
Tel: (800) 747-6897; Fax: (212) 254-1174
E-mail: rubenfeld@aol.com

For information about the Synergist's Code of Ethics, contact:

NATIONAL ASSOCIATION OF RUBENFELD SYNERGISTS
1000 River Rd., Suite 8H
Belmar, NJ 07719 USA
Tel: (800) 484-3250, code 8516

For referrals to Synergists in Canada and the Canadian Synergist's Code of Ethics, contact:

CANADIAN ASSOCIATION OF RUBENFELD SYNERGISTS
112 Lund Street
Richmond Hill, ONT L4C 5V9 CANADA
Tel: (905) 883-3158
E-mail: aturner@yorku.ca

All of these associations support their members' professional growth and promote high standards of professional ethics. They also seek to educate the public about the Rubenfeld Synergy Method and to protect their members' right to practice.

HOW TO LEARN MORE

Claire, T. "Rubenfeld Synergy Method: Touch Therapy Meets Talk Therapy." In *Bodywork*. New York: William Morrow and Company, Inc., 1995.

Field, T., et al., "Tactile/Kinesthetic Stimulation Effects on Preterm Neonates." *Pediatrics* 7, no. 55 (1986): 654–658.

Junglas, M. D. "The Experience of Becoming an Integrated Self Through Rubenfeld Synergy." Unpublished doctoral dissertation, The Union Institute. Ann Arbor: University Microfilms International #9516505, 1994.

Knaster, M. "Ilana Rubenfeld — Our Lady of Synergy." *Massage Therapy* 30, no. 1 (1991): 36–45.

Markowitz, L. "Minding the Body, Embodying the Mind: Therapists Explore Mind-body Alternatives." *Family Therapy Networker* 20, no. 5 (1996): 20–33. *

Mishlove, J. "Ilana Rubenfeld — Mind-Body Integration: An Inner Work™ Videotape with Dr. Jeffrey Mishlove." Berkeley, CA: Thinking Allowed Productions, 1992. *

Pert, C. B., et al., "Neuropeptides and Their Receptors: A Psychosomatic Network." *Journal of Immunology* 135 (1985): 820–826.

Rubenfeld, I. "Alexander Technique and Innovations." In "Dance Therapy: Roots and Extensions." *American Dance Therapy Association* 5, no. 2 (1971): 45.

Rubenfeld, I. "The Rubenfeld Synergy Method, Formerly Gestalt Therapy." Unpublished paper, 1973.*

Rubenfeld, I. "Rubenfeld on the Road" New York: The Rubenfeld Center, Inc., 1973.*

Rubenfeld, I. "Self-Care for the Professional Woman: Beyond Physical Fitness." In *Women and Work*, edited by L. Knezek, M. Barrett, and S. Collins, Arlington, TX: Women and Work Research and Resource Center, 1985. 9–14.

Rubenfeld, I. "Beginner's Hands: Twenty-five Years of Simple; Rubenfeld Synergy — The Birth of a Therapy." *Somatics* 4, no. 4 (1988): 4–11*

Rubenfeld, I. "Ushering in a Century of Integration." *Somatics* 8, no. 1 (1991): 59–63.*

Rubenfeld, I. "Gestalt Therapy and the Bodymind: An Overview of the Rubenfeld Synergy® Method." In *Gestalt Therapy: Perspectives and Applications*, edited by E. C. Nevis, New York: Gardner Press, Inc. 1992.

Rubenfeld, I. "Ilana Rubenfeld - Growing Old Means Forgetting to Retire." A videotaped presentation by Ilana Rubenfeld. In the "Time for Spirit" Video Series produced by W. Whipple. (Copyright jointly by the Omega Institute, New Age Journal and MetaMedia Arts.) Distributed by MetaMedia Arts, (770) 455-0126.*

Rubenfeld, I. "Healing the Emotional/Spiritual Body: The Rubenfeld Synergy Method." In *Getting in Touch: The Guide to New Body-Centered Therapies*, edited by C. Calswell, Wheaton, IL: Quest Books, 1997.

Simon, R. "Listening Hands: The Healing Power of Touch." *Family Therapy Networker* 21, no. 5 (1997):62–73.

Weil, A. *Spontaneous Healing*. New York: Alfred A. Knopf, 1995.

Werblin, J. M. "Sing the Body Electric." *Changes* 10, no. 3 (1995): 30–35.*

* Asterisks indicate availability from the Rubenfeld Synergy Center.

ABOUT THE AUTHOR

Ilana Rubenfeld, a pioneer in integrating bodywork with psychotherapy, has been an influential healer for the past 35 years. Ilana originated the Rubenfeld Synergy Method in the early 1960s and started its professional training program in 1977. Formerly on the faculties of the NYU Graduate School of Social Work and New School for Social Research, she currently teaches at the Omega and Esalen institutes and the Open Center.

Author, humorist, and musician, she has conducted thousands of workshops. She was awarded the 1994 Pathfinder Award by the Association of Humanistic Psychology for outstanding and innovative contributions to the field of humanistic psychology.

Stanley Krippner, Ph.D

35 Shamanism and Healing: *New Light on the Oldest Profession*

WHAT IS SHAMANISM?

The label "shamanism" refers to a body of techniques and practices used to obtain power and knowledge for healing purposes by interacting with "spirit guides," "power animals," "forces of nature," and/or "ancestral entities." To qualify as a shaman, one must voluntarily enter what Harner (1988) calls a "shamanic state of consciousness" using such technologies as drumming, dancing, dreaming, and drugs (what have become, in the English language, the "four Ds of shamanism").

Shamans were the world's first tricksters and magicians, as well as humankind's initial storytellers, healers, psychotherapists, weather forecasters, and performing artists. In other words, shamanism is the world's oldest profession. Personally, I only use the term shaman to refer to socially sanctioned practitioners who bring back power and knowledge from what Kalweit (1988) calls an "alternative domain of consciousness," using this material for beneficial purposes. This is contrasted with priests and priestesses, who may lead rituals but rarely enter altered states: Mediums and spiritualists may enter altered states but rarely exert the control of which the shaman is capable. Sorcerers may enter altered states and exert a degree of control, but they are devoted to the interests of individual clients, not the community as a whole.

In psychological terms, shamans self-regulate their attention, accessing information not ordinarily available to their peers, using it for the benefit of the group that conferred and maintains their social role. The practitioner works for the well being of his or her community and its members by delivering spiritually oriented services that other people are unable to provide (Heinze, 1991; Walsh, 1990).

The shamanic model of healing resembles Western medicine and psychotherapy in many ways, but it also differs from the allopathic model (the currently accepted medical practice in the United States) in that it involves an affinity with the well-being of nature, of one's body, and of the community's spiritual growth. Moreover, shamanic healing encourages people to make life decisions in a way that reflects the ideals of harmony and knowledge. Shamanic models represent a structured and thoughtful approach to healing that attempts to mend the torn fabric of a person's (or a community's) connection with the earth, as well as the splits that frequently occur between the individual and the social group, or between the spiritual and the secular. As a result, shamanism is used for conditions that Western psychotherapy would label depression, alienation, anxiety, irritability, or mind/body ailments, as well as addictive and posttraumatic stress problems.

HOW IT BEGAN

Shamanic practices date back some 35,000 years and seem to have been ubiquitous in the early hunting, gathering, and fishing societies around the globe. In the cultural myths of these tribal societies, there are accounts of three zones: the Upper World, the Middle Earth, and the Lower World. In these societies' Golden Ages, it was said that people traveled between these worlds with ease; there was no rigid division between wakefulness and dreams. If someone could imagine or dream an event, that action was considered to be, in some sense, "real." These cultural myths held that a "fall" took place, triggered by a sin or an arrogant act. The bridge connecting these three zones collapsed; travel between the Middle Earth and the Upper and Lower Worlds became the nearexclusive privilege of deities, spirits, and shamans. Other cultural myths tell of an original Great Shaman, one selected by the deities and possessing incredible powers. The Great Shaman was supposed to have been capable of levitation, flying, and bodily transformation or "shape-shifting." These feats were rarely repeated by later shamans, supposedly because human behavior had evoked divine displeasure. Using illusion and sleight of hand, many later shamans attempted to duplicate the feats of the Great Shaman.

Western anthropologists have commented that second only to the diversity of approaches to health, healing, and sickness around the world are the resemblances of these approaches. Despite diverse languages, cultures, and concepts about the nature of reality, spirituality, humanity, and the human body, there are some remarkable similarities in how both traditional healing practices and allopathic biomedical practices approach wellness and illness. Even though there are relatively few bona fide shamans in the world today, there are still aspects of their legacy worthy of study.

The psychology of shamanism is a growing field as is evidenced by the acceptance of symposia on the topic at the 1987, 1991, and 1994 conventions of the American Psychological Association, the creation of the Society for the Anthropology of Consciousness (a division of the American Anthropological Association), and the publication of a popular magazine called *Shaman's Drum*.

HOW IT WORKS

Over the years, I have visited several indigenous shamans and shamanic healers (of approximately equal gender distribution), principally in North and South America, and have adapted two models to study and explain their healing practices from a Western perspective. The first model was developed by Siegler and Osmond (1974). I have used it to compare and contrast Pima Indian shamanic treatments with Western allopathic treatments, concluding that the flexibility of the Piman model was apparent during the tribe's first confrontations with Europeans (Krippner, 1995.) When it was observed that the newcomers violated sacred objects without dire consequences, the Pima Indians concluded that the Europeans had their own deities and restrictions, hence were not affected by the Piman ordinances. Later, when Piman shamans were told about germs and communicable diseases, they simply subsumed this knowledge under their category of "wandering sicknesses" in which invisible forces "wander" through the body, leaving afflictions in their wake. This flexibility and eclectic stance is characteristic of shamanism generally and may be a principle reason for its purported effectiveness over millennia.

My second model for studying the possible effectiveness of shamanic healing is based on the work of Torrey (1986). Torrey surveyed numerous indigenous psychotherapists. He holds that the nature of any effective treatment, whether conducted by shamans or other practitioners, inevitably reflects one or more of four fundamental principles. Each of Torrey's categories accurately describes my own encounters with shamans:

1. *A shared world view.* The naming process is one of the most important components of all types of treatment. Reaching an agreement on the name of a client's condition is persuasive in convincing the client that someone understands the condition, that he or she is not the only one who has ever had the condition, and that there is a way to get well. The identification of the offending factor may activate a series of associated ideas in the client's belief system producing contemplation, absolution, and general catharsis.

   Depending on the culture, illness is thought to be caused by one or more of three factors: biological events, experiential events, and metaphysical events. The third, downgraded by allopathic medicine, is the very foundation of many other traditions. Not only must the ailment be named, but the diagnosis must reflect the shared world view of the practitioner and client in order to be maximally effective. There is no North American equivalent for *wagamama*, an emotional disorder reported in some parts of Japan that is characterized by childish behavior, emotional outbursts, apathy, and negativity. Nor is there a counterpart to *susto*, a "loss of soul" in certain parts of Latin America thought to be caused by a shock or fright, often connected with breaking a metaphysical precept, with a sorcerer's curse, or with a physical accident. Even within a specific culture, there can be different world views that interfere with treatment, e.g., between upper-class practitioners and lower-class clients, between practitioners whose gender or ethnic backgrounds differ from their clients.

2. *The practitioner's personal qualities.* Rogers (1982) points out that "the shaman may often be a superior individual, in relation to the people of his [or her] community." The shaman's imaginative resources have been emphasized by Achterberg (1985) who considers dreams and visions a source of vital information on human health and sickness.

   Among a shamanic society's symbols and metaphors is that of the "wounded healer," i.e., if a potential shaman has overcome a personal tragedy, sickness, or debilitating condition, his or her community often will bestow respect and deference for this impressive feat.

   There is a consensus among healers, psychotherapists, and medical doctors that some practitioners have personality characteristics that are therapeutic while others do not. Not only are the actual personal qualities of the practitioners important, but those projected onto them by the client are crucial. This process of projection often is termed "transference" by psychotherapists and can be a salient factor in a treatment's success.

Personal qualities that foster recovery from sickness may differ from culture to culture. The shamanic claim to communicate with "spirits," respected by members of their own tribes, would be considered deviant in most Western cultures. However, Boyer, Klopfer, Brawer, and Kawai (1964) reported that Apache shamans received higher scores on tests of mental health than the average members of their society.

3. *Positive client expectations*: There is abundant evidence from many studies that demonstrate the importance of client expectancy; what a person expects to happen in healing often will happen if the expectations are strong enough. Such remedies as lizard blood and swine teeth have no known medicinal property, but if they have worked over the centuries, it is because patients expected them to work. Frank and Frank (1991) conclude that the state of mind conducive to healing depends on a practitioner's ability to "arouse the patient's hope, bolster his [or her] self-esteem, stir him [or her] emotionally, and strengthen his [or her] ties with a supportive group." As a result, efforts to heighten the patient's positive expectations may be as genuinely therapeutic as specific therapeutic techniques. Torrey (1986) has identified several factors that produce client expectations — hope, faith, trust, and emotional arousal. Frank and Frank (1991) have noted that most psychotherapies use emotional arousal as part of the treatment, either at the beginning of therapy, followed by systematic reinforcement of newly developed skills and attitudes, or in the latter parts of therapy, crystallizing gains of the preceding therapeutic sessions.

4. *A sense of mastery*: Frank and Frank (1991) claim that the heightening of the patient's sense of mastery is a direct or indirect effect of all successful therapies. Shamans have used a variety of methods to empower their clients, e.g., pronouncing incantations, singing sacred songs, carrying out symbolic ritual acts, appearing to remove disease-causing objects from the body, placating appeasing spirits, interpreting dreams, and administering herbal remedies (Rogers, 1982). The client's emerging sense of mastery equips him or her with knowledge that can be used to cope with life's adversities. The client may learn self-regulation, dietary and exercise

regimens, and other disease prevention techniques to prevent a recurrence of the ailment.

If there are psychological problems, the client may have learned the proper prayers to counteract malevolent "spirits," the healthy attitudes that counteract depression and anxiety, or the dream interpretation procedures that provide for personal empowerment. Each of these practices has the potential to bolster clients' sense of mastery and self-efficacy by providing them with a personal myth or conceptual scheme that explains deleterious symptoms, and supplies a ritualistic procedure for overcoming them. These myths and rituals combat demoralization by strengthening the therapeutic relationship, arousing hope, inspiring expectations of assistance, and affording opportunities for rehearsal and practice (Feinstein and Krippner, 1997).

Learning and mastery are important components for both "curing" (removing the symptoms of an ailment and restoring a client to health) and "healing" (attaining wholeness of body, mind, emotions, and/or spirit). Some clients might be incapable of being cured because their illness is terminal. Yet those same clients could be healed mentally, emotionally, and/or spiritually as a result of being guided by the practitioner in a review of their life, finding meaning in it, and becoming reconciled to death. Clients who have been "cured," on the other hand, may learn procedures that will prevent a relapse or recurrence of their symptoms.

WHAT THE RESEARCH SHOWS

For many centuries, Western investigators had little respect or regard for shamanic healing, for native rituals, or for altered states of consciousness. In recent years, however, such prominent psychotherapists as Achterberg (1985), Frank and Frank (1991), and Torrey (1986) have found many native practices to contain elements instructive for Western practitioners, including the use of imagination and altered states of consciousness for health maintenance and personal growth.

Kleinman (1985) observed that Taiwanese shamans were most successful when dealing with what Westerners would term acute, self-limited sicknesses, secondary somatic manifestations of psychological disorders, and chronic ailments that were not life-threatening; Finkler (1985) observed that diarrhea, simple gynecological disorders, somatic manifestations, and psychological disorders were most amenable to treatment by Mexican spiritualists. In her description of Malay shamanism, Laderman (1991) describes how practitioners use ritual, dialogue, and music to provide intense personal experiences that mobilize the immune system. Thong (1993) published a collection of case histories of Balinese clients successfully treated by shamans for mental health problems. Torrey (1986) stated that the shamans he observed appeared to have an approximately equal rate of success as that found in the psychotherapeutic literature. He concluded that "many of them are effective psychotherapists and produce therapeutic change in their clients."

REAL PEOPLE AND SHAMANISM

As examples of people who have visited shamans, I have selected two individuals, both living in Nevada, who were helped to overcome substance abuse by Native American "medicine people."

In 1979, I visited Rolling Thunder, a Cherokee-Shoshone shaman living in a healing community named Meta Tantey ("go in peace") in Carlin, Nevada. He introduced me to William, a 25-year-old man who had sought treatment for his alcoholism. Rolling Thunder had placed William on a "cleansing diet" for three months, supplemented by herbal medicines and community support.

That evening, I participated in a healing ceremony that had been arranged for William. For ninety minutes, the more than fifty members of Meta Tantey sang and chanted to the accompaniment of drums. When the drumming stopped, Rolling Thunder introduced me to the group, asking me to give William my personal support. I did this by means of a short guided imagery session reinforcing his desire to abstain from alcohol, the substance that had come close to destroying his life.

After I rejoined the circle, Rolling Thunder stepped forward. Resplendent in a white buckskin suit and a feather headdress, the shaman asked the group members if they had heard the hooting of an owl during my guided imagery session. Various people nodded their heads affirmatively, and Rolling Thunder commented that the owl is a symbol of death or transformation, so William was engaged in a life or death struggle with alcohol.

Rolling Thunder then remarked that the owl had hooted seven times and that seven is a lucky number. On this encouraging note, the shaman began to probe William's body with an eagle feather. When he found a spot which was especially sensitive, Rolling Thunder cupped the area with his hands and seemed to suck a dark fluid from William's body, spitting it into a pail. At the end of the session, Rolling Thunder gave instructions to an assistant to bury the contents of the pail in a remote area.

William was now "purified" and slept soundly that night. The next morning he gave a positive report and, with tears in his eyes, thanked Rolling Thunder and the community members. The following month he left Meta Tantey and, two years later, let Rolling Thunder know that he was still sober.

Stella, in her late thirties when she first contacted a shaman, had tried any number of therapeutic programs for cocaine addiction, a habit she had wrestled with since the age of eighteen. I put her in touch with Fawn Journeyhawk-Bender, a Metis Indian shaman living in Carson City, Nevada where she has created an intertribal healing ranch. Stella's initial regimen involved purification through sweat lodge sessions, an individually tailored diet, and various chants and prayers. After she had been living on Journeyhawk-Bender's healing ranch for two weeks, the community gathered around a campfire while the shaman "journeyed" to the spirit world on Stella's behalf. While there, Journeyhawk-Bender met the "spirit of cocaine" that had "stolen" Stella's soul.

Journeyhawk-Bender tried to cajole this frightening spirit, who took the appearance of a seductive and beautiful, but terribly evil, woman. The "cocaine spirit" insisted that she now owned Stella's soul, and that Stella needed to consume cocaine daily to satisfy both of them. At this point, Journeyhawk-Bender engaged in combat with the cocaine spirit. The group that was present told me of screams, expletives, strange smells, and frightening grimaces on the faces of both Journeyhawk-Bender and Stella.

After about twenty minutes, Stella appeared to pass out.

Journeyhawk-Bender regained her composure, announcing that she had been victorious in her struggle and that Stella's soul had been returned. Indeed, after sleeping around the clock, Stella felt a renewal of energy and a cheerful mood that she had not experienced since her teenage years. Three years later, Stella had not returned to cocaine or any other addictive drug, and felt that Journeyhawk-Bender's "soul recovery" treatment had been effective.

The following case is described in Ingerman (1991):

Edward, a carpenter, sought help from a shamanic healer, Sandra Ingerman, trained by anthropologist Michael Harner. Edward revealed that he had never felt comfortable at any location where he had lived. As a result, he had moved many times, always feeling unsettled and speculating about other places he could go. Ingerman began a "soul retrieval" journey on his behalf, setting her intention to travel wherever she needed to go to retrieve any part of the soul that had "wandered" or been "lost," making it difficult for Edward to feel at home.

Ingerman followed the sound of the beating drum, finding herself at a house near a beach. She passed through the hallway into a cheerful yellow kitchen, seeing Edward at play in the back yard pitching his tent. He appeared to be about nine years of age. Approaching the younger Edward, Ingerman explained that she was sent to bring him home. The younger Edward protested, "But I am at home." Ingerman told him that time had moved on. He was no longer a boy of nine but a man of forty-three. The younger Edward broke into tears. "But I love this place, please don't make me leave."

Ingerman asked the younger Edward where his parents were, and was told that they had moved. "But they can't make me move from here," the younger Edward insisted, revealing that part of the soul that had never left this happy boyhood home. Ingerman conveyed the importance of joining the adult Edward and that, until there was a reunion, neither would truly be happy.

The younger Edward reflected, "Edward really wants me back, does he?" Ingerman assured him that this was the case, and the younger Edward asked how to get back. Ingerman placed his hand in hers and together they waved goodbye to the childhood house, returning to ordinary reality.

When Ingerman shared her journey with Edward, he told her that his father was transferred when he was nine. As a boy, he hated leaving the only home he had ever known. He was sure a part of his soul had stayed at the one home he had truly loved. This soul retrieval exercise was the critical factor in instigating a new sense of security and rootedness into Edward's life.

WHAT TO EXPECT

In shamanic systems of healing, body and mind are seen as a unity, hence there is no sharp division between "physical" and "mental" illness (Frank and Frank, 1991). Pain and other symptoms are viewed as sources of information that can be used in diagnosis, as are the client's dreams, "aura" or "energy field," and unusual life events. As a result, Westerners who visit shamans and shamanic healers might expect to be asked about their dreams, their past medical history, and misfortunes where sorcery or witchcraft might have been at work. The shaman may explore the client's "energy field" in several ways, staring at the client's body, smelling the client's breath, and even tasting the clients' feces and urine.

Treatment procedures used by shamans and shamanic healers vary, but may include suggestions regarding diet, exercise, herbs, relaxation, mental imagery, prayers, purifications, and various rituals (Villoldo and Krippner, 1987). Specific treatment procedures depend upon the diagnosis and the cultural traditions. In many shamanic societies, serious illnesses are felt to be due to the loss of one's soul. A diagnosis of "soul loss" will be accompanied by an attempt to determine whether it has been stolen, "spooked" away from the body, or has simply "strayed" during some other activity (Ingerman, 1991; Kleinman,

1995). Treatment will aim to recover the soul through "soul catching" or similar procedures. The client might be provided with such "power objects" as crystals, feathers, or stones, along with directions as to how to perform a healing ritual to keep the soul from meandering in the future.

Some Western clients are surprised when a shamanic healer prescribes vitamins or recommends a visit to an osteopath. However, shamanism is basically an open-ended system that can be modified, altered, revised, or changed due to the demands of historical circumstances and community requirements. There are shamanic methods of healing that closely parallel contemporary behavior therapy, hypnotherapy, family therapy, milieu therapy, psychodrama, and dream interpretation. Torrey (1986) concludes that shamans and Western psychotherapists demonstrate more similarities than differences in regard to their healing practices.

Symbolic manipulation plays a major role in shamanic healing. The drum may serve as the vehicle with which the shaman "journeys" into the "spirit world." The blowing of smoke toward the four directions may represent an appeal to the "guardians" of the universe's "four quarters." For the shamans and their communities, any product of the imagination represents a form of "reality." As a result, mental imagery and imagination play an important role in shamanic healing, as when a Navajo client is seated on a sand painting or a Toba shaman "sucks" the poisons from a client's body (Achterberg, 1985; Noll, 1986).

The healing community is a part of most shamanic healing, and involves the client's family and friends. Katz (1981) sees rituals of transformation as the essential link in introducing "transpersonal bonding," which enables individuals to fulfill their communal responsibilities. Even when a client must be isolated as part of the healing process, this drastic procedure impresses the community with the gravity of the ailment.

It is typically necessary to bring a gift to a shaman; even if the shaman does not charge for his or her services, the gift is appreciated as a gesture of good will.

HOW TO FIND A PRACTITIONER

Because there is no organized professional association for shamans, I suggest that individuals rely on word of mouth, taking care that they do not become involved with practitioners who charge considerable amounts of money, or who try to manipulate them financially or sexually.

You can also contact the Foundation for Shamanic Studies (P.O. Box 1939, Mill Valley, CA 94942, http://www.shamanism.org) for referrals to reputable shamans. Michael Harner, the founder; his wife, Sandra Harner; and their associates at the Center for Shamanic Studies who run the training program in shamanic counseling, insure that their graduates will be able to assist their clients to receive help and guidance in "ordinary reality." However, one of the assumptions of the counseling service is that there are powerful entities in "nonordinary reality" who can be contacted by the shamanic counselors once they enter their "shamanic states of consciousness" and begin their "journey." The shamanic counselors who become "certified Shamanic Counselors" have been trained to use traditional shamanic skills to help their clients.

Shaman's Drum (P.O. Box 97, Ashland, OR, 95720) is a magazine that contains advertisements from legitimate shamans, some of them licensed counselors and psychologists who have gone through shamanic training and initiation (e.g., Leslie Gray, Ph.D., Larry G. Peters, Ph.D.). However, advertisements also appear for individuals whose credentials are dubious, not only in Western terms but in native circles as well. In the author's experience, the larger the required fee, the greater the possibility that the practitioner is an opportunist. Furthermore, potential clients should be wary of practitioners who demand that someone stop seeing a Western-oriented physician or psychotherapist.

Shamans enter their vocations in several ways, e.g., through heredity, through unusual birth conditions or markings, through "spirit" mediated recovery from illness, during vision quests, or in dreams. The training program for apprentice shamans varies from one part of the world to another, but typically lasts for several years. Usually the apprentices will learn their skills from master shamans who teach them nomenclature (e.g., the names and functions of deities, spirits, and power animals), history (e.g., the tribe's genealogy), technology (e.g., rituals, music, dances), herbology (e.g., the difference between plants used medicinally and those used for sacred purposes), the location of "power places," the identification of "power objects," dream interpretation procedures, and the tribe's mythology.

The apprentice also may obtain knowledge from his or her guiding spirits. These spiritual guides often take the form of a bird or animal, protecting the shamans as they enter potentially dangerous altered states of consciousness, and as they visit the Upper and Lower Worlds. The mastery of drumming, dancing, chanting, and singing often is an important aspect of a shaman's training.

RESOURCES

Articles on shamanism sometimes appear in such scholarly journals as the *American Ethnologist, Current Anthropology, Anthropology of Consciousness*, and *Ethos*. Annual international conferences on the study of shamanism have been sponsored since 1984 by the Independent Scholars of Asia (Suite 3A, 2321 Russell St., Berkeley, CA, 94705). There is an International Society for Shamanic Research; information about this society's Scientific Committee for the United States can be obtained from Ruth-Inge Heinze at the above address.

HOW TO LEARN MORE

Achterberg, J. *Imagery in Healing: Shamanism and Modern Medicine*. Boston: Shambhala, 1985.

Boyd, D. *Rolling Thunder*. New York: Random House, 1974.

Boyer, L. B.; B. Klopfer; F. B. Brawer; and H. Kawai. "Comparisons of the Shamans and Pseudoshamans of the Apaches of the Mescalero Indian Reservation: A Rorschach Study." *Journal of Projective Techniques* 28 (1964): 173–180.

Eliade, M. *Shamanism: Archaic Techniques of Ecstasy*. Princeton: Princeton University Press, 1964.

Estrada, A. *Maria Sabina: Her Life and Chants*. Santa Barbara, CA: Ross-Erickson, 1981.

Feinstein, D. and S. Krippner. *The Mythic Path*. New York: Tarcher/Putnam, 1997.

Finkler, K. *Spiritualist Healers in Mexico: Successes and Failures of Alternative Therapeutics*. New York: Praeger, 1985.

Flaherty, G. *Shamanism and the Eighteenth Century*. Princeton: Princeton University Press, 1992.

Frank, J. D. and J. B. Frank. *Persuasion and Healing*. Third Edition. Baltimore: Johns Hopkins University Press, 1991.

Harner, M. "Shamanic Counseling." In *Shaman's Path*, edited by G. Doore, Boston: Shambhala, 1988.

Heinze, R. I. "Shamans or Mediums: Toward a Definition of Different States of Consciousness." *Phoenix: Journal of Transpersonal Anthropology* 6 (1982): 25–44.

Heinze, R. I.. *Shamans of the 20th Century*. New York: Irvington, 1991.

Ingerman, S. *Soul Retrieval: Mending the Fragmented Self*. New York: Harper-SanFrancisco, 1991.

Kalweit, H. *Dreamtime and Inner Space*. Boston: Shambhala, 1988.

Kleinman, A. *Patients and Healers in the Context Of Culture.* Berkeley: University of California Press, 1985.

Kleinman, A. *Writing at the Margin: Discourse Between Anthropology and Medicine.* Berkeley: University of California Press, 1995.

Krippner, S. "Tribal Shamans and their Travels into Dreamtime." In *Dreamtime and Dreamwork,* edited by S. Krippner, Los Angeles: Jeremy P. Tarcher, 1990.

Krippner, S. "A Cross-cultural Healing Comparison of Four Healing Models." *Alternative Therapies* 1 (1995): 21–29.

Krippner, S. and P. Welch. *Spiritual Dimensions of Healing: From Tribal Shamanism to Contemporary Health Care.* New York: Irvington, 1992.

Laderman, C. *Taming the Winds of Desire: Psychology, Medicine, and Aesthetics in Malay Shamanistic Performance.* Berkeley: University of California Press, 1991.

Rogers, S. L. *The Shaman: His Symbols and His Healing Power.* Springfield, IL: Charles C. Thomas, 1982.

Siegler, R. and H. Osmond. *Models of Madness, Models of Medicine.* New York: Macmillan, 1974.

Thong, D., with B. Carpenter, and S. Krippner. *A Psychiatrist in Paradise: Treating Mental Illness in Bali.* Bangkok: White Lotus Press, 1993.

Torrey, E. F. *Witchdoctors and Psychiatrists: The Common Roots of Psychotherapy and Its Future.* New York: Harper & Row, 1986.

Villoldo, A. and S. Krippner. *Healing States.* New York: Fireside/Simon & Schuster, 1987.

Walsh, R. *The Spirit of Shamanism.* Los Angeles: Jeremy P. Tarcher, 1990.

Weil, A. *Health and Healing.* New York: E. P. Dutton, 1983.

Winkelman, M. *Shamans, Priests and Witches: A Cross-Cultural Study Of Magic-Religious Practitioners.* Tempe, AZ: University of Arizona Press, 1992.

ABOUT THE AUTHOR

Stanley Krippner, Ph.D., is professor of psychology at the Saybrook Institute Graduate School in San Francisco. He is the co-author of several books including *The Mythic Path* and *Spiritual Dimensions of Healing: From Tribal Shamanism to Contemporary Health Care* and the editor of *Dreamtime and Dreamwork.* He is a member of the editorial board of *Alternative Therapies in Health and Medicine* and the editorial advisory board of *Shaman's Drum.* He has visited shamans in Asia, Africa, Europe, North America, and South America.

by Lynette Bassman, Ph.D.

---

36 Sound Therapy:
*Healing with Sound and Music —
An interview with Don Campbell*

WHAT IS SOUND THERAPY?

Sound therapy, also called psycho-physio acoustics, or the Mozart Effect, involves working with the effects of sound and music on the mind, the body, the emotions, and the spirit. Music has the power to reach multiple systems in the mind and body simultaneously, and to move these systems toward wholeness and balance. Sound therapy is helpful for treating a large number of emotional problems, including abuse; accident recovery, pain, Alzheimer's disease, attention deficit disorder, alcoholism, co-dependence, anxiety, schizophrenia, and some forms of depression.

The principles of healing with sound and music are utilized today by psychotherapists, nurses, doctors, and psychologists. (See Chapter 10 and Chapter 13 for more information about music therapy.) There are also practitioners of imagery techniques who integrate music with insight-oriented therapy. The principles of healing with sound and music can also be practiced on one's own. This chapter will focus on self-generated healing with sound and music.

HOW IT BEGAN

Music is basic to religious experience and to many ancient healing arts. Examples include the tarantella dances, David and the harp in the Bible, and the drumming so common to many ancient cultures. In more recent times, Bach's "Goldberg Variations" were commissioned to help someone who had insomnia. The therapeutic use of sound and music has been a part of many cultures throughout history, but so far not much attention has been given to auditory stimulus as health care.

Campbell's interest stems from several powerful healing experiences that he has had with sound. He was classically trained in music in France, and then lived in Japan and Haiti, where he observed firsthand the ritual use of drumming, singing, and dancing as ways of inducing altered states of consciousness for healing. So when he was diagnosed with asthma, which caused life-threatening attacks upon exposure to environmental pollutants in smog-filled Tokyo, where he then lived, he placed himself in the care of a Manchurian doctor. That doctor used hands-on healing techniques that he said would "put the missing tones" back in Campbell's body. Within two months, the attacks stopped and never returned.

Ten years later, Campbell developed a degenerative bone condition and a lump in his left lung. He recalls that he was very depressed, and no longer enjoyed music and art as he once did. One day, while reflecting on his condition, he remembered his experiences in Japan and Haiti, where he learned that sound has the power to transform and heal. He spontaneously began to chant and to tone, until he arrived at one particular tone that felt right. He held that tone for many hours, and felt it "massage him from the inside out." He also listened to certain powerful pieces of music as he continued toning. This experience left him feeling whole and complete in a way that he says was difficult to describe. The illness was healed and has never recurred.

Since that time, he has worked at integrating his classical music training with what he now knows to be the miraculous self-healing aspects of sound. He founded the Institute for Music, Health, and Education as a center for training, education, and research on the healing properties of sound.

HOW IT WORKS

The primary functions of the ear are balance and hearing. Our ears organize far more than just auditory input. The harmonics and rhythms of music affect our emotions. This creates responses in various parts of the brain, including the limbic system (which controls the emotions, among other things), the vestibular system (which controls balance), and the reptilian or hindbrain (which controls the basic rhythms of the body including breath, heartbeat, and respiration). In the neocortex of the brain, we experience the melodies, the meanings, and memories that music evokes within us.

We know that music organizes time and space very efficiently. Music can repattern and recode the body's emotional chemistry. So rather than a quick fix, music and deep listening can transform the whole mind/body awareness.

Following are four categories of healing with sound, with brief descriptions of how they are practiced:

1. *Focused listening.* The ability for music to be central and healing depends upon each individual and how he or she listens. Listening is different than hearing in the sense that, in listening, more focused attention is given to the effects of the music on the body and the mind. How one receives the music is as important as the music itself. An important part of mind/body healing work is taking responsibility for one's own experience and learning to orchestrate it.

   You can begin to introduce music into your life on a daily basis and become attentive to the different effects it has on you. If you are tired at the end of the day, your experience of the music will be very different than if you are fresh and well-rested. We listen differently when we lie down, when we close our eyes, when we sit up, when we are moving, or when we are speaking with someone else.

   Campbell and his colleagues have found that Mozart's music is a safe choice for achieving healthful emotional effects such as stress reduction, increased concentration, and general refreshment. Slower music by Baroque composers such as Vivaldi, Corelli, Pachelbel, Telemann, Handel, and Bach also has very positive effects. Usually vocal music is not used because it has too much of an emotional charge. New Age ambient music such as Campbell's album "Essence" and the music of Brian Eno and Steven Halpern all create a background environment that gives a greater sense of space and unhurried time. It is very healthy for relaxation and for lowering the blood pressure, but may, at times, increase pain perception, so it is not the right music for people in physical pain.

   Some music can serve as a stimulant that helps us stay charged, motivated. This includes many forms of popular music like that of Mannheim Steamroller and Fresh Aire, and some forms of jazz and pop music.

2. *Toning and humming.* Toning is the elongated use of vowels without melody or rhythm. It is a fairly continuous, light, relaxed sound created

with a relaxed jaw. Humming is very similar but doesn't have a vowel sound, because the lips are closed.

The voice is our most useful tool to release stress, balance our brain waves, and actually massage our bodies from the inside out. Lower "aaa" sounds allow the body immediately to begin to relax. A higher, elongated "eee" sound will charge your brain and wake you up.

People can begin with three or four minutes of toning a day. This can even be done while driving a car. There is no wrong way to do it. After four or five breaths, your breathing will naturally deepen. It helps to imagine that you are letting your voice rid yourself of all the stress of the day. Soon you will feel a sense of great well-being, sending the message to the body that all things are well.

Campbell's book *Roar of Silence* (1989) is a seven-week course in toning. There are also a number of tapes that help people get started with a program of toning.

3. *Participation in musical events, both vocal and instrumental:* This includes participating in bands, choirs, or picking up an instrument. For some people who do not play instruments it may mean taking fifteen minutes a day as a sound break, simply by sitting down and enjoying music. Chapter 6 of Campbell's book *Rhythms of Learning* (1991) is all about how to take sound breaks, including giving yourself a lift in the afternoon or relaxing yourself before going to bed. This can take as little as three minutes at a time and has a big impact when practiced regularly.

4. *The use of imagery in music:* The simultaneous use of music and image allows one to move deeper into the unconscious mind/body systems. The most common type is guided imagery, where the imagination is enhanced and the listener can learn to regulate different parts of his or her body by being guided with music. The music allows us to hold our attention on an issue for a much longer period of time. It allows our inner pace to be better regulated. Another use of guided imagery with music allows the person to enter into a lucid dreamlike state where he or she actually begins to receive symbols, impressions, and memories from his or her own body. Imagery allows one to realize there are always unconscious messages ready to appear. Music becomes the vessel that will hold those images for long periods of time so we can begin to learn what our bodies are telling us. The

work of Helen Bonny has been quite prominent in this area. (Please see Chapter 10 for more information on the Bonny Method of Guided Imagery and Music.)

Music is a self-healing device, but it helps if someone else acts as an orchestra conductor while you learn how to play your instrument. The majority of guided imagery work is done in group or one-on-one settings. Often the imagery guide can help you rehearse for situations that you may face in the future. At other times, the work helps you go back to traumas or difficulties from the past and release them from the unconscious.

Music is also an effective aid to meditation. Music holds the thread of the experience together and helps us induce in ourselves feelings of relaxation and well-being. There are many good tapes and books that serve as introductions to different forms of imagery and music.

WHAT THE RESEARCH SHOWS

Campbell has worked with nearly 3,000 students in toning and has found that it allows the body to find its own balance. Within five minutes, the brain waves are balanced, the respiration slows down, body temperature increases, and stress is released. "This is the most effective, simple way for people to center and bring their mind and their body into balance," says Campbell. "And it costs nothing."

Students Campbell has taught over an eight-year period have kept journals. The results are very impressive, he states, but difficult to measure. The problem with doing research on music and sounding is that it affects so many systems simultaneously. In addition, it has different effects on different people and at different times. For example, if a person is in a state of high emotional stress, it will calm them, and if they are depressed, the toning will help charge their body and relieve them. For a given individual, on some days the toning will primarily produce imagery, while on other days the experience is very emotional, or relaxing. "Our amazing bodies do what they need to do through a toning experience," says Campbell.

Dr. Alfred Tomatis is a prominent researcher in France who studies the effects of sound therapy on learning disabilities. In over 100,000 case studies, he has learned that charging the right ear with certain kinds of high frequency sounds allows attentiveness, memory, and communication to improve significantly (Tomatis, 1996, 1991). A French doctor named Berard (1993) cites over

200 cases in which he states that over 93 percent were cured of depression through auditory stimulation.

Campbell (1997) reports that coronary patients who listened to classical music under controlled research conditions reported a happier emotional state, as well as improvements in their cardiac health. Details of these studies and many others can be found in Campbell's book *The Mozart Effect* (1997).

REAL PEOPLE AND SOUND THERAPY

Jack, a 52-year-old salesman, had taken years of psychotherapy and medication in an effort to recover from severe depression dating back twenty years. He worked with Campbell and learned toning. Campbell suggested that Jack hum a long tone for five minutes in the morning and then again in the evening. At first, he was resistant to the idea. Then, suddenly, after trying it he began to see the value of doing this. He used an "ahh" tone to rid himself of tension, "eee" tones to give him energy, and "oooh" tones to increase his ability to concentrate. After three years of this practice, he was able to stop taking medication and only needs periodic maintenance visits with his psychiatrist to talk about issues that arise.

Carl is a recovering substance abuser. His wife was divorcing him. He was suffering from depression, and felt that he needed to work on unresolved issues from childhood. He was in psychotherapy, and anger and fear were emerging in the sessions. He began toning, and found that certain tones helped him to deal with these feelings. He also found that the toning facilitated the meditation he was doing, in conjunction with his work on the eleventh step of Alcoholics Anonymous. Within a few months, the depression had lifted.

Olga is a middle-aged psychotherapist with years of personal psychotherapy experience and training in the insight process. When she had been humming regularly for six weeks, she recovered a repressed memory of being in a bomb shelter in Germany when she was young. She felt a new sense of freedom, and the headaches from which she had suffered for years completely vanished.

∽

HOW TO FIND A PRACTITIONER

As detailed above, much of the health benefit of sound can be derived through self-help techniques. For referrals to practitioners who make use of the principles described here, and to inquire about publications, tapes, workshops, and other educational opportunities, contact the following resources:

THE AMERICAN MUSIC
THERAPY ASSOCIATION
8455 Colesville Rd., Suite 930
Silver Spring, MD 20910
Tel: (301) 589-3300

OPEN EAR JOURNAL
6717 NE Marshall Rd.
Bainbridge Island, WA 98110
Tel: (206) 842-5560

SOUND LISTENING AND
LEARNING CENTER, TOMATIS USA
Billy Thompson, Ph.D., Director
2701 East Camelback, Suite 205
Phoenix, AZ 85016
Tel: (602) 381-0086

HOW TO LEARN MORE

Berard, G. *Hearing Equals Behavior.* New Canaan, CT: Keats Publishers, 1993.

Campbell, D. *The Mozart Effect.* New York: Avon Books, 1997.

Campbell, D. *Music and Miracles.* Wheaton, IL: Quest Books, 1992.

Campbell, D. *Music: Physician for Times to Come.* Wheaton, IL: Quest Books, 1991.

Campbell, D. *The Roar of Silence.* Wheaton, IL: Quest Books, 1989.

Campbell, D. and C. Brewer. *Rhythms of Learning.* Phoenix, AZ: Zephyr, 1991.

Tomatis, A. *The Conscious Ear.* Barrytown, NY: Station Hill Publishers, 1991.

Tomatis, A. *The Ear and Language.* Norval, ON, Canada: Moulin Publishers, 1996.

ABOUT THE AUTHOR

A native of Texas, Don Campbell began his classical musical training at the Fontainebleau Conservatory of Music in France. He later was named outstanding graduate in music education from North Texas State University and continued advanced study at the University of Cincinnati College Conservatory of Music.

Campbell is the author of seven books including *The Roar of Silence* (Quest Books), *Introduction to the Musical Brain* (Magna Books), *Music: Physician for Times to Come* (Quest Books), and *Music and Miracles* (Quest Books). He has contributed chapters to a number of other books as well. His CDs and audio cassettes include *Essence* (Spirit Music), *Healing Yourself With Your Own Voice* (Sounds True), and *The Power of Music* (Nightingale-Conant). He writes a column regularly for *Quest* magazine. He has appeared on over 100 television and radio shows.

Over the years, Campbell's devotion to sound and music has taken him to forty countries where he studied indigenous cultures, taught and worked with children and young adults, and gave his own performances. Campbell is at the center of a vast global network of musicians, scientists, therapists, and consumers who are using sound and music to manage their health and enhance their daily lives. He is the founder of the Institute for Music, Health, and Education, which is presently located in Minneapolis, MN.

Sally Blumenthal-McGannon, R.N., M.A.

37 Therapeutic Touch and Psychotherapy

WHAT IS THERAPEUTIC TOUCH?

Therapeutic Touch (TT) is a contemporary interpretation of several ancient healing practices. Practitioners use their hands to facilitate the healing process by moving them close to, but not actually touching, the client's body, and exchanging energy with the client in an intentional and focused way. In this energy exchange, the practitioner's state of consciousness and intention to help and heal are crucial. The essence of Therapeutic Touch is to enable others to help themselves become more whole.

This approach is effective with almost all clients. It can be helpful in dealing with loss and resolving old pain. It can help clients with marital difficulties and with AIDS. Therapeutic Touch is especially effective in dealing with depression. On an energetic level, people who are depressed have energy fields that are closed, in contrast to a healthy person's field that is constantly interacting with others and with the environment. For anyone who feels shut down, stuck, or depressed, Therapeutic Touch can expand their horizons. For anyone who feels a void, and fills it with too much alcohol, work, sex, food, shopping, or drugs, Therapeutic Touch is an effective tool for healing. Therapeutic Touch is compatible with the twelve-step philosophy. Anybody who comes from a dysfunctional family can benefit from Therapeutic Touch, and begin to feel whole and healed. People who are feeling burned out or who are co-dependent can also learn to feel good about themselves without always putting others first.

People with learning disorders benefit from the calming and "organizing" effect of Therapeutic Touch. Children who suffer from attention deficit disorder and hyperactivity have also been calmed with Therapeutic Touch. Being alone with someone (the TT practitioner) who is calm and centered can calm an agitated or hyperactive individual.

TT can be combined with psychotherapy and with hypnotherapy. It can be done in the last ten to fifteen minutes of the session, so clients are relaxed and feeling better when they leave. Or it can be used at the start of the session, if an individual is very anxious, to help them calm down while remaining open. Therapeutic Touch reinforces clients' own coping mechanisms. Journal writing is enhanced, dreams are often heightened and remembered. Clients' abilities to heal and take care of themselves are encouraged. Resistance is decreased when clients feel safe, as they seem to feel when Therapeutic Touch is part of their healing process. For people who are not comfortable being physically touched, Therapeutic Touch is a wonderful way to reach out on an energetic level. The client feels embraced without feeling invaded or frightened.

TT is not a substitute for medication, but can be used as an adjunct. Sometimes, with the addition of TT to the sessions, the client's own healing has been activated and their medication course is often shortened. Physicians who prescribe the medication frequently are impressed with the short-term use of medications by TT clients, compared to some of their other patients.

HOW IT BEGAN

Although contemporary use of TT is compatible with modern medicine and includes many innovative scientific processes discovered over recent years, its basic technique is as old as human history. These ancient healing practices have been referred to as the "laying on of hands." In some of the earliest cave dwellings, pictures of hands can be found in positions similar to those used in Therapeutic Touch. At the entrance to the Museum of Anthropology in Mexico City, Mexico, there is a mural depicting women from all cultures throughout time, with women on either end shown with powerful symbols emanating from their hands, indicating the use of the hands for healing.

The development of Therapeutic Touch was accomplished through the combined talents of Dora Kunz, a natural healer, and Dolores Krieger, a nurse with experience in meditation and teaching. Dora Kunz was born with a high sense of perception and the ability to see energy around all living things. She left home at age 12 to study with the well-known theosophist, C. W. Leadbeater, and has devoted her life to using her abilities to help and heal others. She has worked with physicians who have studied her diagnostic, and later her healing, effects on patients. Her early work with Dr. Shafica Karagulla is documented in the book, *Breakthrough to Creativity* (1967). Dolores Krieger studied theosophy, meditation, and nursing, and developed the first masters program in healing while at New York University. This program later expanded to offer a doctoral degree as well. Dora was able to teach Dolores how to feel what she could see and together they developed the healing meditation they named Therapeutic Touch. Therapeutic Touch is now taught in over 80 universities in 30 countries and is practiced by an estimated 20,000 professionals in the United States, Canada, and around the world.

HOW IT WORKS

The basic premise of Therapeutic Touch is that universal life energy sustains all living organisms. Life energy has some of the characteristics of a force field. This force field permeates space and is more concentrated in and around living organisms. Therapeutic Touch involves assessing and influencing the client's energy field from head to foot, by holding one's hands 10 to 15 centimeters away from the skin's surface and slowly moving the hands over the client's field.

There are five phases in Therapeutic Touch:

1. Centering. The practitioner becomes quiet. This stillness is a focused state of consciousness like meditation or prayer. Being centered allows the healer and the person being healed to resonate with each other which promotes self-healing within the patient/client.

2. Assessment/scanning. The hands are used to assess the patient's dynamic energy field.

3. Unruffling/clearing. The hands are used again, moving more vigorously from head to foot. This helps facilitate a rhythmic flow of energy in the patient's field.

4. Treatment/balancing. With intent, the practitioner directs energy to the patient, helping to restore order.

5. Evaluation. Treatment is ended and the patient is encouraged to give feedback and to rest. Resting allows the new energy to be integrated.

WHAT THE RESEARCH SHOWS

Harlow's (1958) research demonstrated the universal need for touch in animals. The same findings have been seen in infants. During World War II orphans that were fed and clothed, but left untouched in beds, due to lack of personnel, often died or developed what later became known as "failure to thrive." Nursing research has found Therapeutic Touch beneficial in a number of situations: relieving anxiety in hospitalized patients (Heidt, 1981; Parkes, 1986; Quinn, 1984 and 1989); enhancing spousal sharing and emotional support during childbirth, and aiding the mother in labor (Krieger, 1987); decreasing tension headache pain (Keller and Bzdek, 1986); decreasing premature infants' stress response (Fedoruk, 1985); facilitating personal growth (Sameral, 1992); helping patients to rest (Heidt, 1991); reducing stress in hospitalized children (Kramer, 1990); eliciting relaxation response (Payne, 1989); relieving stress after natural disasters (Olson et al., 1992); and increasing emotional openness (Heidt, 1990). There also have been a number of studies demonstrating the reduction of anxiety for people with physical illness (Heidt, 1981; Parkes, 1986; Quinn, 1984 and 1989).

Newshan (1989) concludes, Therapeutic Touch is a manifestation of compassion. It reaches beyond the physical body and its parts. It connects one with the underlying order of the universe. Therapeutic Touch is a skill that is invaluable in the care of the PWA (people living with AIDS) on many levels, whether to ease the transition in dying or to ease the discomforts in living. It lies at the heart of healing.

REAL PEOPLE AND THERAPEUTIC TOUCH

I once cared for a woman who was dying from abdominal cancer. She was so frightened of dying that she was afraid to go to sleep at night. (This is not an uncommon occurrence.) Each night I stayed with her, I would do TT for her, focusing on the pain in her abdomen. I sent energy to her highest self. One morning when she awoke she said, "Oh shit." I asked her what was wrong and she told me she didn't want to wake up. She was in such a wonderful place, she didn't want to come back. I smiled, said goodbye, and started to drive home when what she said hit me. I drove back and asked her again about what had happened. She thanked me for helping her get to a more peaceful place. I realized then that, even though I had worked on the pain in her belly, my energy, coming from my process of centering, went to her higher self, and she became more peaceful. She died peacefully a few days later.

Liz was married to a man with a life-threatening illness. Her 12-year-old son from a previous marriage needed help in dealing with the impending loss of his stepfather, as did the rest of the family. The stress escalated as Carlos got sicker. Their three-year-old son Martin tended to act out, accelerating everyone's breaking point. Doing Therapeutic Touch for Carlos helped with his symptoms, especially his pain. He could relax better after Therapeutic Touch, required less pain medication, and was more alert and able to interact with everyone after treatments. My office became the only place where all members would open up from time to time. It was a safe place for them to cry, to express themselves, and to recover. Frequently I would do TT for Liz to help her relax. This also made it easier for her to cry and to feel lighter as a result. It also helped her cope with her younger son's tantrums. It was terrifying to them to break through their denial about Carlos's impending death, but the fear of staying stuck prompted them to take risks. Even though it was painful and difficult, they always left feeling better. Carlos was able to die at home, peacefully, with his family around him. They have healed well. The children learned that death is part of life and can be dealt with most easily by being open and honest.

Sandy was referred to me for anxiety attacks. Although she was convinced they had a physical cause, after many visits to the medical clinic without any medical findings, she decided to follow up on her referral for therapy. She told me about her perfect life; her family was perfect, her fiance was the greatest, she loved her job, her future was bright. There was no reason for her to have any problems, especially this kind, she thought. As she sat on the couch, anxiously swinging her foot, she continued to tell me how healthy she was. She worked out fanatically, wasn't anorexic, but had a tendency to feel fat, while appearing obviously thin. She was planning to be married in several months but knew this was not related to her anxiety. Once she agreed that it was within the realm of possibility that she could be anxious about her wedding, she began to realize that perhaps she was a tiny bit anxious about some other things as well. As I did Therapeutic Touch for her, she sighed and sobbed uncontrollably. A lot of her fears, rational and others, came flooding out. I continued to see her for several months until she had gained real control over her concerns and had developed realistic plans to help her with upcoming events.

Jon and Nancy were in a crisis when they came to see me. He was ready to leave her and she was ready to kill him. They responded to the peaceful environment of my office, and visibly relaxed. They appreciated the freedom of being in a safe place where they could be honest, knowing that no one would get physically hurt. I asked them to practice deep breaths while looking at the trees outside my office window. As they started "doing their thing," and losing control, screaming and threatening each other, I would remind them to look at the trees, take a deep breath, and then say whatever they wanted to communicate. At the same time, I calmly sent peaceful energy to them, encouraging them to be strong and healthy. I can do this by taking a deep breath myself, and consciously projecting my field with calm and peaceful energy to the two of them. They learned fair fighting techniques, communication skills, and how to listen. I helped them to learn how to take better care of themselves and how to relax their bodies when they were tense and fighting. I encouraged them to teach their son how to calm down through breathing. This is empowering for all of them, and has created a task they can accomplish with visible results. I believe that the additional technique of changing the energy in the room allowed them to respond faster to the therapy.

Randy and Jeremy had been together for twenty-three years when they tested HIV positive. When Randy got sick, I was their main support person, both through a support group and then one-on-one counseling. Sometimes I would make house calls to do Therapeutic Touch for Randy, who felt so sick and weakened he couldn't get out of bed. Jeremy was very anxious and Therapeutic Touch helped him to relax so he could get some sleep when Randy was napping. They worried so much about each other that it was draining. I helped them to reframe their concerns and learn how to put energy into the way they wanted things to turn out, instead of what they feared.

∞

HOW TO FIND A THERAPEUTIC TOUCH PRACTITIONER

The Nurse Healers Professional Associates, Inc. is a not-for-profit cooperative of health care professionals for the promotion of healing, specifically committed to the practice of Therapeutic Touch. Although Therapeutic Touch practitioners are not licensed or certified, there is a curriculum that the cooperative recommends, based on the Kunz/Krieger method of TT as described in this chapter. For information about Therapeutic Touch practitioners, teachers, and other aspects of the work, contact:

NURSE HEALERS-PROFESSIONAL ASSOCIATES, INC.
1211 Locust St.
Philadelphia, PA 19107
Tel: (215) 545-8079

HOW TO LEARN MORE

Blumenthal-McGannon, S. "Laughing, Crying, Living, Dying, Surviving." An audio-
    tape of a presentation at the Annual Nurse-Healers Conference, Sacramento, CA.
    October, 1993. (Available through the Nurse Healers cooperative.)

Boelli, M. D., ed. *Therapeutic Touch: A Book of Readings.* New York; Springer, 1981.

Fedoruk, R. B. "Transfer of the Relaxation Response: Therapeutic Touch as a Method
    for Reduction of Stress in Premature Neonates." *Dissertation Abstracts Interna-
    tional* 46 (1985): 978B.

Harlow, H. "The Nature of Love." *The American Psychologist* 3 (1958): 673–685.

Heidt, P. R. "Openness: A Qualitative Analysis of Nurses' and Patients' Experience of Therapeutic Touch." *Image: Journal of Nursing Scholarship* 22, no. 3 (1990): 180–186.

Heidt, P. R. "Helping Patients to Rest: Clinical Studies in Therapeutic Touch." *Holistic Nurse Practitioner* 5, no. 4 (1991): 57–66.

Heidt, P. "Effects of Therapeutic Touch on the Anxiety Level of the Hospitalized Patients." *Nursing Research* 30, no. 1 (1981): 32–37.

Karagulla, S. *Breakthrough to Creativity: Your Higher Sense Perception.* Los Angeles: De Vorss, 1967.

Keller E. and V. M. Bzdek. "Effects of Therapeutic Touch on Tension Headache Pain." *Nursing Research* 35 (1986): 101–106.

Kramer, N. A. "Comparison of Therapeutic Touch and Casual Touch in Stress Reduction in Hospitalized Children." *Pediatric Nursing* 16 (1990): 483–485.

Krieger, D. *Accepting Your Power to Heal: The Personal Practice of Therapeutic Touch.* Santa Fe: Bear and Company, 1993.

Krieger, D. *Foundations for Holistic Health Nursing Practices.* Philadelphia: JP Lippincott, 1981.

Krieger, D. *Living the Therapeutic Touch: Healing as a Lifestyle.* New York; Mead & Co., 1987.

Krieger, D. *The Therapeutic Touch: How to Use Your Hands to Help or to Heal.* Englewood Cliffs, NJ: Prentice Hall, 1979.

Macrae, J. *Therapeutic Touch: A Practical Guide.* New York: Alfred Knopf, 1988.

Newshan, G. "Therapeutic Touch for Symptom Control in Persons with AIDS." *Holistic Nurse Practitioner* 3, no. 4 (1989): 45–51.

Olson, M.; N. Sneed; R. Bonadonna; J. Ratliff; and J. Dias. "Therapeutic Touch and Post Hurricane Hugo Stress." *Holistic Nursing* 10, no. 2 (1992): 120–136.

Parkes, B. S. "Therapeutic Touch as an Intervention to Reduce Anxiety in Elderly Hospitalized Patients." *Dissertation Abstracts International* 47 (1986): University Microfilms # 9609563.

Payne, M. B. "The Use of Therapeutic Touch with Rehabilitation Patients." *Rehabilitation Nursing* 14, no. 2 (1989): 69–72.

Quinn, J. F. "Therapeutic Touch as Energy Exchange. Replication and Extension." Nursing *Science Quarterly* 2, no. 2 (1989): 79–87.

Quinn, J. F. "Therapeutic Touch as Energy Exchange: Testing the Theory." *Advanced Nursing Science* 62, no. 2 (1984): 29–42.

Sameral, J. "The Experience of Receiving Therapeutic Touch." *Advances in Nursing* 6 (1992): 651–657.

Additional bibliographic information about Therapeutic Touch is available in many libraries through computerized data bases such as Medline (for medical publications) and CINAHL (for nursing and allied health professionalism publications).

The Nurse Healers cooperative has an extensive bibliography on Therapeutic Touch and related subjects. The group's newsletter is *The Cooperative Connection.*

ABOUT THE AUTHOR

Sally Blumenthal-McGannon, R.N., M.A., began studying Therapeutic Touch twenty years ago, after working as a pediatric ICU charge nurse. She has her master's degree in Counseling from the University of San Francisco. Sally founded the first nursing care hospice in Santa Cruz and later helped to found the Santa Cruz AIDS project. She continues to study with Dora Kunz and Dolores Krieger. She is now in private practice as a licensed marriage, family, and child counselor. She is a consultant for hospices, AIDS organizations, health care providers and others who need help dealing with living, dying, and surviving. She has taught Therapeutic Touch from Alaska to Hawaii, and consults with the International Health Consortium, where she teaches people from around the world.

Deane Juhan, M.A.

38 The Trager Approach to Psychophysical Integration

WHAT IS TRAGER PSYCHOPHYSICAL INTEGRATION?

Milton Trager once said:

> Trager consists of the use of the hands to influence deep-seated psycho-physiological patterns in the mind, and to interrupt their projection into the body's tissues. These patterns often develop in response to adverse circumstances such as accidents, surgery, illness, poor posture, emotional trauma, stresses of daily living, or poor movement habits. The purpose of my work is to break up these sensory and mental patterns which inhibit free movement and cause pain and disruption of normal function. My approach is to impart to the client what it is like to feel right in the sense of a functionally integrated body-mind.

The Trager Approach® is a way of learning and teaching movement re-education. Patients should come ready to absorb a lesson, instead of ready simply to receive a treatment. It is a way of learning to use yourself well, to be a whole person, to have all your pieces and parts well integrated and coordinated, to feel yourself connected to the energies that sustain you. The practitioner's concern is not with moving particular muscles or joints *per se*, but with using motion in muscles and joints to produce particular sensory feelings: positive, pleasurable feelings that enter the central nervous system and begin to trigger tissue changes by means of the many sensory-motor feedback loops between the mind and the muscles.

Unlike various techniques of deep tissue manipulation, Trager does not use extreme pressures or rapid thrusts to create structural change, and it does not produce pain as a necessary adjunct to its effectiveness. Unlike many movement re-education approaches, the client does not need to perform and perfect strenuous or repetitive tasks. Rather, while receiving the table work, the client becomes increasingly passive to the steady, rhythmic, pleasurable motions imparted by the practitioner's hands. Then the client learns to reproduce the pleasuring, relaxing, and spontaneous quality of these gentle movements for him or herself. These mental gymnastics are called Mentastics®. But perhaps what distinguishes Trager from other disciplines is the particular focus and intent of the practitioner's manipulations. Most other methods direct their attention to one or another of the body's tissues — the skin, the fascia, the muscles, the joints, the lymph and blood circulation, overall structural relationships, and so on — and the various properties of these tissues determine the sort of touch and manipulation required by the practitioner. But even though his hands must inevitably contact them while he works, Dr. Trager's focus and intent are not specifically directed toward local conditions in any of these tissues. As Dr. Trager says:

> My work is directed towards reaching the unconscious mind of the client. Every move, every thought communicates how the tissues should feel when everything is right. The mind is the whole thing. That is all I am interested in. I am convinced that for every physical non-yielding condition there is a psychic counterpart in the unconscious mind, corresponding exactly to the degree of the physical manifestation.

Dr. Trager did not espouse a specific list of emotional, cognitive, or psychological conditions for which Trager assures relief. Rather the condition of the body and the condition of the mind are believed to reflect and influence one another in very complex and numerous ways. The Trager work affects the many aspects of this system simultaneously. Typically, an enormous burden of negative emotions, dysfunctional beliefs, and compulsive behaviors are dramatically alleviated when the physical manifestations of discomfort, restricted movement, and distorted body images are resolved.

HOW IT BEGAN

Milton Trager was born in Chicago in 1908. By the age of 18, he was training to be a professional boxer. Mickey Martin, his trainer, used to give him a rub-down after each training session. One day Mickey looked tired, and young Milton said, "Come and lay down on the table, Mickey. I'll work on you." After he had been working for about two minutes, Mickey turned around to him, a little stunned and asked, "Hey, where'd you learn to do that?"

"You taught me, Mickey," Milton said. "I've never done anything like this in my life."

"I never taught you this, kid. But I don't care. Let me tell you, you got hands."

Milton was elated. When he went home, he approached his father, who had been suffering from acute sciatica for two years. "Lay down, Dad," he said, "I think I can fix your legs up." The sciatic pain eased considerably that first session and two sessions later, Mr. Trager was completely free of his symptoms. They never recurred. Milton started going around his Miami neighborhood and down to the beach, looking for aches and pains to work on. He had no idea what he was doing or why it worked, but he got results. People began to seek him out, and the Trager Approach was born.

He quit boxing so that he could take care of his hands. He worked as a dancer and as an acrobat. And he practiced his work. In 1941, he received his Doctorate of Physical Medicine from the Los Angeles College of Drugless Physicians, and was certified by the California Medical Board as a drugless practitioner that same year. He received his M.D. in 1955. In 1975, Dr. Trager found a way to teach his work to others, and the Trager Institute was founded. At present, there are well over 900 students throughout the world, more than 1,000 accomplished practitioners, and 13 instructors. Dr. Trager has demon-strated his work in many hospitals, medical schools, and training centers in the United States and Europe.

HOW IT WORKS

Every individual carries within him or herself an exceedingly intricate comput-er system, a recorder that has no erase button. Whatever experiences have been recorded will always be there, influencing every function of the mind and body. Since it is not possible to avoid a variety of traumas, and since none may be erased once they have occurred, help should be directed toward bringing appro-priate positive feeling experiences to the client. These experiences help directly to influence the mind and body, so that the negative patterns can be alleviated.

All degrees of psychological distress and its physical manifestations have the potential for improvement, as long as the nerve circuits are not destroyed by disease or trauma.

Emotional stress — as has been demonstrated by Dr. Hans Selye in his pioneering studies on stress syndromes — creates long-term changes in the body and the mind. If the appropriate manner of stimulating the tissues is found, this pattern will be released. This is to say that rather than working for local tissue changes, which eventually accumulate to influence physical and mental function, Trager seeks specifically to influence the feeling states in the sensory and the unconscious aspects of the mind that most directly control tissue response, metabolism, postural habits, and behavioral patterns.

In an hour-long Trager session, there are several thousand light, rhythmic contacts. Every one of them is an opportunity to create and deepen the feelings of lightness, freedom, relaxation, ease, and peace. When Trager practitioners encounter stiffened limbs or hardened muscles, their response is never to bear down upon them, to work harder to soften them, or to force them to stretch. On the contrary, the practitioner's response is immediately to become lighter, more sensitive, more searching. They never assert their idea of how soft or free an area should be; they deliberately avoid such assertions and instead project, through the motions of their hands, the questions, "What can be lighter and freer than that? Yes. And lighter than that? Fine. And freer than that?" And so on.

There are several reasons for this avoidance of force. First, heavy pressure on spasmed muscles or forced stretching of stiffened joints normally hurts; the involved area is usually hypersensitive in the first place and is already braced against painful motions. Pain is the opposite of the desired effect, and it seriously interrupts the repetitive rhythmic flow of pleasurable sensations to the mind. More than that, pain automatically tenses the muscles, producing another defensive pattern rather than dispersing the ones that are already there. Secondly, the feelings of lightness and effortlessness simply cannot be imparted by means of heavy pressure and hard work on the part of the practitioner.

Dr. Trager holds that the moment the practitioner tries to relax the tissues, he or she is doomed to failure. Trying is effort, effort is tension, and relaxation is quite the opposite. The practitioner's touch, then, must be as light as the feelings he or she wishes to instill. The point is not to impose a preconceived structural model upon the client's body, but to transmit a pleasurable and continual questioning. "What is freer, what is lighter?" The point is not to arrive finally at a specified goal — after all, we don't know what "freest" or "best" might be — but to instill in the mind of the client the constant renewal of the question, "What is better and what is better?" This is not the imposition of a postural or behavioral model, but rather the initiation of an open-ended growth process, both for the client and the practitioner.

This growth process is of primary importance to Trager practitioners. These questionings and feelings have to be established in their characters, and have to be a part of their minds and bodies, before they can successfully project them into another person's sensibilities. No one can give what they do not genuinely have. This is why the practitioner's cultivation of the mental state Dr. Trager calls "hook-up" — a relaxed, meditative alertness — is crucial to effective Trager work. The state of hook-up is not fundamentally different from a state of deep meditation, even though the practitioner in hook-up is physically active. Achieving this state of active meditation is not an incidental addition to Dr. Trager's work, it is of the essence. Hook-up is the practitioner's source of the enriched and relaxed feelings that he projects, his own contact with the qualities of gracefulness, effortlessness, and non-intrusive presence. "It is," Dr. Trager says, "like floating in a vast ocean of pleasantness," and it is the gentle rocking of that ocean that is imparted to the client's body. Dr. Trager maintains that mind and body are holistically interrelated in the energetic force field that composes all matter and life:

> We are surrounded by a force which sustains everything. You don't have to go beyond the surface of your skin to get it. But people are blocked within themselves, so negative, so tense, that this force cannot enter their consciousness. Once this force comes into them, they are changed people, and will function differently and much better than they have ever done before.
>
> It is the conscious contact with this force, this ocean of pleasantness, which gives the practitioner the pleasurable feelings he projects through his motions into the sensations of the client, and as the client's consciousness is opened to these feelings it is this force which becomes the active source of vitality and health.

The principle is elegantly simple: We learn to love by being loved, we learn gentleness by being treated gently, we learn to be graceful by experiencing the feeling of grace. The goal of a Trager session is no more complex than this —

to bring to the surface of consciousness an awareness of this force, and of the pleasurable and positive feelings that are inherent in it. These feelings will do the rest. As the Maharishi Mahesh Yogi said to Dr. Trager in 1958, "It is natural for the mind to want to go to the field of greater happiness," toward deeper understanding, toward expansiveness, toward connecting with the sources of our being. Trager was developed as a sensory means of redirecting the footsteps of someone who has lost the way.

Dr. Trager contends very firmly that he is not a "healer" or a manipulator of esoteric energies, and that his successes have nothing miraculous about them. The kinds of reflex responses, tissue changes, and behavioral changes he is able to elicit are possible because of the intimate neurological associations between sensory stimulation, emotional feelings, attitudes and concepts, and the body's motor responses to all of them. At this time no one can say with certainty exactly how these sensations, feelings, and actions are materially interrelated, but the fact that they profoundly influence one another is abundantly clear. And it is equally clear that the unconscious forces that control their relationships may be turned back from a vicious circle into a fruitful one.

Dr. Peter Levine, a neurophysiologist, took one of Dr. Trager's early trainings, and discussed possible mechanisms of psychophysical integration with him. Dr. Trager told him that he felt the work had a sound scientific basis, but that it was difficult to explain it and have it accepted. Dr. Levine's response was, "If an accepted scientific theory cannot explain a particular phenomenon, it is not because the phenomenon is unscientific, but because science itself is not appropriately refined."

REAL PEOPLE AND THE TRAGER APPROACH

Elizabeth is a survivor of incest. The violation of her body was like losing ground to an enemy. The battle lay in recapturing what rightfully belonged to her. Trager assisted in her battle. Through gentle, nonintrusive touch, Elizabeth was invited to establish a renewed relationship with her body. She learned that disconnecting from her body served as a defense against painful emotions associated with the abuse. She also found that "waking up" to pleasant and unpleasant feelings led to greater self-acceptance. Trager work helped her to discover her boundaries. She knew what scared her and where it felt safe to be touched. She practiced saying, "No, don't touch me there, but here is okay." She remembered things, too. She wept. She had some bad dreams and some very anxious days. For months, she recalled events and emotions that had been wordlessly trapped in her muscles, organs, bones, and marrow. It was painful, but she feels better now. She knows herself better and accepts herself more — even her long-ago, half-forgotten self. Because of Trager, she made changes in her life. She began to exercise, eat well, relax, enjoy, and to love herself (Mattax, 1990).

Richard, seven years of age, attended a day treatment facility for emotionally troubled children. He was prone to destructive tantrums. Generally, he was a ball of tension, and even his smile was tense and unnatural. He was unable to relax and enjoy himself. At his first Trager session, he constantly asked questions and drummed his fingers nervously on the table. After several sessions, he stopped this repetitious behavior and his body began to relax. At one session, he actually let down his guard enough to close his eyes. When he opened them, he smiled a big, beautiful, authentic smile. He had finally found a situation where he could relax enough to feel safe and happy. When the consulting psychiatrist heard about this incident, she commented that this work was the most important thing the center could do for Richard. The psychologist in charge of the day treatment stated that the Trager work offered "a new lens through which to view children." Disturbed children often communicate through their body language and Trager speaks their language (Goldstein, 1989).

Alice has multiple sclerosis, and she found her way into the Trager professional certification program. When she began, her fellow students could not even touch her feet, they were so sensitive and painful. As a result of the work she received during the training, the acute sensitivity in her feet disappeared, the aching that had plagued her legs diminished dramatically, and she began to feel some spontaneous activity in her weak-ened left thigh. Her overall symptoms went into remission and she was able to postpone the clinical testing and treatment for which she had been scheduled. She states that:

> Most of the issues that came up for me during the Trager class had to do with not belonging, and the fear that things would always recur as they had in the past. I came away with a new awareness that things do not always repeat as they have in the past. It's like the reason my toes and feet were so painful is because every time in the past that my feet and toes have been in those positions I always got a cramp and it was always painful. My body thought that every time my toes pointed they'd cramp. By re-edu-cating my body that this is not always true, some other things started loosening up in my head.

Nancy was oxygen-deprived at birth. She is 39 years old, but she has a mental age of about three. After her first Trager experiences, she demon-strated major behavioral changes. Her repetitious chatter ceased, and her conversational abilities increased noticeably. She began to climb stairs one after the other, instead of one at a time. She began, for the first time in her life, to chew her food. Her father wrote to Dr. Trager and Betty Fuller (director of the Trager Institute) on one New Year's Eve as follows:

> Our daughter has responded in so many ways, showing improve-ment in walking more confidently, chewing her food, also for the first time, being able to swallow in a normal pattern, releasing ten-sions and frustrations in actual conversations, showing determi-nation to communicate with family members. All of these changes are evident in the improvement of skin tone, hair problems, phys-ical, and social happiness. These successes have been noticeable to all family members and friends during this holiday season.

> Nancy has continued to improve. She is now learning to reach out and touch people.

WHAT TO EXPECT

A Trager session takes from one to one and a half hours. The cost of a session ranges from $40 to $100, depending upon the experience and local market conditions of the practitioner. The optimal number of sessions varies, of course, depending on the condition addressed and the client's receptivity to the induced changes. In most instances, five to ten sessions are sufficient to make enough headway and to impart enough skill to the client's use of Mentastics® (described below) to insure a lasting positive result. It can be helpful to have periodic sessions after that as a "reminder" of the feeling states and the new movement patterns. Since both the Trager approach and the capacities of the human system are quite open-ended, further areas and levels of improvement can be pursued as long as there is interest on the part of the client. The gamut can run from resolving acute symptoms, to rehabilitating chronic conditions, to developing optimum performance at the edge of human capabilities. These benefits are cumulative, the results of a learning process.

No oils or lotions are used. The client wears swim trunks or briefs and lies on a well-padded table in a warm, comfortable environment. During the session, the practitioner makes touch-contact with the body of the client, both as a whole and in its individual parts. This touch-contact is done in such a gentle and rhythmic way that the person lying passively on the table actually experiences the possibility of being able to move each part of the body freely, effortlessly, and gracefully on his own. The practitioner works in a relaxed meditative state of consciousness called hook-up. This state allows the practitioner to connect deeply with the recipient in an unforced way, to remain continually aware of the slightest responses, and to work efficiently without fatigue.

After getting up from the table, the client is given some instruction in the use of Mentastics, a system of simple, effortless movement sequences developed by Dr. Trager to maintain and even enhance the sense of lightness, freedom, and flexibility that were instilled by the table work. Mentastics is Dr. Trager's coinage for "mental gymnastics," a "mindfulness in motion" designed to help his clients recreate for themselves the sensory feelings produced by the motion of their tissue in the practitioner's hands. The patient is taught to generate simple, effortless, non-goal-oriented movements that bounce his tissues freely and pleasurably, reinforcing the positive feeling states and the relaxed muscular tones that were initiated in the session. It is a powerful means of teaching the client to recall the pleasurable sensory state that produced positive tissue change, and because it is this feeling state which triggered positive tissue response in the first place, every time the feeling is clearly recalled, the changes deepen, become more permanent and more receptive to further positive change.

It is evident, based upon most recipients' experiences, that the effects of a Trager session penetrate below the level of conscious awareness and continue to produce positive results long after the session itself. Changes described by clients have included the disappearance of specific symptoms, discomforts, or pains; heightened levels of energy and vitality; more effortless posture and carriage; greater joint mobility; deeper states of relaxation than were previously possible; and a new ease in daily activities.

HOW TO FIND A TRAGER PRACTITIONER

All Trager Practitioners must be certified by the Trager Institute in order to practice legally. The Institute has a training program with beginning, intermediate and advanced levels of training, anatomy and physiology specifically geared to the understanding of the Trager Approach. It also requires extensive periods of practice sessions and private tutorials before certification is granted. Practitioners have an ongoing obligation to take a minimum number of continuing education hours after their certification.

Some Trager practitioners are licensed health care professionals in such disciplines as psychology, counseling, nursing, physical therapy, and massage, and normally have no difficulty in providing for insurance payments. Others are trained exclusively in the Trager Approach. In most states, and with many major insurance carriers, there has been no problem with insurance coverage (within any limits specified in the individual's policy) as long as a licensed physician has prescribed Trager treatments. For further information and referrals to Trager practitioners, contact The Trager Institute, 21 Locust Ave., Mill Valley, CA, 94941. (415) 388-2688. The best way to assess a practitioner's suitability for you and your concerns is to talk with them directly.

HOW TO LEARN MORE

Demaree, J. "A Matter of Trust." *The Trager Newsletter* 9, no. 1 (1990): 2–3.

Goldstein, B. "Trager and the Emotionally Troubled Child." *The Trager Newsletter* 8, no. 1 (1989): 4–5.

Hartsong, M. "Trager and Psychotherapy." *The Trager Newsletter* 10, no. 1 (1991): 6–7.

Juhan, D. "The Trager Approach to Psychophysical Integration." *Massage and Bodywork Quarterly* Summer (1994): 29–34.

Juhan, D., G. Quasha, and K. Dychtwald. *Job's Body: A Handbook for Bodywork.* Barrytown: Station Hill Press, 1991.

Levine, P. "Guiding Emotional and Physiological Responses in Trager work." *The Trager Newletter* 9, no. 1 (1990): 6.

Mattax, E. "Reclaiming the Self: Trager as a Gentle Approach." *The Trager Newsletter* 8, no. 3 (1990): 3.

Ricketson, S. "What Practitioners Should Know About Chronic Shock." *The Trager Newsletter* 8, no. 1 (1989): 6.

Stahl, C. "Looking for Stress Relief?" *Advance* (1994): 10–12.

Trager, M. and C. Guadagno. *Trager Mentastics: Movement as a Way to Agelessness.* 2nd Edition, edited by George Quasha, Station Hill Press, 1994.

ABOUT THE AUTHOR

Deane Juhan was born in 1945 in Glenwood Springs, CO, and educated at the University of Colorado (B.A.), the University of Michigan (M.A.), and at the University of California at Berkeley, where he was doctoral candidate in English literature for three and a half years. In 1973, an experience at Esalen Institute in Big Sur changed his career, and he has remained in residence there ever since. First trained in Esalen massage, he developed a private practice and led workshops in massage, as well as seminars in anatomy and physiology for bodyworkers. In 1976, he met Dr. Milton Trager, founder of the Trager Institute for Psychophysical Integration, and he has been a student and practitioner of the Trager approach ever since. He is presently an instructor at the Trager Institute and has developed a series of classes on anatomy and physiology for Trager students all over the United States, in Canada, and in Europe. He is the author of *Job's Body: A Handbook for Bodywork.*

Gerald E. Wintrob, M.A., O.D.

39 Vision and Emotions

WHAT IS VISION THERAPY?

Vision therapy is a program of activities and exercises that can change the way you use your vision. Behavioral optometrists believe that vision is a learned behavior. What happens to your eyes is a result of what you do with your eyes. What you do with your eyes is partly a result of your emotional experiences. Through vision therapy, people learn to understand the deeper connections between their vision and their emotions. It teaches people to make judgments about their spatial world and their relationship to it. It helps people feel grounded and connected to their world, so that they can filter out sensations that are unimportant and process those that they choose to interpret. Vision therapy helps people learn to feel safe in their visual world and to process information in an efficient way with a minimum amount of effort.

In vision therapy, we need to slowly and gently strip people of their visual defenses so that they can be open to learning new ways to use their eyes. Just as people seek, through psychotherapy, to integrate different aspects of the self, in vision therapy there is the parallel experience of integrating different sensory systems. As we work with the kinesthetic, the auditory, the tactile system, and the emotions, the patient gains a greater feeling of completeness or wholeness.

When the patient's sight is examined by a traditional eye care professional, an eye chart is used to measure the patient's vision, in terms of distance and clarity. If a person can't see a certain line on the chart, they are told that glasses are needed. No mention is made of the patient's experience of his or her vision. As a result, visual problems often go undetected. If a doctor treats you symptomatically by prescribing stronger lenses, this treats your blurry vision for far objects, but does not treat the cause of your problem. The vision problem will probably then get worse. In contrast, when a patient undergoes vision therapy for vision problems, the underlying cause of the problem is treated so the vision improves.

My personal philosophy as a visual healer is that in order for any therapy to be effective, it needs to address the whole person. Vision therapy is very successful when it is combined with other modalities. Other therapies I have found compatible in fostering visual healing are massage therapy, nutritional and herbal supplementation, acupuncture, yoga, chiropractic, psychotherapy, expressive arts therapy, movement therapy, and Alexander technique.

HOW IT WORKS

All human beings have a psychological need to feel safe and secure in the world. We develop coping mechanisms that help us create a sense of stability. These mechanisms take many forms in our psyche and they manifest in our vision as well. As we grow and develop, we learn to use our eyes in different ways. We learn different skills that help us to interpret our visual world. The emotional climate to which children are exposed influences the visual adaptations they develop. Children who come from emotionally disruptive homes will often retreat to a narrower and narrower space in which they can feel safe. Their visual systems will develop and modify in such a way that it allows them to create that climate of safety.

As growing children learn to explore their environment, they learn to grasp and grab for different objects, and to pull them toward themselves for visual inspection. They have certain expectations about objects. If the information they gather corresponds to expectations, they will feel validated and be encouraged to continue exploring. However, if a child grasps for an object and it appears to be in a different place from where he or she expects it to be, the child will learn that visual judgments are not reliable. He or she may learn that it is necessary to use other senses to get the needed information. Such children learn not to trust their vision. Self-esteem is adversely affected.

To determine the location of objects in space, and in relation to you, you must be able to accurately point both of your eyes directly at the object. This ability to use both eyes together as a team is called binocularity. A number of visual problems result when this system is not operating reliably and efficiently. These conditions have associated emotional issues.

Overconvergence

Many of us have a tendency for our eyes to either undershoot or overshoot the object we want to see. So we believe that objects are closer or farther from us than they actually are. People whose eyes overshoot or overconverge on the object they are looking at will experience space as being closer than it actually is. It will be difficult for them to know where objects are in space. They will not be able to trust their visual system. This may then affect interpersonal relationships. They may develop the feeling of being closed in. As their stress level increases, they will tend to overconverge their eyes even more. They will tend to shut out their peripheral vision, paying attention only to what is nearby. This, in turn, will cause a retreat into their own personal space and will decrease their level of comfort with the world around them. They may develop a type of "tunnel vision." Children who come from chaotic home lives may develop these behaviors. They close in. They want to shut out the chaos, and experience life where they feel comfortable and safe. The overconverger may also overfocus on things, paying too much attention to detail. When someone comes into the room while they are doing something, like reading, they may not notice. They tend to be perfectionists, not seeing the forest for the trees. People with this visual adaptation tend to hold a lot of their stress in. In school, they tend to be very diligent, spending too much time on the same topic or task. They are physically tight.

Underconvergence

People whose eyes tend to undershoot their target tend to pay more attention to their surroundings. Everything has the same level of importance. They find themselves constantly changing from activity to activity. Underconvergers tend to be scattered, unable to hold their attention on any one item or topic. They are often unable to finish one project before the next one begins. They are unable to filter out what is most important. Things feel overwhelming to them.

Strabismus

Strabismus is a condition in which one or both eyes turn. People with strabismus are unable to point both eyes at the same object at the same time. This condition is obvious to anyone that looks at the person and is often a source of tremendous embarrassment. People with this problem often cover their faces, turn their heads, or shield themselves from the viewer. The strabismic often will hear the question, "Are you paying attention to what I'm saying? You're not even looking at me." Children with this condition may be teased and ridiculed by their peers.

Strabismus is a condition that clearly causes emotional problems, but it also may have emotional causes. According to Dr. Richard Kavner, a behavioral optometrist, strabismus most often develops between the ages of eighteen months and five years (Kavner, 1985). This is the age when children begin to explore their environment and to find their own identity in space. They are establishing an awareness of their bodies as separate from their environment. This is when their sense of reality is formed. We also find that children who do not feel safe in their emotional world may develop an eye turn as a coping mechanism. If one of the eyes turns in, then both of the eyes will be pointed to a spot within a few inches away. This may be the place that feels the safest. It has been suggested that this may be due to "unresolved anger . . . and a tightening of the ego defense." For the patient whose eye turns out, we find "an attitude of resignation and apathy . . . and a giving up of the defenses in a reality situation which appears hopeless" (Groffman, 1978). Heaton points out that children who develop strabismus may have "conflict in the family" (Heaton, 1968). They turn their eyes away from what they don't want to see.

Amblyopia

When the two eyes are not pointed at the same target at the same time, one of the eyes may not be stimulated to develop its "sight" as it should. As a result, the brain learns to ignore the information that comes through that eye. The patient often has a feeling of not being complete or whole because information is only coming in through one eye. I have often heard patients report a feeling of imbalance — both physically and emotionally. They feel that one side of their body is shut off.

If the information coming into the system is distorted, then it may be difficult for a person to get a stable sense of his or her place in space and to feel safe in it. Twenty percent of the visual center in the brain is used for balance and orientation. As a result, people with certain visual deficits will have problems navigating their way through space.

Myopia

Myopia is a condition in which the eyes are too strong. They focus closer than the object being viewed. They focus for such extended amounts of time at near distances that they are unable to relax at far distances, making distant objects appear blurred.

Myopes tend to be introverted and sedentary. They tend to pay enormous attention to detail and read voraciously. When we think of the television image of the intellectual or scientist, they are always shown holding their glasses. Clark Kent was meek, mild-mannered, and bookish. He became Superman when he took off his glasses and went out into the world.

Dr. Frances Young, a psychologist, points out that myopes tend to be achievement-oriented (Young, 1967). Myopes tend to process information centrally. Their awareness of their periphery is reduced. They keep their feelings in and have a difficult time expressing them. Janet Goodrich, a Reichian therapist, has observed that "myopes move through space with chronically stiff shoulders and necks, frozen in a flinching posture." She also points out that "they have limited eye contact . . . [and] cut off their feelings in their eyes" (Goodrich, 1986). According to Dr. Robert Kaplan, a behavioral optometrist, myopia is "a fear of seeing the future, pulling inward to self: 'I am afraid to see what's out there' " (Kaplan, 1987).

Charles Kelley, who did his doctoral dissertation on the psychological effects of myopia, wanted to see if the causes of myopia were emotionally related. He was particularly interested in whether he could cause a patient's myopia to change using relaxation and visualization techniques. He reported that when the mood that he attempted to induce "could be preserved . . . the visual acuity . . . improved greatly" (Kelley, 1962). In vision therapy, we try to help the patient to achieve these levels of visual relaxation as ways to improve myopia.

Accommodative Spasm

Accommodative spasm is when the patient is unable to control the focusing system of the eyes. This is the only visual condition that I am aware of that traditional medicine accepts as being related to emotions. The patient experiences a severe blurring of vision alternating with periods of clearing. Patients with this condition will show an increase in nearsightedness. It can be thought of as an anxiety attack of the eye.

Visually-Related Learning Disabilities

A learning disability is defined as an "extreme difficulty in learning, with no detectable physiological abnormality" (Zastrow and Kirst-Ashman, 1990). There are many different types of learning disabilities that may be related to vision. They can cause the patient improperly to judge spatial relations. Also, they can affect the ability to integrate information from different senses (i.e., vision, auditory, kinesthetic, tactile). They can affect people's ability to orient their bodies in space. Finally, they can cause symptoms when reading, such as headaches and/or double vision, blurred vision, skipping lines, and rereading the same line. This affects the patient's ability to make sense out of what is presented in school. These types of problems have far-reaching emotional implications for the child who is trying to learn using a faulty processing system.

Very often the child with learning disabilities, as well as with many of the other visual deficits that I have mentioned, does poorly in school. No matter how hard the child tries, he or she continues to fail in school. They aren't sure if the reason for their failure is lack of effort or lack of intelligence. As the child continues to try harder and harder, they eliminate the first possibility. Then they must conclude that they are not smart enough. This is a severe blow to the self-esteem. They may feel embarrassed and ashamed. They may begin to act out or withdraw. The learning disability may never be diagnosed. If they are lucky, they may find other ways to express themselves, such as through art or music, which will enable them to bypass the faulty processing system. A standard question that I ask when I take a case history from a patient is, "Do you ever have any discomfort when reading?" When I am examining an adult with undiagnosed learning disabilities, the response I often hear is "No, never." I then ask "Do you ever read?" The answer very often is "No, never."

REAL PEOPLE AND VISION THERAPY

Susan was 23 years old when she came to me for a routine visual checkup. She was a single mother with a seven-year-old son. She had dropped out of high school at sixteen and had immediately gotten pregnant. She presented no real symptoms that she could connect to her vision. She didn't like to read and as a result never did. Upon questioning, it was revealed that as far back as she could remember, she would get very tired when she read. If she continued to read, she would get headaches. She'd had her eyes examined as a child, but no problem was ever picked up. My examination revealed that she suffered from a learning disability and a severe binocular problem. When I told her that this condition was the cause of her symptoms, she started to cry. She told me that she had always thought she wasn't smart enough to remember what she read, and felt that there was no point in pursuing academics, since she thought she was incapable of succeeding at it. She never dreamed that there was a specific cause for her problem.

Jonathan is a 35-year-old accountant. His nearsightedness had continually worsened since he was a child. He wanted to do vision therapy to gain a sense of control for himself and his eyes. Unfortunately, he wasn't able to find time to do his vision therapy adequately and decided to wait six months. He chose instead to start doing a yoga program on a daily basis. He was also being seen by a psychotherapist. One of the aims of his psychotherapy was to make him more aware of his physical body. This was important work for Jonathan because he experienced much of his life in his mind and was disconnected to his physical feelings. Six months later, I examined him again before we started a formal vision therapy program. His prescription had dramatically reduced. He realized that the yoga and psychotherapy had given him a body awareness that he did not have before. It enabled him to feel more relaxed, grounded, and centered in the world and within his own space. We began vision therapy in conjunction with the yoga and psychotherapy with excellent results.

We find that unresolved issues with one parent may cause restrictions in visual awareness in the affected eye. The right eye is referred to by vision therapists as the father eye and the left eye as the mother eye. Ann Marie was a ten-year-old girl who presented with a dramatically increasing prescription in her left eye. Her right eye's sight was perfectly normal — a crisp 20/20. Ruling out all the possible physiological causes of this condition, her relationship with her parents was explored and I enlisted the help of a psychotherapist. Psychotherapy revealed that her mother was very restrictive and controlling. Ann Marie had a difficult time relating to her mother. She wanted to block her maternal images. Her left eye did not want to see. So no matter what prescription she was given, it would suffice for a while and then she needed more. In addition to vision therapy and psychotherapy, she was treated for her visual problem with a colored light therapy called syntonics (described later in this chapter). As a result, her prescription eventually stopped increasing and even began to reverse.

Alison was a 30-year-old art student. Her eyes had difficulty working together but they were cosmetically straight. At the age of three she developed a constant inward turn of her right eye. She had surgery on her eyes at the age of five. It should be noted that a common treatment by the orthodox medical community for a strabismus is to surgically realign the eyes by cutting the muscles. Alison told me that, as a young child, she had a very painful and chaotic home life. She had a lot of difficulty relating to her father and felt very conflicted about it. She felt that the reason for her eye turn was this underlying conflict. As Alison gained more awareness into her emotional problem, she was able to heal her visual deficit.

Billy was an eight-year-old boy with a right eye that constantly turned in. He answered all questions directed to him with one word answers. He rarely turned his head to the side. When asked how he felt, he always answered "fine." His school was very happy with him. He never complained and never made trouble. He was perfectly happy to sit quietly, staring straight ahead. He hated all sports and any physical activity. When he began to work with us in vision therapy, we did exercises requiring him to maintain his balance while performing other activities, in order to make him aware of the two sides of his body and how his body was integrated with his vision. We had him stand on a balance board (an 18-inch square piece of plywood with a much smaller block of wood attached underneath) and pass a bean bag from hand to hand while watching a swinging ball. In this exercise, he is forced to become aware that the two sides of his body are different but, that in order to maintain his balance, he must have everything work in unison — i.e., his eyes, his hands, his torso, and his legs. We were working on his visual problem by addressing his physical relationship to space. We wanted him to feel comfortable relating to objects and people away from his own personal space. It can be frightening to be asked to process visually with an eye that is not normally used. Billy was asked to perform exercises while wearing a patch covering his "good" eye. It was of utmost importance that he felt safe in our office. Without a feeling of trust established between my staff and Billy, he would not have been willing to attempt anything that was potentially risky. By the end of vision therapy, both of his eyes were working together. But of greater importance, he achieved a greater sense of emotional stability. We taught him to take risks in a nurturing environment. He became very engaging and outgoing. He learned how to take chances in many different ways.

Sandy had a tendency to underconverge her eyes. She worked as a printer and had a myriad of symptoms. She suffered from headaches, occasional double vision, and a difficulty concentrating when working. As we began to work together, she realized that her visual condition was much more far-reaching than she had imagined. Six months into vision therapy, she came into the office feeling very happy. She told me that the previous night, she had been asked to be a disk jockey at a dance. This was something she had always wanted to do but which she felt would be very intimidating to her. She felt that she would not be able to keep visual track of all the different things that she would have to be aware of in order to perform adequately. However, she told me that she had done it very successfully. As a peripherally oriented person, it had been overwhelming for her to organize herself and her environment. The goal of her vision therapy was to enable her to process visually by paying attention to more detail-oriented tasks. An example of an exercise she performed was to wear an eye patch, keep her balance while walking on a beam, and call letters off two eye charts on the wall, to the beat of a metronome. The purpose of this type of exercise is that, in order for her to be able to perform so many tasks at the same time, she must learn to allow herself to let go and process each task individually, as well as all of them together. It is important for the reader to realize that an exercise of this level of difficulty is only performed after proficiency has been established in much simpler tasks. Using exercises such as these, she learned to organize her visual space so that excessive stimulation did not feel so overwhelming.

∞

Many people learn ways to compensate for their difficulties and may lead otherwise normal lives. However the choice of a profession is often influenced by an undiagnosed visual problem.

Maria was an adult who came into my office with many symptoms. She suffered from headaches, double vision, and an inability to concentrate at near tasks for extended periods of time. She had just begun an office job that required her to read and write for extended periods of time. Previously, she had been a free-lance photographer. I asked her if she had ever experienced symptoms like this before. She told me she had, but not since she had been in school. Upon examination, I discovered that she had a binocular instability. She had a problem using her two eyes together as a team. It was apparent that she suffered from this problem ever since she was a little girl. To compensate, she went into a profession that did not require her to use her two eyes together. She became a photographer. This way she could make a living, always closing one eye.

∞

Carla came in with no apparent symptoms. She only needed a checkup. Upon examination, it was revealed that she had a constant strabismus. She was unable to point her two eyes together toward the same target in space. I asked her what she did for a living. She told me she was a lawyer. I asked her if she ever had a problem reading and remembering what she read. She told me that she never really read anything. I asked her how she could have gotten through law school with such a handicap. She told me she would tape all of the lectures, play them back to herself, and commit them to memory. She would remember her texts by reading them out loud so that she could hear what she was reading. Relying on her auditory system, she would act as her own lecturer so that she could remember the material. She was very surprised when I explained to her that her strabismus was the cause of this problem and that she did not have to continue this way.

This patient had learned that using her visual system required too much energy and that it was unreliable. It is hard work to establish trust in one's visual system after so many years of relying on adaptations. First, the adaptations need to be removed in order to allow for a more efficient use of the visual system. This creates more symptomatic behavior, as it brings into question patterns which the patient has internalized as just being "me." This creates a great deal of vulnerability. The patient must allow his beliefs to shift from one system to another.

WHAT TO EXPECT

A thorough vision analysis should take approximately forty-five minutes, and should assess a number of visual skills, such as accommodation, binocularity, eye movements, and visual perception. Many practitioners structure their therapy sessions differently. In my office, patients are seen once or twice a week for forty-five minute sessions. In each session, they are given two to three exercises. Each patient is assigned exercises to perform at home on a daily basis. The exercises require less than twenty minutes per day. We see some patients individually and others in a group. Patients who are in a group perform their exercises individually, but in a room with other patients. The doctor is in the therapy room at all times and occasionally is aided by a vision therapy assistant. If the patient needs to be alone during a session, we use other rooms in the office for that purpose.

The patient is also given a syntonics treatment. In syntonics, varying colors, or frequencies of light, are viewed by the patient to help stimulate the internal balancing of the patient's autonomic nervous system. Because the functioning of the eyes is directly affected by the functioning of the nervous system, syntonics has been effectively used to improve the performance of the visual system. A syntonics treatment requires the patient to look into a machine and view a colored light for up to twenty minutes. We find that the syntonics treatment enables the patient to achieve greater gains in vision therapy than would otherwise be expected. As the patient's nervous system is put into balance, underlying emotional concerns may surface. Often patients experience a deep sense of emotional release after such a session. In certain cases, we have the patient come for a series of syntonic treatments before a formal vision therapy program is initiated.

The length of therapy differs widely from patient to patient from a few months to two or three years. Currently the fee is approximately $50 per group visit and is reimbursable by most major medical insurance plans. Some different fee structures exist.

HOW TO FIND A PRACTITIONER

A practitioner of vision therapy should be a doctor of Optometry. Optometrists complete a four-year postgraduate doctoral program. All optometrists are licensed to practice vision therapy, however philosophies regarding vision therapy varies greatly.

The following organizations have listings of member practitioners who practice vision therapy. However, the reader should be aware that not all members will use all the techniques that I have mentioned, nor will they necessarily work on the more subtle relationships between emotion and vision. Therefore it is suggested that you interview the practitioner regarding his or her philosophy and techniques before attempting a program.

THE OPTOMETRIC EXTENSION PROGRAM	THE COLLEGE OF SYNTONIC OPTOMETRY
1921 E. Carnegie Ave., Suite 3-L	Secretary of the College
Santa Ana, CA 92705-5510	Solomon Slobin, O.D.
Tel: (714) 250-8070	1200 Robeson St.
http://www.healthy.net/oep	Fall River, MA 02720
	Tel: (508) 673-1251

COVD INTERNATIONAL OFFICE
Stephen Miller, O.D.
Executive Director
243 N. Lindbergh Blvd., Suite 310
St. Louis, MO 63141
Tel: (888) 268-3770

THE COLLEGE OF SYNTONIC OPTOMETRY
David J. Luke, O.D.
121 North Allen
Box 82
Centralia, MO 65240
Tel: (314) 581-3848

THE COLLEGE OF OPTOMETRISTS
IN VISION DEVELOPMENT
P.O. Box 285
Chula Vista, CA 91912-0285
Tel: (619) 425-6191

HOW TO LEARN MORE

Bates, W. *Better Eyesight Without Glasses.* New York: Henry Holt and Company, 1981.

Berne, S. *Creating Your Personal Vision.* Santa Fe, NM: Color Stone Press, 1994.

Goodrich, J. *Natural Vision Improvement.* Berkeley: Celestial Arts, 1986.

Groffman, S. "Psychological Aspects of Strabismus and Amblyopia — A Review of the Literature." *Journal of the American Optometric Association* 49 (1978): 995–999.

Heaton, J. M. In *Phenomenology and Psychology of Function and Disorder,* edited by R. D. Laing, London: Tavistock Publications, 1968.

Kaplan, R. *Seeing Beyond 20/20.* Hillsboro: Beyond Words, 1987.

Kavner, R. *Your Child's Vision.* New York: Simon and Schuster, Inc., 1985.

Kelley, C. "Psychological Factors in Myopia." *Journal of the American Optometric Association* 33 (1962): 833–837.

Leiberman, J. *Light Medicine of the Future.* Santa Fe: Bear and Company, 1991.

Leiberman, J. *Take Off Your Glasses and See.* NY: Crown Publishers, 1995.

Young, F. "Myopia and Personality." *American Journal of Optometry and Archives of American Academy of Optometry* 44 (1967): 192–201.

Zastrow, C. and K. Kirst-Ashman, eds. *Understanding Human Behavior and the Social Environment.* Second Edition. Chicago: Nelson-Hall, 1990.

ABOUT THE AUTHOR

Dr. Gerald E. Wintrob has his Doctor of Optometry degree from the State University of New York College of Optometry, and a Master of Arts and B.A. from Brooklyn College. He is currently in private practice in the Park Slope section of Brooklyn, NY. He specializes in vision therapy, vision enhancement, visually-related learning problems, and syntonics (color healing). He is currently a member of the faculty at the New York Open Center, the largest urban holistic learning center in the U.S. He has lectured widely.

Richard Rosen

40 Yoga

WHAT IS YOGA?

Yoga is a Sanskrit word, a distant relative of our English word "yoke." It is a very evocative word, its definition in my Sanskrit-English dictionary running on for an entire column of eight-point type. But in the context of the subject at hand, it is usually translated as both "application" and "union." This dual meaning neatly summarizes what yoga is and what it aims to do.

Most uninitiated Westerners dismiss yoga as some exotic Eastern philosophy or religion with nothing much to offer them of any practical value. Nothing could be further from the truth. Yoga indeed has elements of philosophy and religion, though not in the way that we typically think of philosophy and religion in the West. You'll also find some metaphysics (speculations on where we came from, who we are, and where we're all headed), ethical injunctions, and psychology, all rolled into one. But more important, yoga is a pragmatic, experimental application of a variety of time-tested techniques for self-exploration and self-understanding.

I should quickly point out that this "self," in yoga, is not limited to the mind, with its conscious and subconscious contents, its various capacities and potentials, and its often squabbling community of structures. Yoga has what we might call today a holistic view of the self that incorporates, along with our mind, our physical and "breathing" bodies, a "higher" mind or wisdom faculty, and a superconscious principle that embraces and at the same time transcends all of this. The yogis call it the *atman*, or soul.

However rational and sophisticated we like to imagine ourselves, yoga techniques — which include behavior modification and positive affirmation; physical and breathing exercises; the repetition of significant syllables, words, or phrases; visualizations; and meditation — are just as valid today as they were centuries ago in the "mystical" East. The goal of the practice, simply stated, is the union or integration of all these often-fragmented parts of our self, and the direct and joyful experience of our authentic identity.

Most yoga teachers are not, of course, licensed mental health care providers, although experienced teachers have a wealth of on-the-job training with both physical and emotional difficulties, from bad backs and knees to job-related stress and depression. But yoga can be remarkably thereapeutic; in fact, many people nowadays start yoga on the recommendation of their doctor as a supplement to, or a continuation of, a therapy program. Yoga has been effective in helping people who have depression, anxiety, addictions, learning and memory problems, personality disorders, confusion and brain fog, and irritability. It can also help people achieve better overall health, spiritual growth, and self-actualization.

HOW IT BEGAN

Nobody really knows how or when yoga began. Scholars have debated for a long time about the age of yoga and its antecedents, but have yet to reach a consensus. But most everyone will agree that yoga is very old, at least 3,500 years, and that it is rooted in the ritual practices of people who once inhabited a riverside civilization in what is now Pakistan and northern India.

While there is quite a wide range of beliefs and practices that are blanketed by the word yoga — I have a list with over thirty distinct schools, including something called *samrambha-yoga*, the yoga of "hatred" — there are only about six or so schools that could be considered historically important. The first systematic written exposition of yoga, the *Yoga-Sutra* by the sage Patanjali, appeared about 1,700 years ago. This school, known as *raja-yoga*, the "royal" yoga, affirms a stringently ascetic, meditative discipline that, with its central theme of "all is suffering," is not likely to capture the hearts or minds of many people nowadays.

What is popular today in the West, however, with several million practitioners, is *hatha-yoga*, the "forceful" yoga, which first appeared in India only about ten centuries ago. This school has, over the last few years, sprouted a bewildering number of branches. Some of the better known subschools or related approaches include (along with the name of the founder, or leading modern teacher, in parentheses): ashtanga yoga (K. Patabhi Jois); hidden language yoga (Swami Sivananda Radha); integral yoga (Swami Satchidananda); Iyengar yoga (B.K.S. Iyengar); kripalu yoga (Yogi Amrit Desai); kundalini yoga (Yogi Bhajan); Sivananda yoga (Swami Vishnudevananda); viniyoga (T.K.V. Desikachar).

Hatha-yoga is probably most closely associated in the minds of Westerners with its curious physical exercises, called *asanas,* or postures; unfortunately, this has led to a perception, even among many of its adherents, that this approach is merely a kind of calisthenics. Despite the emphasis on the physical body and its forceful training with *asanas* and breathing exercises, *hatha-yoga* has, like all forms of yoga, a spiritual context and intent.

HOW IT WORKS

In this section, I'll limit my comments to two uniquely yogic practices: posture or *asana,* and controlled breathing or *pranayama* (though these practices appear, in various forms, in other spiritual disciplines). Remember that, while yogic practices may have many hygienic and therapeutic benefits, both physical and mental, these are traditionally considered to be only side effects, desirable to be sure, but still secondary to the primary aspiration of spiritual union.

Georg Feuerstein, a well-known yoga scholar, has described yoga as a "technology of consciousness transformation." The yogis believe that the mind, or our normal consciousness, with its constant turmoil, conflicting desires, and often alienating ego-centeredness, is one of the major stumbling blocks to full self-understanding. This habitually limited and limiting mind is what the yogis wish to transform. Their ideal is a mind that is, in the words of the 2500-year-old *Bhagavad-Gita,* the so-called New Testament of Hinduism, "steadfast and still" under the divine guidance of the *atman.* For most people, however, the mind is slippery as an eel, almost impossible to grab onto, and this is where *asana* and *pranayama* come in.

The yogis have long recognized, and based their teachings on, the intimate connection between the body, the breath, and the mind. The body and breath incarnate or "flesh out" the mind, so that the state of the mind, whether positive or negative, is expressed in the bearing, the physical posture, and the general behavior of the body and the rhythm of the breath. But the reverse is also true: If you, for example, outwardly mimic the physical signs of depression — go ahead and try this, by slumping forward and purposefully making your breathing shallow — this can exert a powerful influence on the mind.

The mind may slip through our fingers, but we certainly can lay our hands on its more tangible "sheaths," as the yogis call them, the body and the breath. The postures act first to stretch, strengthen, and align the physical body; this releases habitual tension in the muscles and joints and frees bound energy, which is further balanced or "tuned" by the postures. The yogis want a physical body that is, as Patanjali notes, both "steady and comfortable" (and so prepared for the challenges of *pranayama* and meditation). Next the breathing exercises help to direct awareness inward, away from the distractions and disruptions of the world, and toward the mind (and the soul). By controlling the rhythms and timing of our breath, we can purge ourselves of toxic "bad air" and further expand our store of energy. Moreover, the rhythmic pulsation of the breath calms the turbulent mind and so turns up the inner light of our self-awareness. And finally, the postures and breathing exercises (along with other techniques such as meditation) open us up to the "true knowledge," to quote the *Gita* again, "established in the heart of all."

WHAT THE RESEARCH SHOWS

Yoga is now being used in a surprisingly wide range of preventative and therapeutic applications in the mental health field. The research shows that yoga (usually yoga breathing exercises and yoga-based stretching exercises) is being used with a moderate to high degree of success in the treatment of various psychosomatic and psychiatric disorders (Balodhi, 1986; Goyeche, 1979; Norton, 1983; Shannahoff-Khalsa and Beckett, 1996; Singh, 1986; Wood, 1993), drug and alcohol addiction (Nespor, 1991 and 1993; Sharma and Shukla, 1988), and epilepsy (Panjwani et al., 1995). Yoga is being taught to elderly patients in geriatric mental clinics (Allen and Steinkohl, 1987) and to mentally retarded children, who have demonstrated improved I.Q. and social adaptation (Pathak and Mishra, 1984; Uma et al., 1989).

Yoga has a positive impact (when performed by "normal" volunteers) on such mood states as anxiety, depression, anger, and aggression, and improves concentration, memory, learning ability, self-confidence, physical and mental energy, and contentment. For example, in a study comparing the effects of yoga, relaxation techniques, and visualization on physical and mental energy and on positive and negative moods, yoga proved most effective of the three (Wood, 1993). It was reported to have an "invigorating" effect on perceptions of both mental and physical energy, and increased high positive mood.

Interestingly, yoga is also credited with being a "suitable element of prevention" of professional stress and burnout for workers in the health services (Nespor, 1993).

REAL PEOPLE AND YOGA

Emma, a female in her mid thirties, characterized herself as a "workaholic," always "on the go." The most important thing in her life was her position with a large investment firm. But she felt strangely "disembodied," trapped inside her "racing brain," and a friend recommended that she give yoga a try.

At first, like many newcomers, she had a difficult time in class. Because her sense of balance was poor, she was always tipping over in the postures, unable to keep her feet on the ground; and because she couldn't stop thinking about her job-related responsibilities and deadlines, she often lost the thread of the teacher's instructions, and became disoriented — confusing right and left, front and back.

Over time, though, through her work in the various postures and with the breath, she learned to slow down her brain. She reacquainted herself with her body and improved her ability to concentrate on what was happening in the present moment. One dramatic change was in her balance. When she first came to class, she was terrified of the shoulder stand posture in which the student balances on her shoulders (lifted on a stack of blankets) with the feet pointed toward the ceiling and the back of the torso braced by the hands. After a few months of practicing the posture near a wall, for both physical and moral support, she was able to move into the center of the room and perch confidently and even happily on her shoulders. This newfound physical balance was reflected in her mental life. She was able to create more room in her life for activities outside of her job.

Alan, a male in his late forties, first came to yoga class in a way that is quite typical for men of his age. He was dragged in, mumbling under his breath, by his wife. Like Emma, Alan was also "in his head," abstracted, and didn't much like yoga to start. He had always been athletic, active, but over the years had stiffened up —not only in his body but, as his wife remarked, in his outlook too — and experienced moderate to extreme pain during the stretching exercises. He was also used to fast-moving sports like tennis and basketball, and chafed at the sometimes slower, more meditative pace of the class. To add to these stumbling blocks, Alan was a perfectionist, highly critical of himself and others, and "result-oriented." When forced to confront his own physical limitations, in both strength and flexibility, and when "nothing happened" in class right away, he tried to "bull" his way through the exercises, grunting and groaning like a man carrying a heavy weight in a race to the finish line.

Quite often men like Alan don't last more that a few classes, if that many, but surprisingly, he persisted — his wife claimed that he was too obstinate to give up — and gradually, like Emma, he learned to slow himself down. He was especially helped by some breathing exercises that seemed to soften the tension in his body. At least in class, he became less concerned with "getting somewhere" and "doing things right," and more willing to accept and work within his limitations. Over time, Alan's experience of the postures became less and less painful, and he even began practicing at home, using yoga to work therapeutically with an old back injury and to relieve the pressures of his job with a computer manufacturing firm.

WHAT TO EXPECT

Though there are a good number of instruction manuals and audio and video tapes available, the best way to learn yoga is from a teacher. Most students attend public classes held at local yoga schools, health clubs, or community colleges. I have provided some tips below to help you find a capable teacher.

Occasionally, a student is unable or unwilling to attend a public class; in this case, it is possible to hire a teacher to give you private lessons, but expect to pay considerably more for this at-home instruction. How often you go to a class is largely determined by how much time you have on your hands and what you can afford. I generally recommend that students, for the first month or so anyway, go once a week; after that, you can always add a class or two to your weekly program if you like.

Just like any other skill or art you're interested in learning, the more time and effort you put into your practice, the more quickly you'll improve and begin to realize tangible results. This means that, along with your weekly class (or classes), you should try to commit yourself to a regular home practice. How often is "regular"? Start with once or twice a week for fifteen to twenty minutes a day. Ask your teacher to help you devise a reasonable routine, something that's enjoyable and appropriate for your physical capacities and emotional needs. Then see if you can, over a few months' time, add a day here and ten minutes there, until you're practicing pretty much every day for thirty minutes.

Remember, though, that yoga is what we would call today a lifestyle, and that while regular class attendance and home practice are necessary and admirable, it's important to apply what you learn in these controlled situations — like equanimity, flexibility, and courage — to your everyday, sometimes out-of-control existence. Aurobindo Ghosh, a famous twentieth-century yogi, once said, "All life is yoga."

HOW TO FIND A YOGA TEACHER

There are several ways to find the right yoga teacher for you. Your local Yellow Pages will list teachers and schools in your area. Call up the schools or individuals who are listed and ask them to mail you a schedule of classes, and any other information they have that might be useful to a new student. *Yoga Journal*, the most widely read yoga magazine in this country, publishes a yearly "Yoga Teachers Directory," usually in its August issue, which lists teachers state by state in the United States, as well as in other countries. You can call *Yoga Journal* at (510) 841-9200 for information, or look for the YTD on its Website at www.yogajournal.com. Ask your friends or associates at work to recommend a teacher or school. I'd be surprised if you didn't know someone, or someone who knows someone, who takes a yoga class.

You'll probably want to start with a beginners' class, even though you may consider yourself to be "in good shape." Don't let the stereotype of the skinny little yogi sitting placidly in Pretzel Pose fool you — some classes can be a real workout that will have you begging for mercy. Most beginning classes are ongoing, which means that you'll be joining a more experienced group of students. If this seems intimidating, if you have concerns about looking "foolish," try to remember that just about everybody in the room (including the teacher) once stood in your shoes — or your bare feet — and that they're all fixed on their own "application" and (though there are exceptions) no longer interested in judging yours.

Once you've gathered all your information, talk to someone at each school or, if possible, the teachers of any of the classes you're interested in. Be sure to first find out something about the school's approach: some classes (like Ashtanga Vinyasa) are notoriously vigorous, while others (like Kripalu) are much milder. Be sure you have some idea of what you're getting into *before* you go, to avoid any unpleasant surprises. You'll also want to know (if possible): the average size of the class (more experienced and popular teachers usually have large classes, and so less time to work with individuals, while novice teachers, who might be a little rough around the edges, usually have small classes but more opportunity to give you personal attention); the length of the class (most run between sixty to ninety minutes); the cost of the class; what kind of dress is recommended; and whether the school provides you with an exercise mat or blanket, or if you need to bring your own.

If you have any physical problems or limitations, briefly describe them and see if the teacher seems comfortable working with you. You might ask about his or her training, certifications, and teaching experience. Next, if you're able to sample a few different teachers, try one or more classes with each one. Don't expect miracles. If nothing seems to "happen" after the first class, don't be discouraged. Try again, or try another teacher, or another school, until you find the right situation for you. Give yoga a fair chance.

Once you've settled on a teacher, it's best to study with that one person as much as possible, especially if you're working with a particular problem. This gives the teacher time to get to know you so that she or he can tailor postures and instructions to suit your special needs.

There are a few things to be on the lookout for. *Never* perform any position in class that generates "bad" pain, especially in the knees, lower back, and neck. Naturally, at the outset you'll be feeling some pain — or what I like to call "heightened awareness" — in places like the back of your legs, groin, or shoulders; and while it might be necessary, even honorable, at certain times and in certain places to suffer in silence, you're asking for trouble to ignore or grit your teeth with "bad" pain in a yoga class. Either tell the teacher what you're experiencing and ask for an alternative position, or stop altogether and assume a rest position until the class is ready to move on.

Also, while many teachers make manual adjustments in class — pressing on your back to help you twist, for example — always be certain that you're comfortable with the contact. If the adjustment is too extreme or harsh, or the touch is on what you feel to be an inappropriate place on your body, ask your teacher to please stop.

RESOURCES

The field of literature on yoga is enormous, though much of it is scholarly and not of much interest to the average student. The best contemporary writer on the history and philosophy of the various major yoga schools is Georg Feuerstein, who has written a couple of dozen books on yoga over the past two decades. I recommend in particular *The Shambhala Guide to Yoga* (1996, Boston: Shambhala) as a general introduction or, if you're more ambitious, the more detailed *Yoga: The Technology of Ecstasy* (1989, Los Angeles: Jeremy Tarcher). Once you're familiar with the background, you might want to read an original yoga scripture. I can't think of any more enchanting and edifying book than the *Bhagavad-Gita*, the "Song of the Great Lord," one of the most significant treatises — cleverly cast in poetic form — of the entire yoga tradition. Ask your teacher to recommend his or her favorite translation.

There are any number of instructional manuals on the market, with more appearing all the time. Perhaps the granddaddy of them all, and certainly one of the most influential, is *Light on Yoga* (1979, New York: Schocken) by the well-known yoga instructor, who is now nearing eighty, B.K.S. Iyengar. Two other excellent primers for beginning to intermediate students are *The Runner's Yoga Book* by Jean Couch (1990, CA: Rodmell Press), and *Relax & Renew* by Judith Lasater (1995, Rodmell Press), both available from their publisher, (510) 841-3123.

HOW TO LEARN MORE

Allen, K. S. and R. P. Steinkohl. "Yoga in a Geriatric Mental Clinic." *Activities Adaptation in Aging* 9, no. 4 (1987): 61–68.

Balodhi, J. P. "Perspective of Rajayoga in its Application to Mental Health." *NIMHANS Journal* 4, no. 2 (1986): 133–138.

Goyeche, J. R. "Yoga as Therapy in Psychosomatic Medicine." *Psychother Psychosom* 31 (1979): 373–81.

Nespor, K. "Pain Management and Yoga." *International J. Pyschosom* 38 (1991): 76–81.

Nespor, K. "Twelve Years of Experience with Yoga in Psychiatry." *International J. Psychosom* 40 (1993): 105–107.

Norton, G. R. and W. E. Johnson. "A Comparison of Two Relaxation Procedures for Reducing Cognitive and Somatic Anxiety." *J Behav Ther Exp Psychiatry* 14, no. 3 (1983): 209–214.

Panjwani, U.; H. L. Gupta; S. H. Singh; W. Selvamurthy; and U. C. Rai. "Effects of Sahaja Yoga Practice on Stress Management in Patients of Epilepsy." *Indian J. Physiol Pharmacol* 39, no. 2 (1995): 111–116.

Pathak, M. P. and L. S. Mishra. "Rehabilitation of Mentally Retarded Through Yoga Therapy." *Child Psychiatry Quarterly* 17, no. 4 (1984): 153–158.

Schell, F. J.; B. Allolio; and O. W. Schoenecke. "Physiological and Psychological Effects of Hatha-Yoga Exercise in Healthy Women." *Int J Psychosom* 41 (1994): 46–52.

Shannahoff-Khalsa, D. S. and L. R. Beckett. "Clinical Case Report: Efficacy of Yogic Techniques in the Treatment of Obsessive Compulsive Disorders." *Int J Neurosci* 85 (1996): 1–17.

Sharma, K. and P. Singh. "Treatment of Neurotic Illnesses by Yogic Techniques." *Indian J Med Sci* 43, no. 3 (1989): 76–79.

Sharma, K. and V. Shukla. "Rehabilitation of Drug-Addicted Persons: The Experience of the Nav-Chetna Center in India." *Bull Narc* 40, no. 1 (1988): 43–49.

Singh, R. H. "Evaluation of Some Indian Traditional Methods of Promotion of Mental Health." *Activitas Nervosa Superior* 28, no. 1 (1986): 67–69.

Uma, K.; H. R. Nagendra; R. Nagarathna; S. Vaidahi; and R. Seethalakshm. "The Integrated Approach of Yoga: Therapeutic Tool for Mentally Retarded Children: A One Year Controlled Study." *J Ment Defic Res* 33, no. 5 (1989): 415–421.

Wood, C. "Mood Change and Perceptions of Vitality: A Comparison of the Effects of Relaxation, Visualization and Yoga." *J R Soc Med* 86, no. 5 (1993): 254–258.

ABOUT THE AUTHOR

Richard Rosen has been studying hatha yoga since 1980. He is a graduate of the Iyengar Yoga Institute in San Francisco and, since 1987, has taught public classes in Berkeley and Oakland. He also leads classes in yoga philosophy and pranayama for the Advance Studies Program at the Yoga Room in Berkeley. A regular contributor to *Yoga Journal,* Richard was the magazine's Asana columnist in 1995 and 1996. He lives in Berkeley with his wife and beautiful four-year-old daughter.

Index

A

abandonment issues, 434

abreaction. *See* catharsis

abuse, 122, 363, 400, 434, 490; child, 258. *See also* sexual abuse

accidents, 490. *See also* trauma

acupuncture, 151–56, 158–59; adjuncts to, 159

addiction. *See* drug addiction

aggression, 224, 319, 364, 367–68, 394, 404, 535

alcohol abuse. *See* drug abuse

alcohol cravings, 312

Alexander, Frederic Mathias, 58–59

Alexander Technique, 57–69, 465

alienation, 477

allergies, 80, 258; difficulty detecting, 36; symptoms of, 224–25. *See also* chemical sensitivities

allergy therapy, neutralization, 227

allopathic vs. holistic health, 15–16, 262; diagnosis and, 19; physical-mental dichotomy and, 485

allopathic vs. holistic medicine, 303–4, 324, 400, 402–3, 479; homeopathy and, 262

altered states of consciousness, 43–50; in history of psychotherapy, 45; psychotherapeutic use of, 48–49, 469; require expanded model of psyche, 46. *See also* shamanism

alternative medicine, medical politics and history of, 22–24

alternative practitioners, guidelines for selecting, 8–9, 67, 397. *See also under* specific treatments

alternative treatments: concurrent use of multiple, 11; conditions alleviated by particular, 12–13; failure to inform patients about, 1; guidelines for choosing among, 8, 12–13; psychoanalytic perspectives on, 122.

anger, 87, 152, 224, 363, 364, 390, 471, 535. *See also* rage

anorexia, 314–17, 331–32

antibiotics, negative effects of, 226

anxiety, 88, 89, 115, 120, 122, 146, 177, 302, 306, 312, 315–19, 367, 368, 382, 390, 394–95, 405, 434, 460, 464, 470–71, 477, 490, 501, 533, 535. *See also* panic attacks

appetite. *See* eating disorders; overeating

applied kinesiology (AK), 71–81; emotional recall technique, 74–75

archetypal psychology, 262

aromatherapy, 83–95

art therapy, 166–71

assertiveness, 187

Association for Past Life Research and Therapy (APRT), 436

About the Editor

Lynette Bassman, Ph.D. was born in Norwalk, CT, and received a bachelor's degree in Sociology from Brandeis University. After a brief foray into the food business as a caterer, hospital dietetic aide, health food store produce manager, and apprentice to a Viennese pastry chef, she sought a career in counseling psychology. With a master's degree from Columbia University Teachers College and a Ph.D. from New York University, she has worked as a psychotherapist and a university faculty member. She is currently an Associate Professor at the California School of Professional Psychology in Fresno, CA, and specializes in health psychology.

Dr. Bassman lives with her husband, who is a chiropractor and applied kinesiologist, and her son. She enjoys running, vegetarian gourmet cooking, and reading good fiction. Future publication plans include a book on how and why people deceive themselves about important things like health, relationships and the environment, and the global implications of this self-deception. She can be reached by writing to New World Library at 14 Pamaron Way, Novato, CA 94949 or via e-mail at escort@nwlib.com. She especially welcomes stories from people who have used these and other holistic healing techniques to enhance their mental/emotional wellness, and constructive dialogue with other health professionals.

New World Library is dedicated to
publishing books and cassettes that inspire
and challenge us to improve the quality
of our lives and our world.

Our books and tapes are available
in bookstores everywhere.
For a catalog of our complete library
of fine books and cassettes, contact:

New World Library
14 Pamaron Way
Novato, CA 94949

Phone: (415) 884-2100
Fax: (415) 884-2199
Or call toll-free (800) 972-6657
Catalog requests: Ext. 50
Ordering: Ext. 52

E-mail: escort@nwlib.com
http://www.nwlib.com